In a Rain of Dust

In a Rain of Dust

Death, Deceit, and the Lawyer
Who Busted Big Asbestos

DAVID KINLEY

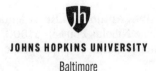

JOHNS HOPKINS UNIVERSITY

Baltimore

Johns Hopkins University Press
2715 North Charles Street
Baltimore, Maryland 21218
www.press.jhu.edu

All photographs and captions by Hein du Plessis
unless otherwise noted.

Library of Congress Cataloging-in-Publication Data

Names: Kinley, David (Lecturer in law), author.
Title: In a rain of dust : death, deceit, and the lawyer
who busted big asbestos / David Kinley.
Description: Baltimore : Johns Hopkins University Press,
2025. | Includes index. |
Identifiers: LCCN 2024038675 | ISBN 9781421451602
(hardcover ; alk. paper) | ISBN 9781421451619 (ebook)
Subjects: MESH: Meeran, Richard. | Cape plc. | Asbestos—
adverse effects | Liability, Legal—history | Environmental
Exposure—history | Apartheid—history | South Africa
Classification: LCC RA1231.A8 | NLM WA 11 HU5 |
DDC 363.738/494—dc23/eng/20250111
LC record available at https://lccn.loc.gov/2024038675

A catalog record for this book is available from the British Library.

*Special discounts are available for bulk purchases of this book.
For more information, please contact Special Sales
at specialsales@jh.edu.*

EU GPSR Authorized Representative
LOGOS EUROPE, 9 rue Nicolas Poussin, 17000, La Rochelle, France
E-mail: Contact@logoseurope.eu

Semper in tenebris lux

Contents

Prologue

Several judges were shaking their heads, exasperated by what they were reading. It was the moment he began to think that they just might win. After years of seemingly endless court battles fighting an unscrupulous corporate giant armed with the best legal team money could buy, an exhausting itinerary shuttling between London and Johannesburg, and countless hours taking victims' statements and poring over hundreds of thousands of pages of medical records, scientific studies, legal documents, and company reports, Richard Meeran could hardly believe it.

Meeran is the lawyer who in the 1990s took on Cape Plc, one of the biggest names in the dirty business of asbestos mining. He alleged that the UK-based company's South African operations had caused the death of thousands of impoverished, predominantly black and coloured workers* and brought disease to many thousands more, all the while knowing of the dangers of asbestos to people's health and welfare. It was a case of willful negligence, coverup, and double standards. Yet despite a body of damning evidence, the whole case turned on arguments over

---

* The terms "black," "coloured," and "white" are used throughout because these were, and still are, terms used in South Africa to denote racial communities and ethnicity (see, for example, Statistics South Africa's *Census 2022*, at https://census.statssa.gov.za/#/). The spelling of "coloured," when used in the South African context, reflects this usage. See Glossary.

arcane and entrenched rules about jurisdiction and the separation of parent and subsidiary corporations. *Where* was the proper place for the case against the company to be heard? In the United Kingdom, where Cape Plc was incorporated, or in South Africa, where its former subsidiary companies had operated? The answer was crucial.

Cape Plc wanted the case heard in South Africa, where the claimants (whose number would eventually swell to 7,500) would likely have no legal representation, as neither legal aid nor lawyers able to act on contingency were then available under South African law. Without legal counsel, any prospects of successfully suing the company were markedly reduced. If, on the other hand, the case was heard in the United Kingdom, as Richard Meeran argued it should be, the litigants could have access to lawyers funded by legal aid, and any finding of negligence might attract a significant award of damages that Cape Plc, as the parent company, had the financial capacity to pay. The problem for Meeran was that a century of established legal precedent favored Cape. Tearing away the corporate veil that protected parent companies like Cape from liability for its own actions or failures in respect of subsidiary operations was a truly monumental task, and yet for the sick, the dying, and the families of the already dead, he felt compelled to give it all he had.

Thursday, June 19, 2000, was a muggy, early summer's day in London as Meeran took his place behind the bar table in the somber and surprisingly understated surroundings of the Appellate Committee of the House of Lords, then the United Kingdom's highest court. The five judges before him—the Law Lords—were considering the reasons why, eight months earlier, three judges of the Court of Appeal below the House of Lords had unanimously sided with Cape. The Law Lords' decision would depend on how persuaded they were by the arguments of the lower court, and as the House of Lords was the court of last resort, its decision would be final.[1]

Meeran was surprised to see senior judges openly show such apparent disdain for fellow members of the bench. Their Lordships' collective head-shaking was indeed a rare sight—and one, as it turned out, that was pivotal in this case. They were not impressed by the Court of Appeal's reasoning (it had failed to take proper account of the evidence presented to it, they said) and duly held, unanimously, that the case against Cape could proceed in British courts. Given the weight of evidence of negligence that he had so painstakingly amassed against the company, Meeran was optimistic about the prospects of a favorable outcome.

Victory was in sight. Or at least so he thought.

≈

The story of how Richard Meeran had reached this point and what happened next is as remarkable as it is unlikely. The plot twists its way through anger and despair, unheralded heroes and despicable villains, unexpected saviors, and peculiar alliances. It mixes corporate skulduggery with political intrigue and the asceticism of law with the raw emotion of righting wrongs. "This is a story I've wanted to be told for some time," Richard said to me when I approached him about it.

I first met Richard in London in the late 1990s, when the Cape litigation was just beginning. Always snappily attired—"trendy," as one glossy business magazine profile put it, "dressed in a black suit and incongruously distressed Prada-like slip on shoes" (it *was* 2001)[2]—he's nevertheless a rolled-up-sleeves lawyer when it comes to the hard graft of litigation. With long fingers often steepled in contemplation in front of a crookedly good-looking face, he has a ready, engaging smile and a slightly disarming intensity when listening to what you have to say. His voice is soft, with a light South London accent, measured in tone, precise and economical. There is no babbling with Richard, no space-filling "ahhs," "umms," or "you knows." What he says is to the point and always worth listening to. He also has a forensically keen eye for both detail and the absurd, which makes him an astute collector of anecdotes and a compelling storyteller.

What he told me back then about the events leading up to his taking on the case in the first place and the events that were unfolding as we spoke was indeed riveting. I was part of what was in those days a small but animated business and human rights movement, and Richard's coalface litigation experiences added authentic bite to the airy pontifications that academics like me were making at the time. The bite is still there. Indeed, in many ways, talismanic cases like *Cape* laid the foundations on which businesses today are pressed to take human rights seriously, even if they don't like it. There's nothing quite like a writ claiming human rights abuses broadcast across media headlines to capture the attention of a corporation's senior management.

When I initially broached the idea with him of committing the Cape story to print, Richard immediately launched a string of yarns about bowel-loosening, two-seater plane rides over the African bush with a cross-eyed pilot; church halls overflowing with desperate asbestosis and mesothelioma victims; depositions detailing the horrors of children playing in asbestos dumps or, worse still, employed to trample asbestos fiber into enormous sacks; women "cobbers," who were often exposed to the worst levels of contamination; and "chissa" boys whose lives depended on how quick they could run after lighting the fuses of explosive charges. He told me about discovering piles of incriminating workers' records in the offices of an abandoned blue asbestos mine; anonymously hand-delivered envelopes exposing smear campaigns against him; the selflessness of some South African doctors alongside the corruption of others; and the obsessive and bitter rivalry between the two sets of opposing lawyers. Two hours raced by. He also hinted at the intense interest that leading South African politicians had in the case ("they used to fly up to London for the day to sit talking in my office") and flagged a deeper story about how a so-called vulture fund (perhaps the most despised form of financier, which says a lot) emerged as the victims' improbable knight in shining armour.

I was hooked.

≈

The litigation began thirty years ago, yet Richard remembers it all as if it was yesterday. Initially, he constructed the case almost entirely on his own (a junior lawyer, Susannah Read, was later to join him). "It was hard, but I loved being steeped in the details," he says. "We had no team of lawyers to do the leg work [as he has now]—just a notebook, tape recorder, and an assistant to help sift through documents and compile evidence."

While it is the legal path of the case that forms the skeleton of this book, it is the stories of the characters populating it that put flesh on the bones, a Frankensteinian exercise that took me more than four years to complete. The formidable task of retracing Richard's footsteps in terms not only of where he went, but also whom he met (where possible), and what he read, said, and wrote, took time, as did the further task of adding in relevant subsequent events and new research that emerged over the intervening years. As these people, places, and records were (and still are) scattered far and wide—in London and throughout South Africa of course, but also in Australia, Scotland, and the United States, reflecting both the transnational nature of the litigation and the global reach of asbestos concerns—the need to find time to travel was as unavoidable as were the proscriptions related to COVID-19 that restricted opportunities to do so.

Chief among these information resources was Richard himself, through whose storehouse of vivid recollections I rummaged in numerous interviews, Zoom meetings, and phone calls, which together amounted to some 200 hours' worth of material. Prompted by these interactions, or sometimes out of the blue, Richard would also pepper me with choice tidbits he'd remembered or found, including articles, reports, transcripts, and press clippings. Some were profound and disturbing, others bizarre and ribald, but all (or nearly all) so compelling as to find their way into the pages that follow.[3]

The book's fleshed-out human stories were also collected via some eighty interviews and meetings (mostly face-to-face), plus many more interactions, with an array of the book's other main players—victims and their families, medical professionals and scientists, occupational health experts, trade unionists, politicians and government officials (both former and current), academics, civil society activists, and lawyers and paralegals involved in the case, as well as Richard's colleagues, friends, and family—all of whom in various ways added depth, color, and vitality.

Delving into these myriad troves yielded many treasures, no matter the daunting task of ploughing through mountains of documents and sifting through hundreds of hours of interviews to find them. But as with tackling a giant jigsaw puzzle, each tiny victory spurred me on to another until eventually the whole image revealed itself.

Amid all the pieces of tragedy, deceit, and courtroom drama surrounding the Cape case there emerged a heartening coalition of hope, a defining force as it were, that helped propel the case forward. For the small South African towns of Prieska, Koegas, and Penge, where Cape's asbestos mines and mills were located, the whole dreadful affair had a galvanizing impact. Black, white, and coloured communities were united in their loss, grief, and determination to see justice done. Asbestos dust is indiscriminate when airborne. It lodges in the lungs of anyone who breathes in the tiny lacerating fibers, regardless of race or riches. Once inhaled, the sentence of death by emaciation and suffocation begins, no matter the color of your skin.

This shared inheritance of Apartheid's capitalist footprint had been building for decades, reaching a peak in the late 1990s, at the very same time as South Africa was wrestling with its newly won freedom from white supremacist rule just a few years earlier. The symbolism of the *Cape* case, Richard realized, was as important to the born-again nation and its people as were the reparations sought by the litigating victims. When the local press started labelling him "son of Africa" as the case began to capture international attention, he thought it reflected merely that his father was born in South Africa (in Pietermaritzburg) and lived there until he was thirty, "but in fact I think it also pointed to a deeper investment in the case in holding Apartheid policies to account," he says. So, the stakes were high.

Glossary

ABSA Amalgamated Banks of South Africa.

ACTSA Action for South Africa.

adit A small mine with a horizontal entry passage.

affidavit In the United Kingdom, a sworn, out-of-court testimony.

AGM Annual General Meeting.

amosite A type of asbestos, colored brown due to high iron (ferrous oxide) content, that is found only in South Africa. Amosite is no longer mined or in commercial use.

amphibole a class of asbestos characterized by the needle-like shape of composite fibers (e.g., amosite and crocidolite asbestos).

ANC African National Congress.

ARDs Asbestos-related diseases; an umbrella term for a suite of medical diagnoses that include, asbestosis, mesothelioma, pleural plaques, and pleural effusion.

ART Asbestos Relief Trust.

asbestos A fibrous silicate mineral, of which amosite, crocidolite, and chrysotile were the principal types used commercially.

asbestosis A chronic lung disease caused by inhalation of asbestos fibers, which cause fibrosis (thickening or scarring) of lung tissue.

barrister (UK) See **counsel (UK)**.

black Individual or community in South Africa, often self-identified as such; sometimes referred to as "African," or "black African."

CALS Centre for Applied Legal Studies, University of Witwatersrand.

CASAP Cape Asbestos South Africa Property Limited, established in 1948 and located in Johannesburg.

"chissa" boys Teenagers employed at mine sites to light fuses of explosives laid by engineers. Once lit they had to run as fast as they could away from the blast site.

chrysotile A type of asbestos, colored white due to high magnesium oxide content. Still mined and in commercial use, especially in Russia and Asia.

cobbing, cobbers Those employed in removing asbestos fibers from host rocks by hand, usually with assistance of a hammer. Their labor is called "cobbing."

coloured Individual or community in South Africa, with mixed white (European), black (African), and/or Asian ancestry, often self-identified as such.

corporate veil Marking a legal separation between corporate entities.

counsel (UK) A barrister who has rights of audience to appear in all UK courts; typically engaged by solicitors on behalf of their clients, to act on the clients' behalf as their advocate in court, most especially when cases reach superior courts in which solicitors do not normally have rights of audience. See also **solicitor.**

Court of Appeal Intermediate court in UK court hierarchy, above the High Court but beneath the House of Lords (now, since 2009, the Supreme Court).

CPAA Concerned People Against Asbestos (Prieska).

crocidolite A type of asbestos, colored blue due to high iron (ferrous and ferric oxides) and sodium oxide contents; significant deposits found only in Australia and South Africa. No longer mined or in commercial use.

CSIR Council for Scientific and Industrial Research (South Africa).

DAC Davies Arnold Cooper (UK law firm).

deposition A sworn, out-of-court testimony in the United States.

environmental exposure Encountering asbestos dust or other dangerous substance outside the workplace.

Forum non conveniens **(FNC)** Inappropriate forum (or jurisdiction) to hear a case when there is more than one forum available.

GASA General Accident South Africa.

HAT Hendrik Afrika Trust.

High Court Court of first instance in the UK for civil cases of importance and significant monetary value; comprising three divisions and sitting beneath the Court of Appeal.

House of Lords Short for the Appellate Committee of the House of Lords, formerly the highest court in the UK curial hierarchy; replaced by the Supreme Court in 2009. Distinguished from the House of Lords as the second (upper) chamber of the UK Parliament.

IBAS International Ban Asbestos Secretariat.

J UK legal shorthand for "Judge," as in Buckley J.

JPP John Pickering & Partners (UK law firm).

LAB Legal Aid Board in the United Kingdom; replaced by the Legal Services Commission, now the Legal Aid Agency.

Limpopo Province in South Africa; previously, known as Northern Transvaal. Includes Burgersfort, Mafafe, and Penge.

LJ Lord or Lady Justice (of Appeal); an Appeal Court judge.

LLJ Lords or Ladies Justices (of Appeal); two or more Appeal Court judges.

LRC Legal Resources Centre, an independent public interest law organization in South Africa.

LSC Legal Services Commission (UK).

MBOD Medical Bureau for Occupational Diseases (South Africa).

mesothelioma A cancerous tumor of the mesothelial (outer) lining of the lungs, heart, or peritoneum.

NCOH National Centre for Occupational Health (1979–2003); replaced the National Research Institute for Occupational Diseases (NRIOD).

NIOH National Institute for Occupational Health (since 2003); replaced the National Centre for Occupational Health (NCOH).

Northern Cape Unofficial name for part of former Cape Province in South Africa. Officially recognized as a province since 1994. Includes Griekwastad, Koegas, and Prieska.

Northern Transvaal Part of former province of Transvaal in South Africa; renamed Northern Province in 1995 and then Limpopo Province in 2002. Includes Burgersfort, Mafafe, and Penge.

NRIOD National Research Institute for Occupational Diseases (1971–1979); replaced the Pneumoconiosis Research Unit (PRU).

NUM (SA) National Union of Mineworkers (South Africa).

NUM/NUM (UK) National Union of Mineworkers in the United Kingdom.

occupational exposure Encountering asbestos dust or other dangerous substance during the course of one's employment.

Per curiam As decided by the court as a whole, as distinct from the reasoning of individual judges.

plaques Thickened, cartilage-like tissue in the lung lining.

PLC/Plc Public limited company incorporated in the United Kingdom.

pleura/pleural A serous membrane that envelops the lungs, comprising an parietal (outer) and visceral (inner) layer.

PRU Pneumoconiosis Research Unit in South Africa; initially established within the Department of Mines in 1953, thereafter under the Council for Scientific and Industrial Research (CSIR) from 1956 to 1971, after which the PRU became the National Research Institute for Occupational Diseases (NRIOD).

Pty/Pty Ltd Proprietary or proprietary limited (company).

QC Queen's Counsel (senior counsel); replaced by King's Counsel (KC) in September 2022; see also **silk**.

R Rand, South African unit of currency.

SAAPAC South African Asbestos Producers' Advisory Committee.

SALAB South African Legal Aid Board.

SAMRC South African Medical Research Council.

SC Senior Counsel (South Africa).

serpentine A class of asbestos characterized by the curly shape of composite fibers (e.g., chrysotile asbestos).

silk Colloquial term for senior counsel in UK legal system (by tradition their gowns are made of silk, those of junior counsel are made of cotton); formally entitled King's (or Queen's) Counsel.

solicitor (UK) Qualified legal professional providing legal advice and support to clients, including in litigation matters. They have rights of audience to appear in the lower courts but not, normally, in the superior courts. See also **barrister (UK)** and **counsel (UK)**.

stay A court order to halt legal proceedings.

tort A cause of action at common law (e.g., negligence).

TRC Truth and Reconciliation Commission (South Africa).

white Individual or community in South Africa, often self-identified as such; typically of European ancestry.

WLC Wits Law Clinic, operating out of the University of Witwatersrand School of Law.

WWB Webber Wentzel Bowens (South African law firm).

Litigation Timeline

1995

February — Lawyer Richard Meeran approached by the National Union of Mineworkers regarding Cape Plc's asbestos legacy in South Africa

1997

February 14 — *Lubbe et al. v. Cape Plc* filed in the London High Court (Queen's Bench Division)

March 7 — Cape Plc issues application to stay *Lubbe* proceedings

July 7–11 — Hearings on stay application before Deputy Judge Kallipetis QC

September 9 — Following written submissions on the effect of *Connolly v. RTZ*, further hearing before Deputy Judge Kallipetis QC

December 9 — Following additional written submissions, further hearing before Deputy Judge Kallipetis QC

1998

January 12 — Stay application granted by Deputy Judge Kallipetis QC; *Lubbe* proceedings halted (first High Court)

February 19	Notice of Appeal against stay lodged in Court of Appeal pursuant to the leave given by Judge LJ
May 13–14	Hearings before Court of Appeal with further written submissions
July 30	Court of Appeal allows appeal and lifts stay on *Lubbe* (first Court of Appeal)
August 27	Cape Plc seeks leave to appeal to the House of Lords
November 9	Claimants' short written objections and observations for the House of Lords lodged (settled by Barbara Dohmann QC and Graham Read)
December 16	House of Lords summarily denies Cape leave to appeal (no hearing) (first House of Lords)

1999

January 18	*Afrika et al. v. Cape Plc* filed in the high court (Queen's Bench Division)
January–March	Further writs filed by Richard Meeran and Anthony Coombs (John Pickering & Partners)
February 5	Cape Plc issues summons claiming abuse of process and applying to stay all actions
March/April	Preliminary hearings before Buckley J in High Court
July 5–13	Hearing of the defendant's stay application before Buckley J
July 30	Buckley J grants stay; all proceedings against Cape halted (second High Court)

August 10	Notice of appeal lodged against stay in Court of Appeal following permission to appeal granted by Buckley J
October	Hearings before Court of Appeal
November 29	Court of Appeal denies appeal, reaffirming stay (second Court of Appeal)

2000

January 10	Richard seeks permission to appeal to the House of Lords, which is granted on February 7
June	Hearings before House of Lords in *Lubbe*, *Afrika*, and other cases
July 20	House of Lords allows the appeal; stay is lifted on all proceedings (second/final House of Lords)

2001

November– December	Negotiations with Cape to settle
December 21	First settlement agreement signed £21 million)

2002

January–April	Establishment of Henrick Afrika Trust (HAT) to manage the settlement
August	Cape Plc's banks decline to offer necessary loans, and settlement collapses
September	Settlement negotiations with Cape Plc reopen

2003

March 13	New settlement agreement with Cape and Gencor concluded (£10.6 million)
May	Individual settlement payout calculations for claimants commence

2004

September	Final settlement payouts are made

CHAPTER 1

David versus Goliath

—*High Stakes*—

SQUASHED UNCOMFORTABLY INTO mismatched office chairs, the two burly miners sitting in front of Richard Meeran meant business. They were members of Britain's National Union of Mineworkers (NUM), and they wanted to know whether Richard could help sue a UK–based asbestos giant, Cape Plc, on behalf of the employees of its former South African subsidiary companies who were now diseased and dying. It was February 1995, and the meeting was taking place in the offices of Leigh Day, a tiny law firm that Richard had joined as a young lawyer a few years earlier. Perched above a Communist Party bookshop at the seedier end of Gray's Inn Road in North London, the rooms were dingy, cramped, and furnished secondhand, but they were being loaned to the firm rent-free, which appeal trumped all other concerns.

However apt the location—the notoriously militant NUM had orchestrated a nationwide miners' strike that consumed British politics and then–Prime Minister Margaret Thatcher for more than a year in the mid-1980s—the union's top brass was not there to talk revolutionary ideology, but rather to discuss a fine-grained

legal point.[1] They knew that Richard was currently representing a Scot named Edward Connelly in a case against mining
giant Rio Tinto Zinc (RTZ). Connelly was claiming that his work
in a uranium mine in Namibia, operated by an RTZ subsidiary during the late 1970s and early 1980s, had caused the la-
ryngeal cancer that he had been diagnosed with in 1986, after he
had returned to Scotland. Connelly, through Richard, was ad-
vancing the novel but contentious argument that the case could
and should be heard in the United Kingdom, where RTZ was
based, despite the injury occurring overseas. The NUM wondered whether the same argument might be used with regard
to victims of asbestos mining in South Africa, with whom the
union was in touch via its sister organization, NUM (South Africa). The Connelly litigation was still in its early stages and facing a torrid time in the lower courts,[2] but perhaps this asbestos
case offered an opportunity for a second bite at the cherry.

Richard was aware of the health-endangering history of mining and mineral manufacturing in South Africa, having recently pursued another UK-based corporation (Thor Chemicals)
operating in South Africa for poisoning workers with mercury
in one of its factories, but he was not familiar with the details of
the legacy of asbestos mining. What his two visitors hinted at
was an appalling trail of destruction. As Richard was soon to
discover, it comprised thousands of Cape's former employees who
were sick, dying, or dead from asbestos-related diseases (ARDs).
Many members of their families and local communities were
also similarly afflicted; little or no compensation was available
to any of the victims under the overtly discriminatory occupational health and safety laws; and Cape Plc itself, having departed the country more than a decade earlier, had washed its
hands of any responsibility. Nearly all victims were black or coloured, with rates of ARDs nearly 200 times the average rate for

the rest of the country.[3] Working conditions had been atrocious, with dust levels so high that asbestos fibers caked miners' faces to the point where they were unrecognizable, even to those who knew them well, when they emerged at the end of their shifts.[4]

What truly shocked Richard, however, were the indications that Cape had known about the health hazards of asbestos for decades and yet had not taken adequate (or any) preventive action to protect its South African workers. Cape "never warned us that it was dangerous work we were doing. . . . I am unhappy with those people who took all those millions and led us to our death," as Hendrik Afrika, one of the lead litigants in the cases that were to follow, put it.[5] Even more damning, there were indications that Cape had actively downplayed any health dangers by suppressing or discrediting scientific evidence and covering its tracks as it did so. Workers and local communities alike had been kept in the dark, dissuaded or prevented from getting medical checks, assured that there was nothing to worry about, and told that if they were having any health problems it was likely due to smoking rather than asbestos dust. Slowly, over many years, and through the tireless efforts of community organizations, local doctors, dedicated scientists, and workers' unions, signs of a massive cover-up were exposed as the numbers of the dead and seriously ill steadily mounted. These "asbestos communities" didn't know the whole story, but they knew enough to make them angry.

The presence of the NUM in Richard's office that morning reflected the path the victims' anger had taken. Political dissent had long been suppressed in Apartheid South Africa, with organizations such as the African National Congress (ANC) being legally banned for thirty years between 1960 and 1990. The many injustices of Apartheid had to be ventilated in other ways, one of which was through trade unions like South Africa's own

3

NUM, representing the interests of black mine workers. Established in 1982 by leading labor and anti-Apartheid activists, including Cyril Ramaphosa (present-day president of South Africa), the union was integral to the formation a few years later of the powerful Congress of South African Trade Unions. Though despised by the government, both organizations were tolerated as conduits through which to negotiate the country's increasingly feverish labor disputes. For the trade unionists, however, these structures were especially significant, amounting to what Thabo Makweya, then a young but leading NUM activist, dubbed "the ANC in disguise." It was "an underground movement of strategic importance" to the whole anti-Apartheid struggle, he adds, underlining the point.[6] Indeed, the long history of black lives and livelihoods sacrificed in South Africa's mines was at the time a readymade flashpoint for the many deep-seated political grievances of the country's repressed majority, to which the human toll of asbestos mining had become an especially dreadful addition.

As organized labor in South Africa gathered strength during the 1980s and early 1990s, it drew on a widening network of overseas sympathy and support. Money poured in from Europe, and senior leaders traveled across the world, gathering intelligence and forging relations with trade unions wherever they went. An alliance between the two NUMs in South Africa and the United Kingdom was an obvious association, providing a channel through which details of the unfolding tragedy of asbestos mining in South Africa were relayed and thence made their way to Richard Meeran's door.[7]

The significance of the fact that the miners' meeting with Richard was taking place barely a year after the historic abandonment of Apartheid, the holding of free elections, and Nelson Mandela being sworn in as the new president of South Africa was not lost on any party. The NUM (SA) was relishing its new-found freedom and power alongside ANC-controlled governments in place, not only at the national level but also in the provinces, including, most particularly, the Northern Cape and Limpopo, where the asbestos mining operations were located. The NUM (UK) was also keen to play its part in helping dismantle Apartheid capitalism and seek out reparations for the harms it had caused to their fellow workers in South Africa. So, the circumstances were ripe for building a bridge between the two unions across which they could share ideas on how best to seek compensation for asbestos's victims.[8]

Doing his bit in this righteous struggle against past and ongoing wrongs appealed to Richard, not just because of his natural disposition to confront injustice regardless of the odds, often biting off more than he can chew, but chewing madly nonetheless. It was also because for Richard racist injustice is a visceral matter and, further, because he himself has strong family connections to South Africa. His own grandmother lived near Cato Ridge in KwaZulu-Natal, where the Thor Chemicals factory had been polluting the river with mercury, which made his suit against that company personal as well as professional.

Race had played a central part in Richard's upbringing. His mother Lilian, an Anglo-Indian, was born and orphaned in India, while his father, Moosa, was born in South Africa of Indian parents. Lilian and Moosa had each migrated to England in the late 1950s in search of work, then met and married. Richard was born a few years later in 1961 in Stockwell, South London. Growing up Asian or African in Britain in the 1960s and 1970s was tough. There was no politically correct filter, not in politics, business, or the law. Least of all were there any checks on racial sensitivities in the school yard. Racism was rife. Brixton, where Richard went to primary school, and Battersea, where he went to high school, were relatively poor neighborhoods in those days, populated by immigrant families and often simmering with pent-up tension.

Richard had just farewelled his teenage years when the first of the Brixton race riots erupted in 1981, but he well remembers his school years as fraught with verbal taunts and physical abuse, including once being pushed off a moving bus during an altercation with a pair of skinheads. He was sporty, which helped, and a bit of a rebel (according to his dad). Most of all, he was witty and smart. All good survival qualities, but also fuel for the fire in his belly, which helped push him through a degree in biochemistry at University College London (UCL) and then a postgraduate diploma in law (the so-called law conversion course)[9] at City University. After qualifying, however, Richard found it hard to put theory into practice. Law firms doing the sort of work that appealed to him were few and far between (they still are), and prejudice was endemic in the profession. His skin color sometimes led to moments of true farce. "After sending my CV to one firm," he recalls, "the partner called me very enthusiastically. He was keen for me to meet him the next day and said he would take me for lunch afterward. But his jaw dropped when he saw me in person. The 'interview' lasted only eight minutes, during which he didn't ask me a single question."[10] Showing mettle that has since become his trademark, Richard duly launched a pioneering and successful discrimination action against the firm in the Industrial Tribunal.[11]

Injustice and unfairness were personal for sure, but Richard also deeply resented their impact on others and was driven to try to do something about it. "I took part in many campaigns and demonstrations, including against multinational corporations" while a student at UCL, he says. Law, he believed, might be a useful tool in a rebel's armory. Goolam, his father's younger brother, had shone a light down that path by becoming a director of the United Kingdom's Commission for Racial Equality before qualifying as a barrister in his forties and later holding judicial positions, first as president of the Employment Tribunal for England and Wales and then serving on the United Nations Dispute Tribunal.[12] "He was a big influence on me when I was younger," Richard tells me when I ask him what pushed him toward law.

≈

As Richard was clearing away the empty teacups and the untouched, slightly stale biscuits after the NUM comrades had left his office, he pondered on all he'd heard. Certainly, he saw many reasons for taking the matter on. The merits of the case and the desperate plight of Cape's former employees and other victims of asbestos mining, most especially. But also, the propitious political circumstances in South Africa, as well as the general goodwill the international community wished the country now freed from the shackles of Apartheid. All of these attracted the bolshie, social justice litigator in Richard. But he was not so rash as to ignore the huge obstacles standing in the way.

First and foremost, there were the legal challenges—among them long established rules of common law that effectively protected parent companies from the legal liabilities of their subsidiaries and shielded UK corporations from being sued in UK courts for their alleged misdeeds in other countries. Notwithstanding the partial successes in the *Connelly v. RTZ* and *Thor Chemicals* cases, the present case was of a different order in terms not only of potential numbers of plaintiffs (many thousands as it turned out), but also the fact that the potential plaintiffs were non-UK nationals, mostly very poor, many illiterate, and all, by definition, gravely ill or deceased and being represented by their families. What is more, the events that sickened or killed them had happened decades ago, and Cape had long since ceased all operations in South Africa. Most particularly, Richard was conscious of a recent failure by US-based victims of asbestos poisoning by one of Cape's subsidiary companies to gain access to the parent company's UK assets, when the English Court of Appeal blocked the enforcement of a Texas judgment for personal injury claims against those assets.[13]

Then there was the matter of the legal liabilities to which Cape was subject. These centered on claims of Cape's negligent behavior regarding its oversight and implementation of health and safety policies as they applied to workers employed by its South African subsidiaries, as well as potentially others affected by Cape's operations, leading to their injury or ill-health. In stark legal terms, the task entailed establishing what duty of care (not to be so negligent) Cape owed, to whom it owed that duty, and whether and how the company had breached such duty, thereby causing damage. Together, these jurisprudential hurdles stood like sentinels guarding entry to the next level of a court-room computer game. Even identifying suitable claimants was challenging, as it necessitated assessing much of the life histories of very ill or deceased individuals who had either worked for Cape or lived close to its facilities. It also required demonstrating that their illness (or death) had been caused by asbestos exposure and that such exposure was occasioned by Cape's asbestos operations either wholly or substantially. Many of those who might fit this bill were poor, illiterate, incapacitated, located remotely, and quite possibly distrustful of lawyers, let alone foreign ones, asking searching questions about their employment, living conditions, and health. Accessing even baseline information, therefore, was going to be difficult and time-consuming.

At the same time, Richard was also educating himself in the science of asbestos, the intricacies of its medical footprint, the processes of its extraction and manufacture, the manner of its commercialization, the history and structure of Cape's corporate operations, and the fine-grained details of South Africa's occupational health legislation throughout the twentieth century. The enormity of the challenge was no less than that which faces all mass tort cases involving powerful and recalcitrant corporations in an industry beset by accusations of gravely endangering the health of multitudes of unwitting employees, customers, and bystanders. Drawing inspiration as well as some trepidation from the massive corpus of litigation against Big Tobacco[14]— the twentieth century's other infamous producer of a deadly carcinogen—Richard was under no illusions as to the size of the undertaking.

With such big undertakings come big bills. Funding, therefore, was another matter of critical concern. Pitted against Cape's deep pockets and a ferociously committed legal team (who would "never surrender" as one of them was later to tell Richard once litigation commenced),[15] Richard's clients were essentially penniless, and his own tiny law firm was still operating on a hand-to-mouth basis as it struggled to establish itself. Whether Leigh Day would be able to secure funding through legal aid was contingent on persuading the Legal Aid Board (LAB) of England and Wales that a group of foreign claimants living thousands of miles away, in a jurisdiction in which the alleged tort is said to have occurred, could and should be funded by the British taxpayer to pursue their case in English courts. It was a very tall order. Yet Richard had little choice, as private-sector litigation funders did not then exist in the United Kingdom. And while conditional or contingency fee (so-called "no win no fee") arrangements had recently been legalized in Britain,[16] that path was not a practical option for Leigh Day, as it had an insufficient capital base against which it could draw to pay for the day-to-day costs of litigation.

Richard needed up-front funding, not merely the promise of recouping costs years down the track. It is true that at the time Richard was more idealistic than practical, caring far less about the money than the cause. He had, briefly, flirted with the idea of doing the case on a no win no fee basis, but the stark reality for him, the firm, and the clients was that without cash-flow funding at the very least, a case of this size and likely duration simply could not be mounted. But luck turned out to be on his side as the window during which these sorts of cases were eligible for legal aid in the United Kingdom was just a handful of years, closing in 2000 around the time the final (House of Lords) judgment in the case was delivered.[17] Richard still had to convince the LAB at each stage of the litigation that their case was both eligible and worthy of funding (no mean task when it went through so many rounds of litigation), but it was a singular opportunity that had to be grabbed with both hands.

Finally, looming over any prospect of taking on the case, were the elemental questions of litigation strategy. How to locate claimants who were both appropriate and amendable to being plaintiffs? How many plaintiffs? Where and when to file the case or cases? And above all, how to address the certainty of Cape and its lawyers raising the formidable twin defenses of corporate veil and proper jurisdiction (or forum) in order to protect Cape from any suit in English courts.

On this last critical point, Richard had already done some left-field thinking in a published journal article.[18] What, he asked, if corporations could be held liable for injuries resulting from their defective *processes*, just as they are held liable, under now well-established law, for injuries resulting from defective products? As negligence is at the heart of both situations, should not the legal consequences be comparable where defect can be traced to the parent company regardless of its location? Even if the logic and simplicity of the argument seemed appealing, Richard knew it was a radical suggestion precisely because it would expose corporate management decisions to unwelcome scrutiny. For this reason, he had sought advice from two senior legal figures on whether his idea had any merit and, more to the point, whether it might succeed in breaching those two redoubtable defenses. He'd done so informally—in conversation with Ken Rokison QC and, through a mutual contact, with recently retired Lord Justice May.[19] Both had listened politely before telling him that while it was a terrific idea, it had little prospect of success.

Nor, later, did Cape and its lawyers give Meeran much of a chance. In characteristically high-handed and dismissive terms, Cape's 1997 annual report published shortly after the case's first trial hearing, declared that the company was currently

> subject to litigation arising out of mining activities in South Africa where plaintiffs are seeking compensation in respect of asbestos-related diseases. The company has received legal advice that there are good prospects of defending these actions as long as the normal rules governing corporate individuality apply. The directors believe, in light of legal advice they have received, that the above-mentioned matters are unlikely to have a material effect in the group's financial position.[20]

This self-assured, combative approach, absent any concern for the victims let alone any signs of responsibility or contrition, set the tone for what became an acrimonious and often ferocious six years of allegations, accusations, professional attacks, and litigation.

≈

Undeterred—emboldened, even, by the audacity of the case—Richard took it on. It was, after all, precisely the attraction of this sort of gross injustice—and of engaging in a David-versus-Goliath contest—that drew him away from his first law job with Brecher & Company, a small commercial firm just off Bond Street in central London. While he credits his time there for helping him understand what really motivates big corporations and how they work, his heart was not then in it.[21] Just how disenchanted he was with the ideas of pursuing profit and making money as life's defining forces became very clear to him in a London court room one cold, cloudy day in early 1990.

He was in court getting ready to represent an extremely wealthy Armenian client (who'd given Richard a lift to court that morning in his Ferrari F40) when two things happened that were to change his life, even if he was not quite aware of it at the time. First, his hearing—concerning a claim for damages in the order of £500,000 for the failed delivery to his client of two Porsche 959s—was briefly delayed when the judge gave priority to an infant settlement hearing. An eleven-year-old girl had sustained serious brain injuries in a road accident after she ran into the path of an oncoming car; the hearing was to seek court approval for an insurance settlement of £50,000. After the matter was dispensed, Richard's client turned to him, bewildered—"That's all the kid gets for losing her future," he said in amazement, "and I'm here demanding ten times that amount for two cars I've never had!" Richard agreed, thinking how he couldn't have put it any better himself.

The second pivotal episode arose from Richard's observations of the solicitor representing the injured girl. His name was Martyn Day, and he was passionate, committed, and confident.

Richard was immediately taken by Martyn's demeanor as much as by the case he was arguing. "As I watched and listened, it was clear to me that *that* was the sort of lawyering I wanted to be doing," he says, reflecting on that morning's events. Fate then stepped in when, a couple of weeks later, his eye was caught by a tiny advertisement in the *Law Society Gazette* for a job with Leigh Day, the fledgling law firm that Martyn Day had established alongside Sarah Leigh only a few years earlier. These two firebrand solicitors, whose dedication to personal injury and public interest litigation and to taking on big corporations rather than serving them, chimed precisely with Richard's inclinations. The firm was suing British Nuclear Fuels Limited (BNFL) at the time for allegedly causing the children of its employees and in local communities to develop leukemia through exposure to radioactive uranium emissions from BNFL's flagship Sellafield plant in the north of England.

The job interview with Leigh Day was rather chaotic. Richard arrived ninety minutes late due to a problem on the London Underground and couldn't make contact to explain and apologize (it was pre–cell phone ubiquity). Martyn then spent most of the interview on the phone to a journalist, barely asking Richard any questions. "But it was clear they desperately needed another lawyer," Richard recalls, "and I'm pretty sure I was the only applicant for the job," though when asked, Martyn claims (somewhat half-heartedly, it must be said) that there was one other candidate. Sarah and Martyn offered him the job, and despite thinking "they were slightly mad" and taking a big drop in salary, Richard leaped on board. The Sellafield cases entailed the longest running civil actions in English legal history at that time. Richard was immediately thrown into the fray, becoming something of an expert along the way on the genetic consequences of exposure to radioactivity (partly on account of his first degree in science), as well as learning first hand what it meant to sue big corporations that were determined to defend themselves at almost any cost. In the end the actions against BNFL failed,[22] but they were the first in a string of so-called toxic-tort suits that Richard and the firm were to pursue against a long list of high-profile corporations in the years that followed.

The fact that the case against Cape would be ground-breaking, *if* Richard and Leigh Day managed to pull it off, simply added to its allure. To be sure, it required ingenuity, even rat-cunning, as well as a thick skin and no fear of gut-busting hard work if the case was to succeed, but something about Richard's droll sense of humor and his steely resolve convinced Martyn and Sarah that he had what it takes. Many years later they expressed to me their respective confidence in him in characteristically distinct fashions—Sarah's generous assessment of Richard's professional attributes, delivered in the cut-glass tones of upper-class English, as "courageous, imaginative, and persistent," being as refined as Martyn's expression of admiration was uncouth: "Yet another of his fucking hair-brained schemes!" But both were sincere, and, as it turned out, both were correct. From those earliest of days, Richard was a good fit for the firm.

Fearless, even foolhardy at times, the three of them were nonetheless conscious of the case's epic dimensions. Primarily, that is, the contest between poor, mainly black victims living in a developing country versus a rich, white-run corporation headquartered in the West. But also, more broadly, all that was at stake. Not just the possibility of some semblance of justice for the litigants and the tens, or maybe hundreds, of thousands like them, but for everyone who has been (and still are) exposed to asbestos, whether from working with it, using it, or simply living with it. The fact, furthermore, that the asbestos industry had become such big business during the Second World War and for four decades thereafter[23] meant not only that companies like Cape were able to defend themselves, but also that they were prepared to do so by giving no quarter.

Long before Richard had even contemplated suing Cape, all major asbestos corporations in the West were painfully aware of how exposed they had become as a direct result of their commercial success. The ubiquity of asbestos in nearly every aspect of modern life—from building materials, brake pads, fire blankets, and oven insulation to mattress fillings, cigarette filters, hairdryers, and tampons—and its sheer quantity—sufficient asbestos cement piping was used in the United States alone throughout the twentieth century "to circle the earth eight times and still run to the moon and back"[24]—represented potential liabilities for asbestos-related health problems of monumental proportions for the producers.

And so it had proved to be. The remediation costs of stripping asbestos from homes, schools, offices, ships, planes, trains, cars, and spaceships were stratospheric, and litigation-inspired payouts made by asbestos companies in the United States (especially) and the United Kingdom throughout the 1980s and 1990s were huge.[25] "Chaos has come to the world of asbestos," as one pair of American scientists declared in 1997.[26] The "crucial irony," as the same authors called it, that enabled, indeed hastened, the health catastrophe was the incontestable utility of this "miracle mineral," as indicated by the extraordinary degree to which it had penetrated (literally and figuratively) our lives.[27]

What Richard knew, and what the asbestos producers feared, was that as public health concerns about asbestos overtook and then dismantled admiration of its usefulness, so the asbestos industry lost control of the narrative. Eventually, no amount of extolling asbestos's seemingly magical qualities and myriad uses could justify or excuse the rising levels of human destruction. As a result, from the late 1960s onward in the West, asbestos mining was banned or severely restricted and its manufacture and use more strictly regulated, leading to a precipitous decline in asbestos consumption in developed countries from the early 1970s.[28]

The fear for companies like Cape was that what it had chosen to do during those game-changing years was not going to fare well under scrutiny. The fact that asbestos was now considered so dangerous in the West that it was, in effect, being regulated out of existence had convinced Cape's executives in 1974 to amend the company's full name from "The Cape Asbestos Company" to "Cape Industries Limited." Cape's chairman, Ronald Dent, fooled no one when he declared at that year's annual general meeting of shareholders that the name change simply reflected the diversified nature of what the company had become. Rather, the real reason seemed obvious when, in the company's annual report for 1974, Dent first acknowledged that "there have been . . . a number of adverse criticisms of the industry and your company on health grounds," before underlining how well founded he knew those criticisms to be by adding: "this company has for many years played a leading part in research into health hazards associated with asbestos and we shall continue our efforts to ensure that our products are made and used safely and efficiently."[29] Just how "leading" that research role was and how manipulatively it was played out in favor of efficiency at the expense of safety were soon to become glaringly apparent to Richard.

≈

More immediately obvious, however, was Cape's flagrant exploitation of the accommodating differences in political and regulatory arrangements between South Africa and the United Kingdom. The introduction of increasingly stringent workplace health and safety standards in the United Kingdom had been a key reason why, in 1968, Cape had suspended the manufacture of asbestos products in its largest British plant in Barking and why, shortly thereafter, Cape closed down all its remaining British factories.[30] Meanwhile, Cape maintained its mining and milling operations in South Africa for another eleven years.

The disparity was due primarily to the absence, inadequacy, or disregard of standards in South Africa at that time concerning maximum levels of airborne fibers, adequate filtration and exhaust systems and the provision of appropriate personal safety gear such as masks and clothing. But it was also due to asbestos mining and milling processes being very different from asbestos manufacturing, such that the former were little known about or understood in the United Kingdom and the West more generally. They "were so separated in time and place," wrote pioneering asbestos researcher Jock McCulloch, "as to render the producers and the users of fibre invisible to each other."[31] In any event, Cape actively campaigned against such efforts as were made in South Africa to improve standards of asbestos regulation or knowledge by using its considerable economic clout in a political system predisposed to discriminating against nonwhites, who comprised the vast majority of its workforce.

Of such blatant double standards, Richard was later eager to pronounce: "We were determined that this case would not be another Bhopal." Indeed, there were many important and, for Richard, especially motivating parallels between the Union Carbide litigation in the United States a decade earlier, concerning a catastrophic gas leak in one of the company's plants in India, and the Cape case. Both involved decades of suffering for thousands of poor people in developing countries, at the hands of

Western-based corporations working with dangerous substances in negligently substandard conditions. Both corporations left decades-long legacies of toxic waste, yet both sought to evade responsibility for the consequences of their actions by resisting all attempts to hold them accountable in the courts of their home states. Richard's present motivation stemmed from the fact that Union Carbide had been successful in foreclosing litigation attempts in US courts, thereby escaping any meaningful sanction and, most significantly, destroying any hope of its victims receiving any meaningful reparation.[32] It was *that* scenario that Richard was vowing not to repeat in the Cape case, no matter the very real risk that he wouldn't succeed. Long-established legal principle stood against him, and the resistance he would face from both Cape and its lawyers was certain to be uncompromising and well funded.

The Union Carbide litigation had foundered on the US courts' strict interpretation of the principle of *forum non conveniens*, ruling that the proper forum (or jurisdiction) in which the case should be heard was India, where the wrongdoing was committed and the damage had occurred, *not* the United States, where the parent company was domiciled. As a result, arguments regarding the company's negligence were never tested or fully aired in the US courts. The same fate for the Cape case, Richard knew, would be just as catastrophic for the victims, as he could see that the strongest part of his case was the evidence of corporate negligence he was already beginning to gather, much more of which he suspected—rightly—was yet to be found. Convincing British courts that England was the only viable forum for the Cape case was a different matter from the task facing the Bhopal victims before the US courts, but still one in which the odds were stacked against him.[33]

Questions of jurisdiction and negligence are not unrelated—the latter being, in part, a determining factor in addressing the former. So the more Richard could educate himself about the mining of asbestos, the science behind its health effects, and the history of both, the more he could show who knew what, when, and where and how they responded.

Coincidentally, Richard was also running another asbestos case in the UK courts, which provided valuable insights into the progression of asbestos science, as well as the limits of the law in providing justice to the deserving. He was representing a group of British women (or next of kin) who had died or were suffering from mesothelioma, having worked for the British pharmaceutical company Boots making gas masks containing asbestos-filled filters from the late 1930s to the end of the Second World War.[34] Unfortunately, their case failed on the ground that the action had commenced outside the statutory three-year limitation period.[35] But while pulling together the facts of the case Richard unearthed some startling evidence of the virulence of asbestos poisoning, most especially its lethality even when patients were exposed to it only briefly.

The incidence of mesothelioma among the women was astronomically high: 67 out of the total workforce in the Boots factory of 1,200, at a rate some 250 times greater than the incidence of the disease in the wider community at that time. In part this was explained by the extremely high levels of asbestos dust to which the workers had been exposed for lengthy periods. But there was also evidence of the disease presenting after relatively short periods of exposure. One deceased woman on whose behalf Richard was acting had worked at the Boots plant for only six weeks, he noted, "yet at post-mortem was found to have a lung fibre count of 50 million fibres per gram of lung tissue," as compared to a mean asbestos fibre count in the general population of women in the same age group of approximately 2,000 per gram.[36] "It seems inconceivable," as Richard notes ruefully, "that any effective dust control measures were taken in relation to her."[37]

What struck Richard as especially significant about these results was that the type of asbestos used in the gas masks was crocidolite (blue asbestos), processed, what is more, in Cape's UK-based factories (in Barking, East London, and Hebdon Bridge, Yorkshire) and possibly sourced from Cape's crocidolite mines in the Northern Cape (although most likely sourced from CSR's Wittenoom mine in Western Australia).[38] The massive incidence of mesothelioma among the Boots workers and the excessive asbestos fiber counts found in their lungs indicated not only the toxicity of crocidolite fibers, but also the inherent danger of their physical makeup of incredibly fine, needle-like crystals (characteristic of amphibole asbestos)[39] that evaded the human body's normal upper respiratory defenses to lodge deep in the lungs of those exposed to them. Workplace, or occupational, exposure to blue asbestos was, therefore, manifestly hazardous.

The fact that environmental exposure to crocidolite could *also* lead to such grave consequences was made clear to Richard in yet another contemporaneous UK asbestos case. The plaintiffs in that case had successfully sued an asbestos processing factory in Leeds for negligently causing significant quantities of asbestos dust to escape its premises and failing to dispose of piles of raw asbestos collected in and around the factory's loading bays. The two plaintiffs were never employed in the factory, but having lived nearby from the 1920s to the 1940s and, as children, having often played around the open loading bays, they had been environmentally exposed to high (and in one case, lethal) levels of asbestos contamination. In finding for the two plaintiffs,

Justice Holland pointedly referred to environmental exposure such as they had sustained in the immediate vicinity of the defendants' premises as having "effectively replicated . . . factory conditions in terms of dust emission."[40]

The combined and coincidental impact of these two cases in Richard's thinking was profound, even if he didn't fully realize it at the time. For while he knew that Cape's operations in South Africa focused almost entirely on the especially hazardous amphibole asbestos variants—crocidolite (blue) in the Northern Cape and amosite (brown) in Northern Transvaal/Limpopo—he was not yet aware how significant the matter of environmental exposure was to become in formulating the case against the company. Nor did he know that such exposure would be the result of so many African children innocently playing with piles of the soft, fluffy mineral.

CHAPTER 2

First Encounters

—Life and Death on Asbestos Street—

THE NATIONAL INSTITUTE FOR Occupational Health (NIOH) occupies an austere, thick-walled Victorian building on the edge of Constitution Hill, a bedraggled section of downtown Johannesburg. It feels like an old medical school, with an ever-present whiff of the preservative formalin in the air. The heels of its boffinish occupants click along corridors of polished stone, voices echoing under high ceilings, as they pass by walls displaying graphic posters of "Asbestos-Related Diseases" and heavy doors announcing "Asbestos Lab" and "Pathology Department." Behind these doors are secure cool rooms with rows of buckets of mine workers' lungs stacked against the walls and white-coated scientists peering into computer screens hooked up to supersized electron microscopes as they count dust fibers and other foreign particles embedded in human tissue samples. It is a formidable enterprise, no matter how genial the staff.

Richard was to become very familiar with these surroundings and people over the coming months and years as he took on the huge task of building a legally convincing case against Cape. It was here—in the National Centre for Occupational Health

(NCOH), as it was then called[1]—that he met a cadre of redoubtable scientists and medics, several of whom were to become crucial players in the development of the case, as well as close friends. "Their care and dedication to helping those whose health has been damaged by simply doing their jobs was truly inspiring," Richard says of them.

It was in April 1995 that Richard first met one of those scientists, Dr. Marianne Felix, whose work on the health impacts of asbestos in the mining communities around Penge in Northern Transvaal (now part of Limpopo Province) was groundbreaking, in terms of both gathering hard scientific evidence and dispensing soft-hearted compassion. It was through her work that Richard learned of the sheer scale of the damage.

Marianne had spent years collecting data from asbestos mining communities in Northern Transvaal for her doctoral thesis. She'd documented in detail the dreadful legacy of death and disease that the asbestos industry had left behind,[2] much of which she had later published in journals and book chapters. Summing up the situation neatly, Marianne entitled one such piece "Risking Their Lives in Ignorance," in which she made the chilling observation that the piles of asbestos tailings in and around Mafefe (west of Penge) were known as "dumps of death," such were the rates of lung disease and death among local communities.[3] Most striking of all was her recording of the elevated instances of disease resulting from environmental exposure—that is, in people who had never worked in the asbestos mines or mills but rather merely lived within their vicinity. Not only did this demonstrate the far and indiscriminate reach of asbestos-related diseases (ARDs); it also became a critically defining theme of the case against Cape. In the mid-1990s, Marianne was still heavily engaged with these communities, even though asbestos mining had, finally, ceased in Penge in 1992. So her input was vital to

Richard's asbestos "education" and to his establishing relations with victims and potential litigants.

Backing up the raw medical evidence she'd gathered, Marianne's calm, deliberative demeanor[4] convinced Richard of the depth of the crisis these people faced, even if he was unsure whether and how he might help them. Armed, however, with this apparently damning evidence and fueled by the injustice of it all, Richard flew back to London determined to see what he could do.

≈

His resolve stiffened on the flight home as he reflected on what he'd learned, and as soon as he landed, he threw himself into a whirlwind of research across an array of relevant disciplines: geological—the physical structure and chemical composition of asbestos fibers; medical—which parts of this composition made the fibers so damaging to human health; political—what role had Apartheid played in the perpetuation and promotion of the asbestos industry in South Africa and how was he to negotiate the new post-Apartheid political landscape; corporate—what were Cape Plc's assets and where were they located; and, of course, legal—what were the legal problems and possibilities standing between him and the victims getting their hands on any of those assets by way of compensation? It was demanding in terms of breadth and depth, but it appealed to his obsessive disposition, which had, coincidentally, been nationally publicized a couple of years earlier, when he was the subject of a rather unforgiving media piece. "You and Your Family," published in the *Daily Telegraph*, documented the lives of a series of "obsessives," one of whom was Richard with his supposed addiction to work. Describing sixteen-hour days, frequent work trips overseas, and his being "fidgety" when *not* working, his wife told the reporter that work "is the one thing he would always rather be doing above everything else."[5]

Life at the time was indeed hectic. Richard's wife, Munoree, had recently given birth to their second child, Nadia, sister to Jahan, who was six years old. A doctor specializing in thoracic trauma surgery at Guy's Hospital in London,[6] Munoree was struggling with a life-long autoimmune disease that had been exacerbated during her two pregnancies. Quick-witted and well-spoken, with a sweep of dark hair over bright eyes and a cherubic smile, Munoree's tiny frame was battered by the illness and the added stress of an initially difficult relationship with Richard's parents, who were her only family in the United Kingdom in those early years. She is Tamil and Hindu, born and brought up in Pietermaritzburg in South Africa's KwaZulu-Natal Province, and had met Richard when he was visiting his family in the same town in 1987. She and Richard had then married, almost on a whim, only six weeks after meeting one another, in a Johannesburg magistrate's office with two criminal defendants they'd just met roped in as witnesses and without telling any friends or family. Both families were shocked by the suddenness and secrecy of the tryst, added to which was the disquieting unhappiness of Richard's father's Muslim family over the fact of Munoree's Hindu heritage.

From a very young age, Munoree had shown extraordinary determination and enterprise. When visiting her chronically ill father in the hospital as a child, she'd been intrigued by the grand and exotic names on doors and corridors: "'Gynaecology,' 'epidemiology,' 'pathology'—I'd jot them down in a notebook and look them up when I got home. It was then that I decided to become a doctor," she tells me when I ask her about her career. Such fortitude as well as precocious talent were now put to good use as she knuckled down, focusing on the kids while still managing to support Richard and juggle her own career.

Munoree shifted jobs to the more regular hours of a doctoral research position in genetic disorders at Great Ormond Street Children's Hospital (albeit still demanding and "very gory" she says, in that matter-of-fact way of medics), which allowed her to take on the bulk of parenting responsibilities, and both she and Richard economized after the huge drop in his salary. "We had each other," she recalls of those tough times, adding that "if anything, it made our relationship stronger." Richard's "boots and all" approach to this new case was therefore predictable, most especially to Munoree, who noted, in characteristically understated fashion in the above-mentioned *Daily Telegraph* article, that on the rare occasions they ever shared a meal together, "Richard would read legal documents, which was very tedious." Even today, when I ask Richard what he does to relax, he replies, "I'm not really one for relaxing, generally."[7] To which Munoree adds, "No surprise there," as she overhears our conversation.

Like an intellectual hunter-gatherer, Richard began to forage for information and evidence near and far, with trade unionists and the medical profession proving to be especially important and productive sources. The National Union of Mineworkers in South Africa (NUM [SA]), for example, reached out through a letter from Fleur Plimmer, the union's health and safety coordinator, offering to help Richard "in every possible way" and pointing him toward the director of the NCOH (and Marianne Felix's boss), Tony Davies.[8]

Tony, like Marianne, had strong links with the asbestos mining communities in Northern Transvaal, where he, together which his wife, Deirdre, a nurse, would embed themselves six months at a time offering free medical services to poor black workers and their families in the small mining towns of Steelspoort and Burgersfort. Tony and Deirdre's work providing basic diagnoses of ARDs through regular medical checks and x-ray readings was invaluable, not only to their patients who were otherwise denied or unable to access such care, but also for compiling a record of the state of occupational health among the communities in which they lived. Driven by a strong sense of selfless altruism born of their Catholic faith, their mission chimed well with Richard's decidedly secular dedication to fighting injustice. Over the years that followed, Tony and Deirdre became close friends with Richard, as well as passionate and committed allies in the case against Cape.

It was during this period that Richard came across a damning report documenting the long history of the atrocious conditions in the Penge asbestos mines, written by Gerrit Schepers, a highly regarded physician and former professor of medicine at the University of Pretoria. Schepers had been engaged by the South African Department of Mines in the 1940s to inspect working conditions across the sector and to assess any associated health risks. After one inspection conducted at Cape's Penge mine and mill site in 1949, Schepers wrote:

> Exposures were crude and unchecked. I saw young children completely included within large shipping bags, trampling down fluffy amosite asbestos which all day long came cascading down over their heads. They were kept stepping lively by a burly supervisor with a hefty whip. I believe these children to have had the ultimate asbestos exposure. X-ray revealed several to have radiologic asbestosis with cor pulmonale [enlarged right (pulmonary) side of the heart] before the age of 12.[9]

Astonished by these words, Richard subsequently wrote to Schepers, who by then had moved to the Virginia Institute of Forensic Science and Medicine in the United States, asking him about the relative levels of occupational health and medical care provided to black and white employees he had seen in the Penge mines and mill at that time. Schepers' reply was excoriating.[10]

"White workers," he wrote,

spent 95% of their daytime in offices or dust-controlled enclaves in the mill. The black men and women and children were exposed to all the dust that could be generated in drilling, blasting, mucking, cobbing and crushing asbestos.

At the mines and mill the White workers lived in proper houses and were paid enough to be able to afford proper food and some luxuries such as automobiles. The Blacks were crowded together in shanty town hovels, paid low and subsisted mainly on sour milk and maize porridge. Their water came from a communal tap or from the river. The Whites had installed water and sewerage. There was no doctor for the Blacks.

Schepers then detailed how white workers were subject to annual physical examinations and chest x-ray screening, while no such provision was made for black workers.[11] Only if they became "perilously ill" were black workers x-rayed, he noted, but even then only by way of inferior resolution imagery, "virtually ensuring that no asbestosis would be detected." He signed off his letter with a biting rhetorical question: "This does not sound like the Whites and Blacks received equal conservation health care, does it?"

While Schepers's commentary was aimed at the dastardliness of the Apartheid-fueled working practices in the asbestos industry, it also pointed to a fundamental problem facing Richard in making the legal case for Cape's negligence. For if black (and coloured) asbestos workers were so poorly provided with medical services, how and, importantly, from where was he to assemble the necessary evidence of their ill-health and death caused by exposure to asbestos dust? "If I yell out at night there's a reply of bruised silence" is a line in Midnight Oil's anti-asbestos protest song "Blue Sky Mine," which was getting a lot of airplay at the time.[12] It resonated sharply with Richard as he contemplated his own predicament trying to replace silence with evidence.

The NCOH medics were, once again, key to helping him tackle the challenge. Tony Davies was able to point Richard toward existing epidemiological research data on ARDs in white communities and what extrapolations could be made regarding ARDs in black and coloured communities. One academic study showed how South Africa had by far the world's highest incidence of mesothelioma (a virulent and invariably lethal cancer of the lung lining, peculiarly associated with asbestos exposure), based solely on the numbers of white South Africans diagnosed with the disease.[13] Another whites-only mesothelioma study focused on the cohort of births in and around Prieska in the Northern Cape between 1917 and 1934. The place was significant, because this was where Cape's blue asbestos mining and milling had been located, having started operations in the area in 1893. The data from this study, published initially in 1990 and updated in 1992, were stunning, for while South Africa's mesothelioma rates were the worst in the world, those in Prieska were the worst in South Africa. "The cumulative mortality rate for mesothelioma in the revised statistics," the study concluded, "is 1,000 times higher than the cumulative rate calculated for all South Africans."[14]

What was truly alarming about these data was that they essentially excluded those who were most exposed to asbestos fiber contamination and therefore most likely to suffer from ARDs. Indeed, the authors of the first-named study above estimated that an additional 1,000 cases among black and coloured people were being missed *every year*, on account of poor or nonexistent medical oversight—meaning that the true figure for mesothelioma victims was very likely significantly higher.[15]

Tony also provided Richard with the raw data from his own research, which was then either ongoing or unpublished. For instance, Tony was in the midst of setting up clinics to survey some 2,200 former miners, all of whom were black, in a remote part of Northern Transvaal, where the Penge asbestos mines were owned by Egnep, a Cape Plc subsidiary. Noting that "no [medical] service had ever been provided for occupational health in the region," Tony was later to inform Richard of the study's findings. Of those former miners and mill workers exposed only to asbestos, Tony found 71 percent of the men and 90 percent of the women presented with asbestosis.[16]

The gendered distinction between these dreadful statistics reflected the peculiarity of the above-ground jobs typically assigned to women at the mine sites; only the men were employed below ground in the mines themselves. Above-ground work, such as "cobbing"—breaking apart asbestos-bearing rock by hand—was undertaken almost exclusively by women and children, in conditions that were intentionally dry (it made the task easier) and therefore filled with airborne fibers. Inside the mines conditions were kept intentionally damp, again because it aided the task at hand, namely drilling, but which also reduced the airborne fiber count.

Appalling though these data were, they did not altogether surprise Tony. They were consistent with his previous work, the results of which he had presented at an international conference on occupational health in Haifa, Israel, in October 1985. Drawing on the records kept by South Africa's National Asbestos Tumour Research Panel, Tony showed that the incidence of country-wide tumor cases occurring in five-year blocks from 1955 to 1985 had risen eighteen-fold across both white and non-white communities. Further data derived from 30,000 autopsy files of miners held by the NCOH during the same period showed "that the prevalence of lung cancer among asbestos miners was 20% as opposed to 6.6% among gold miners."[17]

Tony Davies and Marianne Felix were also instrumental in introducing Richard to André Pickard, a general practitioner in Prieska and a physician in the town's hospital, who had been witness to a remarkable, decades-long record of ARDs within the community. Whereas the asbestos mined in Penge was mainly (brown) amosite, the mines around Prieska were (blue) crocidolite asbestos, which distinction was to prove significant, even if not yet fully understood. While both types are amphiboles (that is, shard-like in structure) within the asbestos family,[18] scientific and medical evidence demonstrated conclusively the heightened lethality of blue asbestos and its strong association with mesothelioma.[19]

Marianne supplied Richard with a copy of her handwritten notes taken when she had recently interviewed Pickard and his wife, who was a qualified nurse. They had moved to Prieska as a young couple in 1941 and together had practiced there for more than fifty years. During that time and especially in the early days, André told Marianne that mesothelioma was rife.[20] And while there existed no formal statistical evidence to support his claim that 20 percent of the town's population had mesothelioma, it is not inconsistent with the fact that over the years he had seen thousands of mesothelioma cases, having himself recorded some 300–400 mesothelioma cases annually throughout the 1940s and 1950s. Fully three-quarters of these cases, he noted, were due to environmental, as opposed to occupational, asbestos exposure.

It is perhaps this observation that was most disturbing. Cape's asbestos mill had been situated on the northern edge of the town, next to the coloured community's church and close to the town's coloured school. Raw asbestos ore, shipped in by rail from the Koegas mines 140 kilometers to the northwest, was crushed, cleaned, sorted, packed, and stored in and around the three-story high mill. The mill was Prieska's biggest building, and asbestos was everywhere—beaten into the road surfaces, mixed into the mortar in people's houses, lining the playgrounds of all three of the color-segregated schools, and packed into surfaces of the town's rugby pitch and golf course, as well as floating on the surface of the Orange River, which marked the town's northern border. It was also, of course, an ever-present component of Prieska's air.

The atmosphere in and around the mill itself was incredibly dusty—workers' hair and clothes were daily caked in asbestos fiber—which inevitably led to substantial and persistent contamination of the whole town. The mill had had a roof vent installed to suck out (some) of the dust, but that, as André Pickard indicated, succeeded only in blowing it into the path of the prevailing, northwest winds, which duly swept the asbestos dust across the rest of the town.[21] The mill ceased operating in 1964, though it was still used as a storage facility until at least 1972.[22] But by then, as both Pickards made clear, the damage had been done, accounting for the markedly high rates of environmental ARDs among people who had *not* worked at the mill, but merely suffered the misfortune of living nearby.

It was the phenomenon of environmental asbestos exposure and its extent among communities living near the mines and mills that caught Richard's attention. One of the first things he'd learned when he began taking on corporate negligence cases in South Africa was that the country's occupational health laws provided no state-based compensation to those *not* employed in the relevant industry, no matter how badly damaged their health or how clearly the damage was caused by the relevant industry.[23] So here, with these environmental asbestos victims, the only path toward possible remediation existed outside the statutory regime in the common law, where they might sue in the tort of negligence. This meant identifying both the negligent party (the "tortfeasor") and the grounds on which they had acted negligently, conditions that Richard was now in the process of trying to satisfy. The two conditions were in fact inseparable. The main challenge in identifying Cape as the tortfeasor lay in successfully making the case for its negligence in respect not only of those people who had worked for the company or its subsidiaries, but also those who had never worked for either.

≈

To succeed in the tort of negligence, plaintiffs must show that (1) they are owed a duty of care by the defendant; (2) the duty was breached; and (3) as a consequence, they suffered damages. As it seemed likely, even at this early stage, that a significant number of claimants would not be former Cape (or Cape subsidiaries') employees, Richard was mindful that their case could falter at the first hurdle, as the company would almost certainly argue that it owed them no particular duty of care—as distinct, that is, to Cape's position regarding former employees, to whom it seemed the company did owe a duty of care. However, even here Richard could see that Cape would likely contest these workers' claims on the grounds that they were employed by Cape's South African subsidiaries rather than directly by Cape itself.

To convince the courts that Cape owed a duty of care to both categories of claimants, Richard knew that he first had to establish the company's proximity to the claimants and to the actions they claim to have been damaged by. Such proximity, in turn, depended on his demonstrating that by virtue of its levels of oversight and control, Cape knew of the health hazards posed by the asbestos mining and milling operations of its subsidiaries to workers and to nonworker neighboring communities alike *and* that it failed to take adequate precautions to protect those workers and those communities. The task, in other words, was to show that the parent company, Cape Plc, headquartered in the United Kingdom, effectively presided over levels of occupational and environmental asbestos exposure in its South African businesses that it knew were dangerous to human health. It was to that end that of the five plaintiffs in whose names the first legal action against Cape was eventually commenced in England a year later, in February 1997, three had been asbestos Cape mine workers (from Penge) and two had merely lived in the vicinity of a Cape asbestos mill (in Prieska).[24]

Before getting to that point of filing the case, however, Richard's next step was to gather evidence that directly linked the records of rampant ARDs compiled by Marianne Felix, Tony Davies, and André Pickard to Cape's actions or inactions. Gerrit Schepers's testimony certainly helped, but Richard needed more. That meant getting into the communities themselves, meeting victims and potential claimants, seeing the former mine and mill sites, and finding and following paper trails of evidence and information.

So, in late February 1996, with a jam-packed itinerary in his hand and a hold-all over his shoulder, Richard headed back to the late summer heat of South Africa on the first of what was to become a series of intense, two- to three-week fact-finding trips undertaken throughout 1996. He'd always felt comfortable in South Africa for reasons beyond the fact that his father was born and grew up there. When a journalist interviewed him during one of these trips, for example, he confessed:

> I feel very at home here. . . . Everyone can feel they belong. There is no problem with identity. In the UK, everything is so orthodox. Here there is not so much of a stigma attached to being different. My father is Muslim, my mother is Christian, my wife is Hindu, and my sister has married a German Buddhist. I didn't have an orthodox upbringing.[25]

Glad to be back where unorthodoxy "is much more acceptable," he landed in Johannesburg early in the morning and headed straight to the NCOH for a quick catch-up with Tony and Marianne who also introduced him to the NCOH's director, Ian Webster, whose earlier work with the center's Pneumoconiosis Research Unit (as we will see in the next chapter) was to become hugely significant in the case. Immediately thereafter, he was ferried across the city to the NUM's headquarters in Marshalltown, past the striking bronze *Miners' Monument* on De Korte Street, symbolizing the wealth and prosperity that the mining industry has brought to South Africa on the back of its black miners.

At the NUM, Richard met with the ever-accommodating Fleur Plimmer and a pair of occupational health workers' representatives from the two asbestos mining provinces.[26] From these three, he was able to hear firsthand experiences of the history of asbestos exposure in the respective communities and the current state of people's health and well-being. The three were also instrumental in providing Richard with contact details of whom to see when he visited the old mine and mill sites in the two provinces.

But before heading out into the veld, Richard made the short trip from Johannesburg north to Pretoria to meet with his first victim of mesothelioma. It was a profound experience in more ways than one. There were some indications that Cecilia Van Schalkwyk might be a prospective plaintiff no matter that she had never worked with asbestos. It appeared that her condition was a result of her regular visits to an asbestos mine in the Northern Cape, when she brought lunch to her miner husband and sat with him for a few hours as he dug the asbestos rock out of the hillside. This had been when she was a young fit woman who was later to establish a kick-boxing school with her husband and long before she was diagnosed with mesothelioma at the age of forty. She and her husband were from the bush and both were white Afrikaners.

In an early example of the many times Richard found out how wrong one's assumptions can be in the social and political melting pot of South Africa, he'd misjudged the Van Schalkwyks when he later admitted to being wary of taking on a prospective client with their background, knowing that the vast majority of Cape's asbestos victims were poor and black or coloured. But that was before he met Cecilia's lawyer, Benedicta Monama—a young black woman who was as formidable as she was unexpected—at the Pretoria office of the Legal Resources Centre. "It was a salutary warning against stereotyping," he noted in his diary that evening. The Van Schalkwyks themselves turned out to be most genuine, down-to-earth people, who despite their tragic circumstances wanted to do anything they could to assist other victims. Cecilia expressed particular sorrow for the plight of black workers whom she knew had been exposed to the worst levels of contamination. "She died within weeks of our meeting," Richard recalls. "Her husband was distraught."[27] It turned out that the mine in which Mr. Van Schalkwyk had worked was not owned by Cape, so, to his great frustration, Richard was unable to assist him in respect of any claims made on behalf of his wife's estate.

Corporate ownership aside, such encounters were to become standard fare for Richard as the case progressed—tragedies borne stoically by asbestos victims struggling to come to terms with what had happened to them, why it had happened, and who was responsible. They were so common, indeed, that years later at public meetings about the case (after it expanded beyond the original handful of litigants to become a class action of thousands), Richard had become used to seeing masses of people trudging into church and community halls of local mining towns to hear him speak, "clutching pieces of paper confirming their own illnesses or the death certificates of loved ones," hoping they provided sufficient evidence for them to join the litigation. "It was heartbreaking," he says, "but also overwhelming given their desperation and hopes for what the case might achieve."

≈

Leaving behind the cityscapes of Pretoria and Johannesburg, Richard next headed north for his first visit to an asbestos mine site. Remote and by then almost deserted, Penge had been home to Cape Plc's principal source of amosite asbestos. Attempts had been made to rehabilitate the site by plugging mine entrances and covering abandoned asbestos dumps with a few centimeters of topsoil, but the efforts had been incomplete, and the region's semi-tropical downpours had washed away much of the dirt cover. It was to be a short visit, made even shorter by the difficulties in getting there. A storm disrupted Richard's original plan to fly up, so he and Victor Uys—the pilot-turned-driver—took to the road instead. Zack Mabiletja, a local environmental activist, was waiting for them at the police station in

Penge. Ebullient and affable, Zack had driven down from Mafefe, an hour or so northwest, as he was keen to help Richard in any way he could.

Zack's whole life has been steeped in asbestos. His father owned an "adit"—a small asbestos mining plot, typically dug by one person or family, who would then sell their output to a corporation (such as Cape), either directly or through a broker. His mother used to work at the mine, bringing along her young children, including Zack, so that she could keep an eye on them while giving them something useful to do. None of them had any idea about the health hazards they faced until many years later, after the mining operations had closed. Zack recalls the horror of watching so many of his peer group falling ill and dying, while "miraculously," he later told me, none of his own family had succumbed. At least "not yet," he added somberly.[28] After leaving school, Zack had become a schoolteacher from which job he resigned in 1988, when he first met Marianne Felix in Mafefe and decided to join her efforts in documenting the health crisis unfolding in his community. "The asbestos problem politicized me," he says, by way of explaining his life-long environmental activism and why, thirty years ago, he was happy to show Richard around the old mine sites.

There was, in truth, little to see. A dilapidated mine shaft tower (at one of the bigger mine entrances), a few derelict buildings and accommodation blocks, and mounds of bare earth. But if you looked closely, fluffy brown asbestos fiber was readily visible, either sticking out of rocks in the asbestos ore tailings dumps or nestling in clumps on the ground where the old stockpiles of sorted fiber used to be located. Zack explained that while the region's generally wet and humid climate might be beneficial in terms of reducing the quantities of airborne asbestos fibers, the same conditions were responsible for eroding the soil coverings of old dumps and washing fibers off the mine sites into the local rivers and streams. The asbestos problem, it was clear, was not just historical, but ongoing.[29]

From the amosite asbestos mines of Penge in the north, Richard then traveled south via Johannesburg to the crocidolite asbestos mines around Prieska, which were also owned by Cape. The weather was a little kinder on this occasion and his short onward flight from Kimberley to Prieska was all booked and ready to go when he arrived at the airport. He did a double-take as Johan Jooste, the pilot, strode out to meet him, not only on account of his size—"He was a huge, barrel-chested Afrikaner such that I wondered how he'd fit into the cockpit of the little two-seater Cessna we'd hired"—but also because he was strabismic. Nervously, Richard helped wheel the plane out of the hangar, climbed on board, strapped himself, in and donned a pair of headphones, meanwhile wondering what would happen if he was called on to use any of the dual controls laid out before him. In the end, Richard needn't have worried *too* much, with Johan merrily chatting away as they bumped through the hot air turbulence radiating off the scorched scrub below and successfully negotiated the stray livestock wandering across the beaten-earth airstrip as they landed.

"Welkom to Prieska" was daubed in white paint on the side of the corrugated tin shed that passed for the airport terminal, beside which Mrs. Pickard was parked and waiting to provide her own welcome to Richard. He had exchanged letters with the Pickards, and he'd also spoken to Mrs. Pickard on the phone, but none of this helped Mrs. Pickard when she was faced with the sudden dilemma of which of the two men walking toward her was the London lawyer. "Was he the small brown guy or the tall, broad, and bearded Afrikaner? Neither were likely candidates—in the end she opted for Johan" is how Richard retells the incident, adding that while she was mortified, he laughed it off with "Don't worry, it happens all the time!"

Dr. André Pickard's decades-long account of a community ravaged by ARDs included his own and his wife's personal heartbreak. Their eldest son, Henri, a surgeon with five children, had died of mesothelioma at the age of thirty-six. He had grown up in Prieska until he left to study medicine at the University of Cape Town and thereafter emigrated to England to practice. Having never worked with asbestos, Henri was a classic case of environmentally acquired mesothelioma.[30] His mother was to become another when she died of the same disease in 2000, some four years after greeting Richard at the airstrip.

Angry as well as heartbroken, the Pickards' attempts over many years to warn the authorities of the health dangers of asbestos were summarily dismissed. "Don't make a fuss," André was told by one government official in the Ministry of Health. André's fury and frustration are evident in almost every line of one of his first letters to Richard: "I hate these mining companies," he wrote when describing how he and others were bullied by them and by anyone won over (or bought) to their side, including politicians, government officials, and doctors. "A book should be written about all the sadness it has caused," he exclaimed before imploring Richard to "come to Prieska . . . come and see!"[31]

What Richard did see was a small dusty town of lattice-work streets, including one named "Asbestos Street" at the western end of which the mill had been located. The mill had been dismantled more than twenty years earlier; now, only a large concrete slab on which the principal crushing and sorting shed had been built remained. Uncovered blue asbestos fibers were still visible strewn across the bare earth between the mill and the adjoining coloured school and church. The rest of the town was not far, rows of houses standing just a short distance across the road. How could anyone avoid inhaling the characteristically tiny, sharp fibers of blue asbestos when so much of it had been milled so close to where people lived, learned, played, and prayed, Richard thought to himself.

The town and its inhabitants continued to struggle against the legacy, not only in terms of people's health (Dr. Deon Smith, André's colleague, told Richard that he was still seeing between ten and fifteen mesothelioma cases per year), but also their livelihoods. Following Cape's closure of the mill in the mid-1960s and, by 1979, all the asbestos mines in nearby Koegas, the town lost its main employer and with it many people's only source of income. In an apt representation of the dreadful irony of this relationship with the mineral, a lump of blue asbestos on prominent display in a flimsy glass cabinet near the entrance of the local municipality offices in the town's center was dubbed the "killing stone" by Lillian Valacia, Prieska's mayor during the later years of the case.[32]

As Richard was ushered into the municipality offices and stood gazing at this peculiar artifact, it dawned on him just how much of the townsfolk's hopes for redemption, having been dashed so often and for so long, now lay with him and whatever case he was able to mount. It was, to be sure, a daunting responsibility, but one that he now better understood, having visited both Penge and Prieska.

≈

With the unwavering support and assistance of the medics and occupational health specialists at the NCOH and following a series of further South African trips to meet with an expanding range of asbestos victims, lawyers, activists, politicians, and journalists (the case was beginning to attract attention, being seen, increasingly, as a trial against colonial capitalism), Richard was assembling a cohort of potential claimants with relevant profiles and in whose names the case could be filed. His initial encounters with researchers at the NCOH had blossomed into a web of fruitful collaborations. "Working with them was a revelation," Richard says, "because their professional objectives were so closely aligned to mine. They too wanted to help the sick and to stop corporations acting in ways that made people so sick." And "they were all so passionate about it," he adds.

Even though Tony Davies was about to step down after eleven years at the helm of the NCOH, he had set the tone for the institution in the new post-Apartheid era, most especially that in its scientific endeavors it would not be cowed by the self-serving interests of mining corporations. Nominally heading into retirement, Tony was in fact to continue his selfless humanitarian efforts to help sick miners in Limpopo for another decade. His work, together with that of Marianne Felix, was to form the basis of much of the medical history and data concerning Cape's amosite asbestos operations in Penge on which Richard relied in his action against the company. Marianne's work had also extended south into the crocidolite asbestos mines of the Northern Cape. There, she made contact with the matron at Prieska hospital who pointed her toward people in the local community who were suffering from ARDs, including those who had never worked in asbestos mines or mills.[33] In addition to gathering information that helped Richard to understand the dimensions of the health calamity that was asbestos's legacy, these efforts led to instructions from a handful of individuals to pursue legal action as plaintiffs.

These few would turn into many in the years to come, as there was no shortage of people in Penge or Prieska keen to tell their stories to Richard and his colleagues, no matter how difficult and often harrowing was the experience for those giving and those taking the statements. Withered and emaciated, many struggled to lift themselves out of a chair and were breathless after crossing a room. Men looking thirty years older than their true middle age describing in soft, rasping tones how they toiled in the hot and humid mines, shirtless and maskless, digging or drilling holes, and hauling ore-filled cocopans (small trolleys on rails) up to the mine head. Women, gaunt and glassy-eyed, recounting their work as cobbers and still traumatized by the realization that not only had they been poisoned, but so had their babies strapped to their backs and their toddlers playing around them, whom they'd brought to work to care for.

When I was in Prieska in March 2023, I met one of those toddlers. Fildah Bosman, now eighty-three years old, with a husky, singsong voice, dancing sepia eyes, and a wide toothless smile, had lived with her family next to the Koegas mine. Among her earliest memories is one of running her fingers through mounds of the silky, cobalt blue fiber as her mother worked nearby. "I was between three and five at the time," she said, "and before that my mother used to breast-feed while she was cobbing." Though still big-hearted and effervescent, even while relating stories about sitting on top of bags of raw asbestos when hitching rides on open-topped trucks travelling between Koegas and Prieska, Fildah told me that these days "inside is all dead. I have a pain behind my lungs that stops me lifting my arms when I try to hang up the washing."[34]

Other victims told Richard of clouds of asbestos dust enveloping them as they operated the ore crusher (which mechanized cobbing) at the mill, or packed raw asbestos into porous hessian sacks out of which plumed wafts of dust-clogged air, or loaded full sacks onto trucks or train carriages for haulage. Masks were hardly ever provided but were in any case quickly discarded because they were so ineffective. Neither protective clothing nor workplace showers were made available, so workers carried asbestos home each day impregnated in their own clothes, layered on their skin, and matted into their hair.

Most disturbing of all were the repeated accounts of how ubiquitous asbestos was throughout their communities. Asbestos dust was deposited on the biltong (dried meat) they hung outside their homes and on windowsills inside; it showed up in rivers and lakes (turning them aqua-blue in the case of crocidolite); it was permanently suspended in the air, providing stunning, ethereal sunsets; and its fibers were mixed into the mortar of their brick houses or crushed into the bare dirt of their children's school yards. Matter-of-factly, people remembered how, as kids, they played with the slagheaps of asbestos tailings, twisting clumps of the silky fibers into balls or crude figurines and, like Fildah, fooled around on top of sacks of asbestos stacked high on the back of trucks.[35]

Extraordinary though these scenes were—part Dickensian horror, part surreal fantasy—they were not always immediately usable for Richard. Many of the victims he interviewed lacked corroborating documents, such as complete employment details or adequate medical records, or their recollections were hazy, dulled by age and illness. Many others had died, so their tales were being told second hand. All that said, it was a discrete group of five individuals who sought to instruct Richard and it was in their names, as plaintiffs, that he filed the case in February 1997. They were Rachel Lubbe, Nkala Maile, Matlaweng Mohlala, Catherine Nel, and Sebushi Selwana.

Each of these initial five plaintiffs satisfied criteria necessary to implicate Cape, albeit in different ways. While all suffered ARDs, two had been diagnosed with mesothelioma and three with asbestosis. Two had been asbestos workers and were therefore oc-

Lubbe and Others v. Cape Plc (1997): The Initial Plaintiffs

Rachel Lubbe: Female, white (Afrikaner), South African. Environmental and occupational exposure.

Rachel was born on February 11, 1940, on a farm east of Koegas, Northern Cape. From 1940 to 1947 she was environmentally exposed to asbestos from the Koegas mine. From 1947 to 1956 she attended school in Prieska. From 1959 to 1975 she was employed as a secretary at Cape's Koegas mine. She also lived in Koegas between 1959 and 1984. Rachel was diagnosed with mesothelioma in March 1996. She died on June 29, 1997; she was fifty-seven years old. Thereafter, she was represented by her husband, Schalk Lubbe, as administrator of her estate.

Nkala Maile: Male, black, South African. Environmental and occupational exposure.

Nkala was born on or about March 1, 1933, in Mmutlane, Limpopo. From 1945 to 1957 he worked as a truck driver, lasher (loading asbestos ore onto trolleys or trucks), team leader, and senior team leader at Cape's Penge mine. During this twelve-year period, he lived in the mining compound and went home once a fortnight. His first symptoms of tiredness began in 1994. He was diagnosed with asbestosis in November 1995. Nkala died on April 15, 1998; he was sixty-five years old. Thereafter, he was represented by his wife, Mamabolo Phala, as administrator of his estate.

Matlaweng Mohlala: Male, black, South African. Environmental and occupational exposure.

Matlaweng was born in 1939. Starting at the age of twelve, he worked at the Penge mine packing asbestos fiber into sacks with his bare hands for fourteen years. During that time, he lived in the mine hostel. He was diagnosed with asbestosis in July 1995.

Catherine Nel: Female, white (Afrikaner), South African; suing on behalf of the estate of her late husband, Matthys Nel (who died before the case commenced), male, white, South African. Environmental exposure.

Matthys Nel was born in Prieska on or about November 9, 1936. He lived near Cape's asbestos mill in Prieska from 1936 to 1950. He was diagnosed with mesothelioma in July 1995 and died on November 15, 1995, aged fifty-nine. His brother, Jacobus, grew up in Prieska during the same period and died of mesothelioma in England in 1986. His mother also lived in Prieska all her life and died of the same disease in 1974. Matthys never worked at the mill or in the asbestos mining industry, nor did Jacobus or their mother. See also Pauline Nel, below.

Sebush Selwana: Female, black, South African. Environmental exposure.

Sebush was born on October 27, 1925. Her only known exposure to asbestos occurred while she worked as a domestic servant from 1963 to 1979 for a mine manager at Cape's asbestos mill in Penge, who lived next to the mill. During that period her duties included washing the manager's work overalls. She was diagnosed with asbestosis in October 1995.

≈

These five were joined, shortly after filing, by a sixth plaintiff:

Pauline Nel: Female, white, British; suing on behalf of the estate of her late husband, Jacobus Nel (who died before the case commenced), male, white, South African. Environmental exposure.

Pauline was the sister-in-law of Catherine Nel (above). Pauline met and married Jacobus when he came to practice as a doctor in England during the 1950s. Jacobus was born in 1932 in Prieska, where he lived near Cape's asbestos mill until 1951. He was diagnosed with mesothelioma in 1984 and died in 1986 at the age of fifty-four.

cupationally exposed, while three were environmentally exposed, having never worked in the asbestos industry but had lived near an asbestos mill. Two were deceased and represented by their next of kin (this was to become three when the lead plaintiff, Rachel Lubbe, died shortly before the case's first hearing); three were from Penge, two from Prieska; two were men and three women; and two were white, while three were black.

This composition of plaintiffs was no accident but rather a carefully thought-through strategy on Richard's part, aiming to reflect the breadth and depth of interlocking medical, social, racial, geographical, and geological components of the case. Another important consideration was that they all fell within the three-year statutory time limits for instituting personal injury torts claims that operated under both UK and South African law. For while their claims were based on injuries sustained decades earlier, the United Kingdom's Limitation Act 1980 and South Africa's Prescription Act 1969 impose the three-year time bar only from the date on which an individual becomes aware of their injury, by way, for example, of a definitive medical diagnosis, which was the case for all five litigants.[36]

With each of these plaintiffs, Richard was certain as he could be that he'd be able to satisfy the third of the three limbs upon which any case of negligence needs to be established—namely, that harm or damage had been suffered. He was less confident, however, regarding satisfying the first (duty of care) and second (causation) limbs of the negligence trifecta, as both presented substantial legal and factual barriers. Both were also inextricably connected.

As to the first limb, Richard needed to demonstrate that Cape owed one or more duties of care regarding the manner in which it did business. This meant establishing that Cape—the parent— had owed duties of care to its employees and employees of its subsidiaries,[37] as well as to people living in the immediate vicinity of its South African operations. In these respects, the long-established common law rules of proximity (to employees) and foreseeability (of harm to others) that constitute the "neighborhood principle" demanded that Richard provide evidence of the nature of the duties owed to both employees and neighbors, together with details of the care that ought to have been afforded to each group.

As to the second limb, Richard had to address the intermediate matter of causation that sits between duties owed and harms suffered. This meant showing how Cape Plc in the United Kingdom had breached its duties in ways that caused the harms sustained by the plaintiffs in South Africa arising from Cape's actions (or inactions) taken while being aware that they were likely to lead to such harms.

There was no doubt in Richard's mind that in terms of substantive law (that is, what would follow the settling of the question of which jurisdiction, whether the United Kingdom or South Africa), the battle with Cape and its lawyers would be fought on two questions: "*What* duty of care?" and "*How* broken?" The key to answering these questions convincingly and winning the legal argument lay in establishing what Cape knew about the health hazards of asbestos dust at the time the plaintiffs were either working for it or its subsidiary companies or living near their facilities and what Cape did or did not do with that information to protect them from harm. What roles, in other words, did Cape, the parent company, play in the creation of these environmental conditions and in the supervision and implementation of health and safety provisions in its South African subsidiary asbestos companies? And was Cape Plc sufficiently proximate to warrant the imposition on it of a duty to safeguard the health of those South African workers and residents?

≈

In formulating answers to these questions, Richard already had some foundations to build on. He'd begun to dip into the enormous body of medical and scientific evidence gathered during the relevant years up to 1979 (when Cape departed South Africa), so he had a good idea of the incidence, and therefore levels of awareness, of ARDs among asbestos communities themselves. Asbestosis, or fibrosis of the lung, resulting from prolonged periods of heavy asbestos exposure, was rife, as were pleural plaques, a hardening and thickening of the lungs' pleural lining, again resulting from long-term exposure. There was also strong evidence that mesotheliomas, or cancers of the pleura of the lungs, abdomen, or even heart, were peculiarly associated with crocidolite exposure, including after relatively brief periods of exposure.[38] What was less obvious was how much the executive management of Cape's subsidiaries, and most especially of Cape itself, knew of these health effects and their likely or possible causes throughout the years up to 1979 *and* whether they shouldered any responsibility to address them.

There were clear signs of both. In the United Kingdom, for example, as far back as 1928, health officials from the local government where Cape's Barking asbestos factory was located had raised concerns over high levels of asbestosis in the town, calling it a "difficult and serious problem."[39] Such pertinent and public reporting could hardly have escaped the attention of Cape's management. Furthermore, the company's own chief medical officer, W. J. Smither, had written a scathing report after returning from a visit to South Africa in 1962 on working conditions at Cape's asbestos mills in both Penge and Prieska, noting, in respect of the latter, that "men . . . were working in a rain of dust."[40] The report demonstrated not only the parent company's awareness of the severity of the health risks but also its active (and therefore proximate) role in monitoring health and safety standards in its South African plants.

These were important leads, but what Richard really wanted was definitive evidence of Cape's failure to act accordingly to protect the health of its workers and local communities in South Africa. Which is why his meeting with Laurie Flynn at this time was so fortuitous, for it was Laurie who provided Richard with smoking-gun evidence to these ends. Introduced to him through UK trade union connections, Richard had by then already read Laurie's 1992 book *Studded with Diamonds and Paved with Gold*, a trailblazing exposé of the destruction of people and the environment done by mining companies across southern Africa. A charismatic, larger-than-life Scots journalist and documentary maker, Flynn had spent years following the trails of corporate malpractice in the mining sector, from Britain to Africa.

Affable and possessing an almost chameleon-like capacity to talk to anyone anywhere about anything, he'd spent time in the asbestos communities in the Northern Cape and Northern Transvaal, visiting mines and mills and interviewing workers and site managers (sometimes with one of his film crew dressed up as a priest in order to gain access that would otherwise have been denied them), while gathering some chilling reportage along the way. In a chapter of Laurie's book dedicated to the asbestos industry and what it knew about the health impacts of its product, two things caught Richard's eye.

First, Laurie's pithy reference to the fact that it was "sometime in the late 1960s and early 1970s when medical evidence moved from being merely incriminatory to being overwhelming." To which Laurie added in brutally poetic fashion while musing over the sector's failure to act on that evidence: "What sort of civilization was it that defecates in its own bed? What sort of companies were they that had specialised and detailed knowledge of the dangers of this dust and left it to blow around the desert lands and injure local people who knew nothing of the threat that faced them?"[41]

The second item of note was altogether more sinister. Tucked away in a footnote, Laurie cited an earlier piece of his published in the highly respected *New Scientist* in 1982, entitled "South Africa Blacks Out Blue Asbestos Risk."[42] What rang alarm bells for Richard was Laurie's annotation that "this edition of the magazine was withdrawn from circulation in South Africa under pressure from the mining companies, who threatened the local distributer with legal action."[43] After getting hold of a copy of Laurie's article (by then freely available outside the country and now, once again, inside it, too), Richard could see why it had so spooked the asbestos companies. It detailed instances of their active interference and even suppression of scientific research; it named names, including "compliant" scientists and scientific bodies, as well as government departments; and it pointed the finger at a shadowy, menacing figure named Fritz Baunach, who presided over the euphemistically named South African Asbestos Producers' Advisory Committee (SAAPAC), which did much more than dispense advice. Like a suffocating pall, it (and Fritz Baunach) hovered over all asbestos-related research conducted in South Africa and beyond, circulating messages that stressed asbestos's virtues and downplaying or dismissing any health risks, to a degree that would make proud any autocratic state's office of propaganda.

Laurie confirmed all of this and elaborated on the extent of the malign influence when Richard met with him in London in the spring of 1996. He also gave Richard a copy of a seemingly innocuous four-page document prepared by Ian Webster of South Africa's Pneumoconiosis Research Unit, entitled "Report on the Progress of the Mesothelioma Survey as at 30 April 1962," concerning some 2,000 asbestos workers and local residents in Northern Cape and Northern Transvaal. Richard had not previously seen a copy of this report in the records then held by the NCOH for the simple reason that it had been removed from them.[44] Its content had so inflamed the asbestos companies that the SAAPAC had attacked the report's findings and ordered its suppression (and subsequently stripped it altogether from the NCOH archives), as well as defunding the project with immediate effect. What had prompted this hyperactive response were the report's twin killer (literally) conclusions: (1) that the survey showed ARDs are contracted from environmental as well as occupational exposure to asbestos dust, and (2) that the "alarmingly high number of cases of mesothelioma of the pleura" suggests the condition is peculiarly associated with inhalation of crocidolite, again not limited to industrial exposure only.

This looked like a smoking gun, as in both conclusions the report was referring to asbestos mines and mills owned and operated by Cape.

CHAPTER 3

Breathless

—An Alien Invasion—

"IT MAY SEEM INAPPROPRIATE THAT I should introduce this topic by discussing a swimming bath, but the similarities between a swimming bath and the lung are indeed striking."

These are the opening lines used by Ian Webster of South Africa's Pneumoconiosis Research Unit (PRU) in a short paper he wrote entitled "The Effect of Dust on the Lung."[1] He continued by equating the gas-exchanging surface area of an average pair of adult human lungs to the surface area of a good-sized suburban swimming pool (seventy to eighty square meters) and comparing the latter's "skimmer which prevents larger particles such as leaves reaching the bottom of the pool" to the human "upper respiratory tract [which] has an epithelium consisting of numerous hair-like structures that beat at over 100 times per minute," wafting larger particles back up the throat to be coughed out. So far, so good. The comparison also holds true when smaller particles evade these first levels of defense and reach the bottom of the pool or the alveoli of the lungs. A suction brush or automatic pool cleaner will sweep up the debris in the pool, while our alveolar macrophages do much the same thing deep in our lungs by ingesting miniscule foreign bodies and transporting them away from the lungs through the lymphatic system.

But, alas, here is where the correspondence breaks down. For while "we can clean out the baskets and backwash the filter of a swimming pool, the regional lymph-glands cannot be cleaned" when the macrophages fail to degrade the foreign bodies they've ingested. Normally, such failure does not occur. Nearly everything (including bacteria and viruses) that gets to the point of being commandeered by our body's macrophages will succumb to their scavenging prowess in a process known as "phagocytosis." It is a formidable defense mechanism, deserving of our utmost admiration, Webster suggested, but only if the lungs are looked after properly. "Unfortunately," he added, "Man does not look after his respiratory tract."

The remainder of his paper was dedicated to describing the pathology of lung diseases caused by what he labeled "nuisance dusts," the irritating properties of which are critically exacerbated to hazardous levels by the ways that corporations mine, mill, and manufacture certain minerals and the carelessness with which they put people in harm's way while doing so.

Ian Webster was an accomplished and committed occupational health specialist (he was still working when he died, aged eighty, in 1998), with a capacity for adding a dash of popular vernacular to explaining his work. With a degree in medicine and an abiding interest in pathology, he was dedicated to his science in a commendably nerdish way typical of white coat-clad intellectuals.[2] Somewhat timid and averse to confrontation, he was not well suited to the rough-house tactics of corporate apparatchiks determined to protect their industry from any uncomfortable truths that scientific research might present them. When Richard met with him in March 1996, he already had a copy of Webster's incendiary 1962 report, the ill fate of which Richard was keen to talk about. Throughout the two hours Richard spent with Webster, he found him to be careful, cagey even, reluctant to say much at all in response to Richard's repeated questions about the asbestos industry's interference in the integrity of scientific research.[3]

In truth, Ian Webster was somewhat enigmatic in his declared perspective on the role the asbestos industry played in his life's work. Seemingly affronted and frustrated by such overt interference, while at the same time pragmatically accepting the reality of the industry's financial and political clout. The intrepid Jock McCulloch was probably closest to the mark when he described Webster as having endured "a terrible struggle" for most of his professional career trying to reconcile the dilemma. McCulloch had used these words in a comment added by way of introduction to a written record of an interview he'd conducted with Webster in December 1997.[4]

Throughout the interview Webster, who by then was eighty years old, was frank about those in both the business and scientific communities he blamed for having "blocked" asbestos research and irritated (maybe even angered) by those who "wanted to vet all PRU publications on asbestos." At the same time, however, he also pointed to others in the industry who he believed were more enlightened in having "accepted the link," or been "sympathetic to the idea of a connection," between mesothelioma and crocidolite mining and manufacturing. He named names, including, specifically, those who had worked for Cape Plc, which was all very different from his guarded responses to Richard's questions a year earlier. It also contrasted sharply with Laurie Flynn's experience when interviewing Webster in the early 1980s. Probing (again) the propriety of the asbestos industry's interference in his scientific endeavors, Flynn had elicited a peculiarly defensive response from Webster, including flat denials that his or his colleagues' work was ever vetted, restricted, or otherwise compromised by "editorial" inputs from asbestos industry representatives.[5]

Webster's equivocation was a symptom of a malaise that went to the very heart of the case that Richard was compiling against Cape. A malady of manipulation of scientific process and deceit in the delivery of its results that had consigned thousands of Africans to stunted lives and early deaths. A disease driven by corporate greed and carelessness, aided by an accommodating political environment. Ian Webster's career was also a casualty of the asbestos enterprise, very different, to be sure, in terms of scale and gravity to that suffered by the asbestos communities in the Northern Cape and Northern Transvaal, but a casualty nonetheless. When I pressed Richard on what he thought might explain Webster's behavior, he agreed that Webster was no doubt intimidated by the industry's bullying, not just of him directly, but also of others undertaking similar research.[6]

Most particularly, Webster had watched the chastening spectacle of fellow South African medical scientist Chris Wagner's professional defenestration, following the publication in 1960 of a ground-breaking article of which he was the lead author. The article had provided, for the first time, incontrovertible empirical evidence of the link between crocidolite asbestos exposure and pleural mesothelioma.[7] Erstwhile colleagues at the PRU, as well as brothers-in-law, Wagner and Webster didn't get along. That, however, didn't detract from the lessons Webster learnt from the excoriating and almost wholly unjustified criticism that the asbestos industry directed at Wagner in an orchestrated campaign to discredit him and his research. Such was the virulence of the assault (including, it was rumored, threats of assassination) that Wagner felt compelled to leave Africa altogether. Just two years after publication of his article, he resigned from the PRU and accepted a position as director of the Pneumoco-niosis Research Unit at Llandough Hospital in Wales.

The price Ian Webster paid for deciding to stay in his home-land and keep his job was different, if no less wrenching. It was to bend to the asbestos industry that helped fund his research at the PRU and to yield to the authority it thereby claimed for itself to vet the PRU's work insofar as it related to asbestos. At least that is how it appears. The industry's response was made clear to Webster even before he submitted his 1962 report, most especially that it would suppress its publication and immedi-ately suspend the industry's funding of the PRU.

These potentially devastating actions seemed to have caught Webster and his team by surprise (in his report, Webster refers to them in masterful understatement as "untoward reactions"[8]), which they were able to overcome in part only by accepting that funding would resume on condition that their work in the area would be renamed and, essentially, reconceived. The "Mesothe-lioma Survey," which gave rise to the 1962 report, was rebranded "An Investigation into Possible Air Pollution by Asbestos Dust," and doubts were cast on the strength (or even existence) of the link between asbestos and mesothelioma based on the data then collected. Both ploys were designed specifically to distance sug-gestions that asbestos dust—most especially that of crocidolite or amosite—might be carcinogenic.

This Faustian pact seems to have been behind the extraor-dinary, above-mentioned denials Ian Webster made to Laurie Flynn, when asked whether he thought there was anything improper about the direct and active involvement of asbestos corporations in the supposedly independent research on the occupational health hazards of their operations. It also goes some way toward explaining Webster's rethinking of the un-equivocal forebodings raised in his 1962 report when, in an article published in the *South African Medical Journal* in 1973, he stated: "It is difficult to postulate a direct relationship between crocidolite and the development of mesothelioma," and further, that it is also "difficult to conceive of amosite . . . causing malignancy."[9] With regard to both asbestos types, Webster "postulate[d]" that "another factor" must be associated with the asbestos fibers "before malignant change occurs."[10]

Many years later, Webster was to claim in a sworn deposition in a US case involving Cape that his intentions at the time had been noble—that he had consciously "reduce[d] the impact" of the evidence of his own research to "buy time" for "the asbestos industry to make the conditions safer for its workers and to stop environmental pollution." Doing so, he said, would "allow me to influence the industry to inject more effort into improving conditions." Noble or not in their intention, his actions were nevertheless naive and misguided, as he himself conceded later in the same deposition. When asked whether "the industry use[d] that time to the [desired] optimum benefit," he replied sheepishly, "I don't think to the optimum benefit, no."[11]

As it turned out, the mere possibility of a break in the direct link between asbestos and mesothelioma as suggested by Webster was just what the industry was looking for—a scientific "get-out clause" that provided it with sufficient plausible deniability to continue business as usual.[12] The fact that the South African Medical Research Council (SAMRC), under which authority Webster worked, also backed these skeptical views added more grist to the asbestos industry's mill. Indeed, SAMRC had gone even further, proclaiming in an August 1970 statement sensationally headed "ASBESTOS DUST IS NOT LETHAL" that "it is doubtful whether the inhalation of asbestos dust alone would cause cancer tumors to develop in the lungs."[13] Consequently, it went on to say, "it is important to place the health hazard constituted by asbestos dust into its correct perspective"—that depended on the view that the carcinogen is to be found elsewhere, including "tobacco smoke, a mineral or a virus of sorts," as SAMRC helpfully suggested.

What perhaps is most remarkable about these scientific and medical salvos against the serious concerns of asbestos exposure is that they came so soon after a major international conference on pneumoconiosis held in Johannesburg in April 1969. Three full days of the conference were dedicated to symposia on asbestos and asbestosis, during which these very same concerns were repeatedly and robustly aired, including, specifically, the damning association between crocidolite and pleural and peritoneal mesotheliomas.[14] In fact, the SAMRC's 1970 statement was expressly premised on combatting what it labeled "the alleged dangers of asbestos" as "discussed" during the 1969 conference, adding, for good measure, that "asbestos is not the 'killer dust' it is often made out to be."

History, as it turned out, was not on SAMARC's side. Richard knew this well, not only from evidence subsequently collected by Tony Davies and Marianne Felix during the 1980s and 1990s, including both the incidence of mesothelioma in Northern Transvaal and the reasons why it was overlooked,[15] but also evidence gathered by a host of other scientists and researchers documenting an incontrovertible causal link between asbestos (most especially crocidolite but also amosite) and mesothelioma.[16] One of these other researchers was Jonny Myers, a straight-talking environmental and occupational health epidemiologist at the University of Cape Town. His comprehensive review of asbestos-related diseases (ARDs) in South Africa published in June 1980 concludes with the unforgettable injunction that "with a carcinogen . . . there can be no bargaining on the part of those irrevocably exposed to it from a medical point of view." Nor can "society decide for a few of its worker-members that . . . they should die a premature, nasty death" in order that society as a whole might enjoy the purported benefits of asbestos's many uses.[17]

≈

It's not hard to understand why the asbestos industry in South Africa was so unnerved. Even clinical descriptions of the havoc asbestos fiber causes once inside our bodies read like horror fiction: "It invade[s] human tissue like a sci-fi alien," *Time* journalist Peter Hawthorne wrote, after hearing local doctors describe their patients' symptoms while reporting from Prieska during the Cape litigation.[18] Allowing such shocking details to permeate the consciousness of the general population, let alone be brought to the attention of those who were daily exposed to asbestos, was sure to have a dramatic impact on the industry's commercial viability. That much had already been made clear to asbestos corporations by the negative reactions to their product in the West throughout the 1960s and 1970s, as medical evidence became more widely known and understood. So, they seemed determined to fight a rearguard action in South Africa to save the industry there from ruin, no matter what the cost to the health of their workers, families, and local communities.

The health implications were indeed grim. Prime among the dangerous dusts discussed by Webster in his "swimming pool" paper were asbestos fibers, the inhalation of which causes a range of ailments. These include, most notably, asbestosis and mesothelioma. Asbestosis manifests as fibrotic scarring or thickening of lung tissue caused by the body's valiant but unsuccessful attempts to eliminate minute asbestos fibers that have reached the lungs' lower lobes. The multitudes of normally thin, lacey air sacs (the alveoli) that constitute the lungs' enormous gas-exchanging surface area are thereby occluded or fused such that both oxygen uptake and carbon-dioxide expiration are irreparably damaged. All this happens inside the lungs and affects their parenchyma, or functional tissue, in ways that are explicable even to non-medically educated.

What flabbergasts us non-medics (well, it did me, at any rate) is that asbestos fibers can pass *through* the lungs into the pleural space between them and the inner lining of the chest. Here the damage they cause is different and, if anything, more drastic. Designed both to permit and promote the smooth expansion and contraction of our lungs, the two pleural linings are supposed to glide smoothly across each other with every breath we take. The tiny cavity between them should be entirely free of any foreign bodies, most especially ones that are sharp and almost entirely non-biodegradable. It takes little imagination, therefore, to appreciate the lacerating discomfort (and more) when the pleural cavity is compromised. Think of it like sandpaper against silk, or grit under your eyelid, though that short-term irritant only hints at the incapacitating and long-term harm done when asbestos fibers traverse our lungs' mesothelial lining.

Referred to as "translocation," the process involves only those asbestos fibers that are small enough in length and, especially, diameter. By small we mean microscopic. Measurements registered in terms of microns (μm), or thousandths of a millimeter (or millionths of a meter if you prefer). Some—at the larger end of respirable fibers capable of translocating in this way—are 10 to 20 μm long and 1 to 2 μm wide, while the smallest and most penetrative fibers measure less than 5 μm in length and under 0.25 μm in diameter.[19] To put these figures into some context, we are talking about dimensions closer to those of bacteria (typically 1 to 10 μm long) than, say, the width of a human hair, commonly measured as roughly 100 μm. Ultrafine asbestos fibers are not only more than 400 times narrower than a human hair, but are also so short that you can fit more than 20 of them in a row across the cut end of that same human hair.

Shape too is important. The "rod-like rigid fibers" of amphibole asbestos varieties (namely, crocidolite and amosite) are more aerodynamic and more deeply penetrative than the "curly and flexible" fibers of serpentine chrysotile (or white) asbestos,[20] especially at the larger end of the spectrum of respirable asbestos dust.[21] Chemical makeup is also a factor in the relative durability, or biopersistence, of fibers, since the more resistant they are to our bodies' defenses, the more time they have to wound, poison, or kill us. All asbestos fibers are depressingly durable once embedded in our viscera, but the amphibole fibers (again) are the hardiest. Bearing a biological half-life (measured in decades) significantly longer than that of serpentine fibers (measured in months), they are never fully broken down or eliminated by our macrophagic defense mechanisms within a normal human lifetime.[22]

It is this combination of size, shape, and chemistry of particular asbestos fibers that makes them so lethal. The deeper they pierce human tissue, the more damage they do. The translocation of those asbestos fibers that are small and fine enough, sufficiently aerodynamic or sharp enough, and tough and durable enough is a process as extraordinary as it is ruinous. Such fibers pass through the lungs, across their visceral lining and into the pleural cavity by hitching a ride on fluid (mainly water) exchanges across the semi-permeable pleura—what scientists call "pulmonary and pleuro-pulmonary interstitial fluid dynamics."[23] One of these dynamics is osmotic, driven by differing chemical concentrations on either side of the pleura. The other is hydraulic, driven by a pressure gradient on one side that pushes fluid across to the other.[24]

Once there, between the pleura linings of your lungs and your chest wall, the fibers grind like sand in gears. They aggravate and tear the delicate pleural membranes, prompting a macrophagic storm, which despite its inability to eliminate the fibers, can isolate and engulf the foreigners, thickening the walls of the pleura or building hard plaques, "like a worn-down bar of soap," as epidemiologist and pathologist Gill Nelson described them to me, which can hinder or even obstruct breathing.[25] The clinical presentation of plaques appears ominous—clusters of cartilaginous nodules adhering to the lung wall—but it is in fact the solid lesion-mass of pleural thickening that is the more harmful as it slowly expands its rigid grip around the lungs. It can take between ten and thirty years for such thickening to reach the stage where it impairs breathing, but as and when it does, the symptomatic sensations are frightening. Sufferers told Richard that their chests felt compressed, their breathing reduced to labored wheezes, and they often panicked when struggling to get enough air into their lungs.[26] The fact that pleural thickening is also often accompanied by effusion—the accumulation of fluid—in the pleural cavity, as well as by fibrotic scarring inside the lung architecture itself, adds to these debilitating sensations.[27]

It is in the pleura that the deadliest of asbestos-related diseases are most commonly found. Pleural mesothelioma occupies a special place in the pantheon of such diseases on account of both its singular etiological association with asbestos (most notably crocidolite) and its insidious malignancy. Once diagnosed, patients have "a dismal prognosis," as medics bluntly state,[28] such is the speed with which this cancerous neoplasm replicates and incapacitates its host organs. Lungs are literally squeezed shut, as though a fist were closing around a sponge, with the time between diagnosis and death typically ranging from four to eighteen months. Chests collapse, and the tumor masses encasing the lungs grow large enough to be observable and palpable in the chest wall, simultaneously pressing against the thoracic spine and distorting its shape in characteristic scoliotic form.[29]

As awful as these circumstances are, they are not what kills you. Once again, it is the body's response to this mutant invader that creates the complications leading to death. "Macrophages play a dichotomous role in cancer, where they promote tumor growth but also serve as critical immune effectors of therapeutic antibodies," as stem-cell biologists put it.[30] And while both roles may have good intentions, as it were—trying to isolate and/ or eliminate the original foreign bodies (i.e., asbestos fibers)— by the time a malignant mesothelioma has formed, the body's defense mechanisms have reached levels of uncontrolled overdrive. Toxic, pus-filled fluid (the residue of the macrophagal and antibodies' battle against the invading fibers) quickly accumulates inside the pleural cavity, flooding upward and eventually enclosing the whole lung. This effusion, alongside the expanding mass of the tumor itself, any preexisting pleural thickening, and, quite possibly, the presence of alveoli flattening asbestosis *inside* the lung give the organ no chance of survival. In the end, patients slowly suffocate, drowned by their own body's frustrated efforts to eliminate the tiny, toxic intruders.

This ghastly image of "progressive asphyxiation" has been known to medical specialists from the earliest days of the identification of ARDs. Pathologist William E. Cooke's break-through autopsy examination of the lungs of Nellie Kershaw, a thirty-three-year-old asbestos factory worker in Rochdale, Northern England, who died in April 1924, made that much clear. Swamped with razor sharp asbestos fibers and disfigured by scar tissue, her lungs were almost entirely encased in dense fibrous adhesions such that they were "to a large extent airless," according to

Cooke.[31] His conclusion that Nellie Kershaw had died from "pulmonary asbestosis"—thereby giving the disease its name—was consistent with the diagnosis of "asbestos poisoning" that W. J. Joss, Nellie's physician, had provided when she was still alive.

By the 1990s, it was well established how extensively ARDs could affect the human body. Mesotheliomas, it was clear, are not restricted to the pleura surrounding the lungs (though they remain the predominant site) but are also found in serosal membranes encasing other organs, including, most notably, the heart (pericardium), the testes and ovaries, and abdominal organs (peritoneum). The latter arises from the ingestion of asbestos fibers—an ever-present hazard for asbestos mine and mill workers and their families who consistently reported layers of dust covering every surface in their homes as well as workplaces—which then translocate to the peritoneum in much the same way as they do from within the lungs to the pleura.

This dual-entry system is further enhanced by the fact that the fibers making it this far into the body are then liable to enter the lymphatic system, as indicated by Webster,[32] the macrophagal response having been frustrated in its effort to eliminate the fibers. Once there, and maintaining their extraordinary biopersistence, fibers can be carried directly into the blood stream via the finely tuned interchange of filtered fluids between the two systems that otherwise protects the body from harmful trespassers.[33] It is in this way that asbestos fibers reach the gonads as well as kidneys, liver, spleen, pancreas, fetal tissues via the placenta, and the gastro-intestinal tract.[34]

While there is clear medical evidence of asbestos fibers deposited in all these organs,[35] the primary sites for mesotheliomas remain the linings of the lungs, abdomen, and the heart (by way of its proximity to and close interaction with the lungs).[36] For asbestosis and other ARDs, the sole site is the lungs. The gruesome fact of the matter is that the most penetrative asbestos fibers are also the most lethal, such that we seldom see just how far they can go. Certainly, they are capable of reaching just about every corner of the human body—in addition to which the cancers they cause can reach those few organs denied to them (metastasizing mesothelioma, for example, can reach the brain)[37]—but your life is typically ended by complications encountered at the primary sites (of lungs and heart), where the asbestos burden is greatest, before serious damage is incurred further afield.

≈

Courtesy of the good offices of the NCOH, and especially Tony Davies and Marianne Felix, Richard was now seeing the (barely) living evidence of this carnage in South Africa as he met with and interviewed former asbestos workers and residents in asbestos towns. He'd also read the above-mentioned ground-breaking 1960 article by Chris Wagner, C. A. Sleggs, and Paul Marchand in the *British Journal of Industrial Medicine* linking mesothelioma to crocidolite asbestos exposure in South Africa's Northern Cape, which provided him with further insights to the pain and suffering these victims were enduring. This remarkable article—which remains to this day the most cited scientific work in the field of occupational health[38]—is unsparing in its graphic detailing of the clinical effects of the disease. With regard to Case 1 of the thirty-three cases of diffuse malignant mesothelioma that were the basis for the study, the authors report:

> A radiograph [x-ray] taken at a mine hospital on August 18, 1955 showed a massive, right-sided pleural effusion, and 3,000 ml [3 liters] of fluid was withdrawn. He was admitted to the Witwatersrand Native Labour Association Hospital on August 24, 1955, and two days later aspiration yielded 1,000 ml [1 liter] of thick

gelatinous pus "which could be pulled out in threads." He was treated with frequent aspirations and instillation of varidase [medication for suppurating wounds] but without improvement and he died on February 15, 1956.[39]

The patient was a thirty-six-year-old black male mine worker from the Northern Cape who also showed signs of asbestosis.

Case 4 in the same study was a fifty-six-year-old white female social worker from Griquatown in the Northern Cape, "who could only have had a short exposure to asbestos as a child and probably a further slight exposure as a young woman." X-rays of her lungs taken between July 1955 and July 1956 showed a marked deterioration of her right lung capacity from something like 90 percent to almost nothing (less than 10 percent) over the year—the lung simply disappeared in the x-rays. She too suffered from pleural effusion "of straw-coloured fluid . . . contain[ing] mesothelial cells," and despite extensive remedial treatment, she died in January 1957.[40]

In other cases, the authors refer to an autopsy revealing "the right chest occupied by a huge whitish tumour . . . extending through the diaphragm onto the superior surface of the liver" (Case 14) and to thoracotomies (chest surgeries) on living patients, successfully stripping "hard as rock" pleural thickening from upper lung lobes, but failing to remove "a hard craggy mass" (Case 15) or "grossly thickened pleura" (Case 22) adhering to the lower lobes. Pleural cavities are described as "obliterated" (Cases 16 and 24), and in all cases the authors report effusions of "pints" of yellow fluid, many containing "malignant cells."[41]

Indeed, so symptomatic of ARDs (and of mesothelioma in particular) are these extensive effusions that the insertion of "a tap" through the chest wall to drain the fluid became well-known and feared among local communities as a calling card of the grim reaper. So dreadful a prospect was the near certainty of an untimely death when a tap was prescribed that many years later Charles Schoeman at Prieska Hospital told me that some sufferers simply avoided seeking out medical help. A sad reflection of preferring hope based on ignorance above expectation drawn from knowledge. "They fear the diagnosis and treatment more than the disease itself," said Schoeman, whose wiry frame and indefatigable, almost serene, manner reflect his dedication to providing medical care to the people of Prieska since 1990.[42]

While the intricacies of this biological warfare may have been entirely unknown to South African asbestos workers, their families, and the local communities in which they lived, they were all acutely aware of the consequences as they watched their health deteriorate, their bodies fail, and their livelihoods—and eventually their lives—disappear under the onslaught. Inhabitants of the affected towns in Northern Transvaal and the Northern Cape were uniquely exposed to the worst asbestos types—the deeply penetrative, translocating amphibole fibers of crocidolite and amosite asbestos, then mined almost exclusively in South Africa. The destructive force was brutal for all sufferers and their families, but in some cases it was truly horrific.

Shirley Celanto lives in a small brick cottage on the edge of Prieska. Her hair is in curlers when she greets us at the door, framing an open face with soft, benign features that belie all that she has endured during her sixty-nine years.[43] After ushering us into her living room, which is disconcertingly dark compared to the searing glare outside, we perch on chairs around a small dining table above which hangs a haunting black and white photograph of her sister Stephanie, staring blankly from her sickbed, set up in the very room where we're now meeting. I'm with Cecil Skeffers, a longtime asbestos activist and one of the founders of Prieska's Concerned People Against Asbestos in the late 1990s.

Cecil had also worked with Richard for many years throughout the Cape litigation and knew the lay of the land—figuratively as well as physically—of his community's gruesome relationship with asbestos. Cecil had earlier primed me with some details of Shirley's background and I'd also instantly recognized the portrait of "Stef" as one of Hein du Plessis's celebrated photographs documenting Cape's asbestos victims and their families (see photo gallery).[44] But still, I was simply not prepared for what unfolded over the next hour as Shirley calmly laid out the full extent of the tragedy that had befallen her and her family over more than four decades.

Her family had been wiped out by asbestosis and mesothelioma. Her mother and father had died at forty-four and forty-eight years old, respectively, as had her two brothers (aged forty-nine and sixty-two) and her two sisters, one aged thirty-six and Stef, aged forty-four. Shirley had been a teacher but had to give that up to care for Stef when she was diagnosed with mesothelioma in 1998. She and Stef were both single mothers (Shirley with two children and Stef with three), so Shirley soon found herself the de facto mother of five children as well as Stef's full-time caretaker, so rapid was her sister's deterioration. Following Stef's death eighteen months later in March 2000, one of her brothers also died of an ARD, and she became mother to his three children. On her own, with eight children and no job, Shirley says that she was "cross and upset," often "fighting with the Lord" over her predicament. Her words seem thoroughly inadequate were it not for the emotion with which she delivers them.[45]

Having lived all her life near the asbestos mill in Prieska, Shirley recalls a childhood playing on the asbestos dumps surrounding the mill with her siblings "and lots of other kids," and how she realized only when she was twenty-eight years old that asbestos was dangerous after her mother fell ill and died shortly thereafter. By the time Shirley first saw and heard Richard at the town hall meetings in Prieska in 1999, there wasn't a family in the town that hadn't been ravaged by ARDs, even if few were as eviscerated as was hers. Generations of people in communities across the Northern Cape and Northern Transvaal/Limpopo had been poisoned by asbestos fiber dust, whether through occupational or environmental exposure or both.

≈

The roots of occupational medicine can be traced back as far as Hippocrates in ancient Greece, who documented occupational health hazards as disparate as mutilated limbs of soldiers and lead poisoning in miners.[46] Even the more systematic and scientific discipline that we recognize today has a long history. Italian physician Bernardino Ramazzini's work on diseases and ailments associated with a wide range of working environments (from cobblers, tailors and bakers to porters, mirror-makers and miners) in the seventeenth century earned him the sobriquet "the father of occupational medicine."[47]

Mining has always been notoriously prominent in the field, due not only to the inherent structural dangers of working underground but also to the irritating dust, metals, and chemicals one encounters in such cramped and enclosed spaces. One hundred years before Ramazzini, German minerologist Georgius Agricola described the primitive and ineffective ventilation methods employed in the gold and silver mines of central Europe, which caused miners to have "difficulty in breathing and destruction of the lungs."[48] Roman philosopher and keen social documenter Pliny recorded mercury poisoning as so common among mercury miners during his time (first century BCE) that only slaves were engaged in the mines, as no Roman citizens would risk their own health doing the job.

All that said, it was not until the dawn of the Industrial Revolution, when the scale of occupational health hazards expanded exponentially, both in terms of severity and the numbers of people affected, that the discipline began to attract the levels of attention it has today. The appalling working conditions of factory workers, miners, and mill workers throughout the 1800s triggered the interest and growing concerns of welfare groups, lawmakers, social researchers, and sympathetic industrialists and engineers, together with those of medical experts, eventually spawning a new, overarching specialty of "occupational health." Part scientists, part sociologists, practitioners in the field are concerned not just with workers' diseases and afflictions and how to treat them, but also, crucially, with how to prevent them or minimize their occurring in the first place.[49] As such and to do their job properly—especially in places like Apartheid South Africa—they have to possess considerable political acumen alongside unimpeachable integrity. It is a combination, evidently, that can be very difficult to establish let alone maintain. The various tribulations of Chris Wagner, Ian Webster, and Tony Davies had already made that much clear to Richard.

The breadth of knowledge and skills over which occupational health practitioners must exert command to be effective was also reflected in the work of Sophie Kisting whom Richard met during these early years. From her base at the University of Cape Town, this softly spoken, nerves-of-steel, occupational health clinician and researcher had worked closely with the NUM, helping it negotiate access to asbestos workers' medical records held by the mining companies. Thereby, and with the consent of the workers, Sophie and her colleagues in the university's Industrial Health Research Group had been able to undertake independent (or at least additional) examinations of these records to determine whether there existed grounds for compensation claims to be made. Such examinations were also significant at the time for what they revealed about the working conditions at the mine and mill sites. And it was for this reason that the asbestos companies had been wary and reluctant to provide access, even though they were obliged to conduct such health checks by statute.[50] Navigating these political thickets later expanded to Sophie supporting the NUM push, successfully, for the establishment in 1995 of South Africa's first commission of inquiry into health and safety in the mining industry since the early 1960s.[51]

What Sophie learned about dealing with asbestos companies and the government authorities often beholden to them helped explain how the health catastrophe she was documenting in the asbestos mining towns of Northern Transvaal, the Northern Cape, and Mpumalanga provinces had come about and why it had been left to fester for so long. All this Sophie was able to pass on to Richard, together with an insistence that addressing this calamity required an unswerving commitment to ethical professional practices, not least from the scientific and medical communities investigating and treating it. This clarion call—which Sophie and fellow occupational health specialist Leslie London described at the time as necessary because of health professionals being "squeezed" by neoliberal forces "prioritis[ing] trade over the environment"[52]—was fast becoming a defining feature of the case being built by Richard. It corresponded closely with what Sophie (this time with co-author Lundy Braun) cautioned as the need to "go beyond technical solutions . . . to recast our understanding of disease causality by integrating historical knowledge about social and political conditions that produce disease with biological understandings of the pathogenicity of asbestos fibers."[53]

In the United Kingdom, the first examples of occupational health and safety legislation appeared with the passage of series of so-called Factories Acts beginning in 1802. Initially aimed at protecting the exploitation and abuse of children in textile factories by setting standards such as maximum working hours (twelve per day), sufficient ventilation, cleaning premises (two quicklime washings per year), and accommodation (no more than two per bed), they were widely unenforced and routinely evaded. The establishment of a Factory Inspectorate in 1833 did, however, bring some welcome rigor to upholding the laws, especially after the engagement of workplace inspectors was extended beyond factories into mines, quarries, and mills throughout the nineteenth century and eventually to almost all workplaces by the latter half of the twentieth century.[54]

While it was a chief inspector of factories who had stated in 1898 that asbestos had "easily demonstrated" health risks,[55] it was not until 1931, following a damning government "Report on the Effects of Dust on the Lungs and Dust Suppression in the Asbestos Industry," that any legislation specifically addressing the problem of asbestos in the workplace was introduced in the United Kingdom.[56] Nominally designed to set limits on permissible levels of airborne dust contamination in asbestos factories (including Cape's in Barking, London), the Asbestos Regulations (1931) were dismally inadequate in practice. The limits themselves were merely guidelines and in any case were so generous to the factory owners (there was, for example, *no* maximum limit set for the shortest and most dangerous fibers measuring less than 5 μm)[57] that they provided little or no protection to their employees. Not a single conviction was recorded under the regulations during the entire period they were in force (until 1969, when they were revised and somewhat strengthened by a new set of regulations).[58] Such laxity underscores both how ineffective they were and how accurate was the damning assessment that the reason asbestos corporations offered any support for their introduction in the first place was "not to protect the health of their workers," but to provide themselves with a semblance of cover against legal action (for doing something rather than nothing at all).[59]

Cape Plc, alongside Turner & Newall, and British Belting & Asbestos (the so-called Big Three), had been a powerful broker in terms of the asbestos industry's influential relationship with the British government at that time, the results of which Richard could see reflected in how Cape had conducted its business in South Africa. "Lessons well learnt," as he put it to me years later.[60] And so they were. It must be stressed that in the United Kingdom, decades before the ground-breaking Wagner, Sleggs and Marchand study on mesothelioma in 1960 and the suppressed Webster report in 1962, the factories inspectorate report in 1898 and William E Cooke's revealing publications of details of the Nellie Kershaw case in the 1920s had unambiguously described how grave were the health effects of exposure to asbestos fibers. Yet, neither of these earlier key events in the history of ARDs registered much beyond medical and occupational health circles, and insofar as they did, they were ignored or dismissed by the industry and governments alike.[61]

Lucy Deane—coincidentally, Britain's first female inspector of factories—who wrote the 1898 report, did not mince her words. "The evil effects of asbestos dust" she noted, are evidenced in "ascertained cases of injury to bronchial tubes and lungs medically attributed to the employment of the sufferer." These cases, she continued, "instigated a microscopic examination of the mineral dust by HM Medical Inspector [which] clearly revealed . . . the sharp glass-like jagged nature of the particles, and where they are allowed to rise and to remain suspended in the air of the room in any quantity, the effects have been found to be injurious as might have been expected."[62] Such "expected" injuries comprised the plaques, pleural thickening, and asbestosis that were later to be documented by Cooke in his two *British Medical Journal* articles in 1924 and 1927 on the cause of Nellie Kershaw's death, which he labeled "lung fibrosis" and subsequently "pulmonary asbestosis." Mesothelioma, at this stage, was unknown, so it was not included, but these stark, publicly aired accounts of debilitating and life-threatening ailments were surely serious enough not to be swept so contemptuously under the carpet. And yet that is, in effect, what happened to them.[63]

≈

Late one evening, nearly one hundred years later, Richard was reading Lucy Deane's words back home in London at a kitchen table surrounded by the detritus of a family dinner he'd promised to clear up but hadn't quite got around to doing so. What forces are at work, he wondered, that can effectively silence such powerful words for so long and across two continents? Whatever the answer, he knew the very same forces would soon be aligned against him and his clients in the lawsuit he was about to file against Cape.[64] He also knew he was tough, determined, and as near inexhaustible as any lawyer can be, but would it be enough? The answer eluded him as he belatedly attended to the dishes and shuffled off to bed.

CHAPTER 4

Mining the Miracle Mineral
—*Playing with Fire*—

MMELE'S DAY BEGAN EARLY. Dawn's haze was lifting above the hills as he walked the five minutes from his hut in Cape's mine compound at Penge to the mine shaft entrance, or adit. Throughout the eleven years he had been employed at the mine from 1965 to 1976, Mmele had worked across a range of jobs in the mining process, from drilling holes into the rock face underground for dynamite blasting to packing milled amosite asbestos fiber into sacks and loading them onto trucks for delivery to ports and railway stations. In between, he'd also driven trucks transporting the blasted ore from the mine site to the milling machines for crushing and sorting. When working underground, he remembers, "The dust would fly off the rocks onto my clothes, hair, and skin. I was never provided with protective clothing or a mask and would inhale dust and fibers all the time." Even above ground, the dust was everywhere, "on our food and on my bedding." And "when the [milling] machines were cleaned, which was at least once a day, the dust would fly into the air and settle on me."

While pausing for a moment to contemplate the irony of clean machines at the expense of dirty lungs, Richard notes that the consequence of all this for Mmele was his diagnosis twenty-three years later with asbestosis in the first degree, having suffered for decades "from very severe chest pains, coughing with tiredness and shortness of breath."[1]

Extreme and prolonged exposure to asbestos dust remained a drastic hazard in Cape's mines even after mechanical compressors replaced the hand-packing of raw asbestos fiber and masks were provided to mill workers. "The compressor itself raised dust as it stamped the fibers into the bags," one of Mmele's Penge colleagues recounted, "like a thick cloud in the air." The masks "were not effective, for the dust was too fine and managed to go through to my nose where it was clearly visible when I removed the mask. When we complained about the levels of dust to the boss, we were told to drink milk to help clear out the asbestos."[2]

≈

What was so special—even magical—about this particular mineral that made mining it so compelling, despite its long trail of human destruction?

Richard knew that the challenge he and the victims faced in bringing their case against Cape was made all the more difficult by asbestos's illustrious past. Its remarkable qualities were known to the ancient Greeks, Egyptians, and Persians, who wove it into cloth and pottery for added strength and built it into housing materials for insulation.[3] Most of all, its earliest uses centered on its resistance to fire. Commonly used to make wicks for candles or oil lamps, it was also worked into crematorium cloths by the Romans, who recognized its utility in preserving the ashes of their incinerated dead. While it was originally regarded by many as a vegetable as distinct from a mineral, it was this characteristic of incombustibility above all others that attracted awe and wonder.

This seemingly miraculous feature of asbestos remained its key appeal when it began to be mined and milled on an industrial scale in the late 1800s. But it was soon followed by widening appreciation of its extraordinary durability and tensile strength (greater than steel, no less),[4] weavability,[5] and high resistance to chemicals, water, and electricity. Together, these qualities elevated its status to a commercially attractive product.

It was this development—the realization of asbestos as a profitable commodity—that motivated the forces now ranged against Richard, as indeed they had long been ranged against anyone or anything that threatened the industry's viability.

Recognizing the broad utility of an exceptionally strong and fire-retardant material in the turn of the century's rapidly industrializing economies driven by engines and machines powered by coal and steam, asbestos companies were appearing across Europe ready to mine and mill asbestos wherever it was found and to manufacture products made from it back home. Lagging in ships and factories, insulation in homes and offices, and brakes and other friction-prone parts in trains and (slowly emerging) automobiles, in addition to fire prevention and control (such as fire blankets) everywhere—the uses for asbestos were seemingly endless. The Cape Asbestos Company was one of the early movers in the commercialization of asbestos, being incorporated in the United Kingdom in 1893 following the rediscovery of substantial blue asbestos deposits in 1890 in the Northern Cape (hence the company's name) by an intrepid Cornish miner named Francis Oates. Dubbed "the father of the Cape Asbestos Company," Oates was determined to exploit that which had been merely noted ninety years earlier by Hinrich Lichtenstein, a German geologist, who made the original discovery of masses of "lavender" blue asbestos in the hills surrounding Prieska and along the Orange River.[6]

≈

As the dimensions of the case expanded, so Richard needed help to gather information and sift through it looking for key documents and paper trails that might help construct the case against Cape. Susannah Read, a smart, determined young lawyer recently graduated from law school, was the first to join what would eventually become a sizeable team of lawyers, paralegals, and administrative assistants. While these committed individuals were spread across (and often traveled between) Leigh Day's London office and another bespoke office established in Prieska, Susannah was steadfastly London-based. Wary of flying, Susannah never made it to South Africa, though this did not diminish the contributions she made to building the case from the ground up. Turning her attention to Cape the company—its history, people, and motivations—one of the first things she reviewed was an obscure eighty-page hagiography published by Cape in 1953 to celebrate its sixtieth anniversary, which Richard had recently unearthed.[7] For the two of them the document offered a wealth of relevant information both in what it said and in what it didn't say.

The pioneering spirit of the company's founders was laid out, including such intriguing tidbits as the "discovery" (by a European Caucasian, that is) of an entirely new asbestos variety peculiar to Africa. A clump of brown asbestos—later named "amosite," after the acronym for Asbestos Mines of South Africa—was found by a farmer in 1907 among a "witch doctor's" hoard of old bones, artifacts, and curios near Penge in Northern Transvaal.[8] There were also plenty of promotional references to asbestos's "freakish" properties and its many beneficial applications that promised commercial returns for the new company. What was glaringly absent in the booklet was any acknowledgment, let alone discussion, of the dangers that asbestos posed or might pose to human health in Cape's mines or factories.[9] Perhaps, Richard mused, one ought not to expect the company to rain on its own parade in a publication like this. But still, given what was then (in 1953) already known or, at the very least gravely suspected, about the medical impacts of exposure to asbestos dust, glossing over the matter so completely showed how comfortable and confident Cape was with maintaining its profitable and carefree status quo.

The profitability of asbestos and the industry's confidence that came with it had been secured by the two World Wars. The vast quantities of fire and brimstone hurled by all sides throughout both conflagrations assured soaring demand for asbestos products to protect, insulate, and strengthen the huge numbers of increasingly powerful vessels, vehicles, and machines used in combat. Demand was further increased after the wars when the battle-tested uses of asbestos were converted to civilian pursuits, reaching into almost every corner of our lives, albeit with little or no understanding outside medical circles of the dangers it posed. That something so innocent as the fake snow falling on the sleeping faces of Dorothy and friends in the 1939 movie *The Wizard of Oz* was in fact 100 percent pure chrysotile (white) asbestos underlines the levels of ignorance at that time.[10]

From a total worldwide production of all types of asbestos of 31,487 metric tons in 1900, global tonnage figures rose to 193,000 in 1920 and 1.3 million in 1950. Worldwide production peaked at 4.75 million tons in 1979, after which it remained above 4 million tons per year until 1990, when it began steadily tailing off. Asbestos production in South Africa largely mirrored this trend line, rising from 158 tons in 1900 to an all-time high of 380,164 tons in 1977, before falling to 6,272 tons in 2003.[11]

The South African output, however, differed in one crucial respect. Whereas chrysotile comprised the bulk of the global asbestos output (between 90 and 95 percent), most of South Africa's asbestos output was amphibole—that is, asbestos characterized by the needle-like shape of composite fibers, as in crocidolite and amosite, which typically accounted for two-thirds of its total output, with chrysotile comprising the remainder.[12] Thus, while during these peak years South Africa accounted for less than 10 percent of global production of asbestos, it produced nearly all the world's supply of crocidolite and amosite, being home to the world's largest deposits of the former and the only known deposits of the latter.[13] Cape was a major player in South Africa's production of both types of asbestos. In 1976, for example, Cape was responsible for 29 percent of crocidolite mined in the country and all of its amosite, according to the data epidemiologist Jonny Myers managed, with some difficulty, to get hold of for that year.[14]

The Second World War and its aftermath were indeed profitable years for Cape, with its fortunes growing exponentially between 1938 and 1953, during which time the company's assets increased by more than 800 percent. Reflecting on the reasons behind its commercial success, Cape's sixtieth anniversary booklet had this to say:

> The successful introduction of its products to a hesitant market is the first prerequisite to a company's progress and growth; this objective attained, there remains an unabating struggle to maintain and advance the position achieved. During the past sixty years The Cape Asbestos Company has been successfully engaged in these battles and will continue the fight with the certain knowledge that both the raw materials from the mines and the manufactured products from the factories are indispensable to modern industry.[15]

Self-assured bravado, to be sure. But behind the pomp one cannot help thinking there lies a deeper message, one that portrays
an element of concern—an awareness (in 1953) of the health
dangers and medical disquiet about asbestos and therefore the
need to "struggle," "battle," and "fight" with skeptics and naysay-
ers. Above all, perhaps the expressed "hesitancy" of the market
refers to creeping doubts among consumers (that is, nearly everyone) about the safety of this magic mineral fast becoming so
ubiquitous in everyday life.[16] Or at least, that is how it seemed
to Richard when reading these words in 1996.

There was in fact plenty of evidence of this corporate
schizophrenia, as Richard and Susannah were finding as they
dug deeper into Cape's history. The company's enthusiastic promotion of blue asbestos began early with an advertisement in the
Engineer on July 9, 1897, extolling it as "much lighter than other
varieties and the fibre is longer and stronger"; it was also said to
provide the "most efficient, convenient, durable and lightest non-
conducting covering extant" for boilers and steam pipes.[17] By
1951 the company had begun to publish its own house journal,
Cape Asbestos Company Magazine, filled with internal staff
matters (promotions, plaudits, and parties) and corporate news
about new plants, operations, and market opportunities. Occa-
sional references were also made to new regulations, including
on health and safety matters. But these were typically addressed
with glib assurances that "dust extraction equipment throughout the mills prevents asbestos from being released into the atmosphere" and accompanied by staged photographs of black and
white mill workers wearing masks (albeit, curiously, alongside
other images of maskless black miners digging and drilling ore
underground).[18]

Keen to trumpet asbestos's virtues so loudly as to drown out
any countervailing concerns, Cape resorted to elaborate stunts

such as the "experimental firing" of a three-storey "test building" erected in a factory yard in Cowley, West London, in May 1957.[19] Fitted with "asbestolux" thermal insulation lining and watched by an audience of 600, who were provisioned with a buffet lunch served in a big marquee and entertained by a jaunty ditty written specifically for the occasion, entitled "Fire House Blues Calypso,"[20] the building was set alight using 2 tons of timber, 20 gallons of kerosene and dozens of rubber tires. It burned for nearly an hour, reaching a maximum temperature of 2,450 degrees Fahrenheit.

The building's steel-frame and asbestos lining survived intact, and the fate of the several combustible objects placed behind a protective asbestos curtain erected inside the structure was almost as impressive. A telephone directory was "slightly charred," a box of frozen peas "defrosted"; an aluminum saucepan containing water and fresh eggs yielded "water warm; eggs lightly coddled." The guest of honor was a member of Parliament, accompanied by a senior official from the Ministry of Labour's Department of Safety, Health and Welfare, and the deputy chief inspector of factories.[21] A running commentary throughout the conflagration was provided by Cape's sales director of building products, fittingly named P. A. Denison.

In the four pages of the company magazine devoted to this extraordinary event, readers were assured not only that "the smoke was quickly cleared," but also that "Nurse David was on duty in her First Aid Tent, and that Peggy Edwards attended to the needs of thirsty reporters and photographers in the Press Tent." All in all, the article concludes, "a very thorough and worthwhile exercise."[22]

For the wider audience of potential customers, Cape and the whole of the asbestos industry were quick to use television and newspapers to promote the life-style benefits of asbestos as well as its practical utility. Modern asbestos products were said to add "dignity and charm" to homes and were "designed to last a lifetime. A trouble-free lifetime," to which promise a certain Mrs. Adams in one 1950s American TV commercial responds brightly, "and it's never given us any trouble at all."[23]

The collective clout of asbestos companies also extended to capturing supposedly dispassionate media, such as when the *Times* published a four-page "Special Report on Asbestos" on November 28, 1967, comprising articles by eight journalists, interspersed with advertisements from major asbestos corporations (including Cape) and other supporters of the industry.[24] One of the articles parrots the standard industry line that "if reasonable precautions are taken there is no reason why asbestos should have any adverse effects on its users." Another—written by the paper's unnamed "Medical Correspondent" no less— pronounced that while "increasing appreciation of the public health hazards of many modern industrial processes [is] laudable" and that "in certain instances the health risk may be such that the process must be given up," they were adamant that "there is no indication that asbestos falls into this category." They then rounded off their commentary with the terrifically peremptory conclusion that, as the sector had "introduced . . . improved ventilation and dust suppression," the matter was now "settled . . . so far as the medical profession was concerned [as] the industry set about putting its house in order and complying with medical recommendations."

Even then, in 1967, these words were recklessly optimistic at best or cravenly complicit at worst, but they illustrated to Richard just how wide and powerful was the reach of the industry's influence. Cape's own advertisement in the *Times'* four-page spread evidenced both the foundations of such authority and the confidence it bequeathed. "In Britain alone," it pronounced, "thirteen million cars and trucks rely on their asbestos-based brake linings to stop them safely," which, according to statistics compiled by the British government's Department for Transport, meant just about every vehicle on the road at that time.[25] Such market monopolization, it seems, warranted the company's catchline "CAPE.ABILITY: when nothing else can cope . . . Asbestos can!" Asbestos products were shamelessly promoted as safety-enhancing—tough, strong, and above all, fireproof— no matter the industry's awareness of the sinister capacity of their products to kill and maim.

There were some who sought to justify such selective promotion of asbestos in terms of cost-benefit analyses—"that human life in all its complexity involves the balancing of myriad benefits versus risks," as medical scientists Douglas Henderson and James Leigh put it (while forcefully rebutting the proposition).[26] It was to this end that in December 1968 Cape's medical officer, W. J. Smither, suggested that the asbestos industry accept a limited proposal for "a carefully worded label" on asbestos products "that might read something like: 'In the interests of fire prevention, this board contains 20 percent asbestos. Handle with care.'"[27]

The NCOH's Ian Webster also employed this balancing approach in the short paper he wrote in May 1976 (mentioned in the previous chapter), in which he counseled readers to view the health hazards of asbestos in *true* perspective.[28] After accepting that asbestos causes asbestosis and mesothelioma, he nevertheless maintained that "it is a hazard which can be, and is being, controlled in our mines and mills." Further observing that "an asbestos-containing product is useful and with proper care is safe," he asked, "How many children have died in fires because an asbestos blanket was not available?" Webster's bewildering remarks and the drawing of such an invidious false equivalent between dying miners and endangered minors are perhaps explained by his acknowledgment in the same paper that his work on asbestosis and mesothelioma was "co-sponsored by the asbestos mining industry."

For an especially vivid example of the terrible trade-off everyone everywhere was then being urged to accept regarding asbestos, it is to *The Wizard of Oz* (again) that we might turn. This time to the scarecrow costume worn by actor Ray Bolger, which was impregnated with asbestos fibers to protect him from his character's frequent run-ins with fire.[29] Clearly, most people at that time, whether inside or outside Hollywood, were unaware of just how terrible the consequences of the trade-off were, but *that* is the crucial point. For those who did know did not act, or did not act appropriately or quickly enough.

≈

With the hindsight of thirty years, Richard could see clearly that the emperor was indeed wearing no clothes. The intervening years had yielded such overwhelming and widely disseminated medical evidence of the ferocity of asbestos's assault on the human body that legal and political pressure had turned against the industry. But to make a case against Cape that would stick, Richard had to consider carefully the state of knowledge *at that time* (i.e., during the 1960s and 1970s) of the cost-benefit analysis of asbestos utility to society and, significantly, its reasonable interpretation decades later. Reflecting on this critical point Richard confesses: "Though it didn't seem possible that we could overstate our case given how horrible these [asbestos-related] diseases are, we knew that a big part of Cape's argument would rely on its lack of knowledge, or at least awareness, of the seriousness of ARDs and—bizarrely—whether in fact exposure to asbestos was their root cause."[30]

While the 1960s and 1970s were certainly golden years for Cape, they were also the years when massive strides in medical analyses of the nature and causes of ARDs were being made. These two forces could hardly co-exist for long, as it proved for Cape after it divested all its South African asbestos operations in 1979. Richard was betting on finding evidence not just of the tension between these opposing forces but also of how the profit-motive was actively used to deflect or suppress medical impera-tives. He'd already encountered clear evidence of the state of medical knowledge in South Africa regarding the health effects of asbestos, most notably in Wagner, Sleggs, and Marchand's ground-breaking article in 1960, linking mesothelioma to occu-pational *and* environmental exposure, as well as Ian Webster's Pneumoconiosis Research Unit (PRU) report in 1962 under-lining the same causative association. Further, Richard had unearthed what looked like compelling evidence of Cape man-agement's awareness of these damning accounts, as reflected in its concerted efforts to tarnish and even suppress such find-ings and others like them, as well as harassing their authors. But what, in addition, was critical to the case was establishing the state of such knowledge and awareness in the United Kingdom generally and, specifically, in the minds of Cape's London-based management and board members.

Why? Well, because Richard knew that his case hinged on showing not only that Cape Plc, the parent company located in the United Kingdom, maintained a supervisory or controlling role over health and safety matters in its South African subsid-iaries. He also had to show that it knew, or at least should have known, about the health risks workers in those subsidiaries and their local communities were routinely exposed to and that it, the parent company, had not acted accordingly to eliminate or adequately mitigate such risks.

Cape had a number of operations in the country, including the asbestos mines in Koegas and Penge and the mill in Prieska, all of which were managed and operated directly by Cape Asbestos Company Limited (Cape UK) from its headquarters in London until 1948.[31] On June 3 of that year, Cape created an entirely new company—Cape Asbestos South Africa Proprietary Limited (CASAP), a wholly owned subsidiary of Cape UK—to manage all Cape's interests in the country, including its mining and milling operations in Northern Cape and Northern Transvaal.[32] In terms of the case, this event was especially significant as the intended defendant was Cape UK, thereby permitting the argument that the case should and could be heard in UK courts. For injuries and illnesses sustained by employees, casual workers, and others in South Africa *before* June 3, 1948, the road was therefore open to arguments establishing Cape's direct responsibility.

After that date, however, Richard anticipated that Cape UK would mount a strong argument that it could not be held liable for any harms sustained in or around its South African operations, as they were then managed by the CASAP, not Cape UK, and were operated by local subsidiaries: Cape Blue Mines, Amosa, and Egnep. Thus, according to this line of argument, any litigation brought against Cape UK in British courts would have to be restricted to claims regarding harms incurred before 1948, which would, necessarily, involve very few living claimants and fewer still whose ailments could be confidently traced back to Cape.[33] And any claims regarding harms incurred after 1948 would have to be directed at CASAP (or its subsidiaries) to be pursued in South African courts.

To counter these arguments, Richard needed to compile a near watertight case showing that despite the formation of CASAP, key decisions, both directorial and supervisory, were still being made by Cape UK after 1948 *and* that in making those decisions the parent company knew, or could be presumed to know, that the working conditions in its South African installations were hazardous to human health and yet failed to take appropriate action. In short, Richard had to establish that from its London headquarters and/or through its UK directors and management, Cape was still effectively in charge of its operations in South Africa and, therefore, that responsibility for any negligence in their performance that led to people's injury, illness, or death lay with Cape UK. It was a tall order, requiring some seriously forensic research and a good deal of creative analysis to pull it off.

As the volume of work expanded, so the space in Richard's already cramped office further contracted. The floor soon became an obstacle course of teetering piles of box files and papers, and the walls plastered with spider web threads linking post-it notes, photographs, and map locations of Cape's business empire and personalities. Richard, and later Susannah, also started an annotated "Cape Chronology" spanning the company's history and key events, which eventually ran to thirteen typed pages lines with scratchy, red-inked, hand-written notes and exclamation marks in the margins (and was a godsend for me when I happened on it twenty years later). With the old sash windows in Leigh Day's office thrown open during the English summer days of 1996—a dubious ploy to encourage air to circulate as it also ushered in the noise and fumes of one of North London's busiest roads—the two lawyers accumulated and ploughed through the mountain of materials.

From Richard's initial forays into the archives of Companies House (the UK's registrar of companies) to obtain copies of Cape's annual reports, he knew that shortly after CASAP was formed in 1948, Rupert St. G. Riley, a Cape director in London, was dispatched to South Africa to become its first managing director.[34] The significance of Riley's appointment was made clear in Cape's 1953 celebratory booklet, which recounted the move as intended "to strengthen Cape's position in South Africa and by centralisation to give greater administrative flexibility," while underlining the fact that Riley "retained his seat on the London Board."[35] Furthermore, the Board, and Riley in particular, would have been well aware of the scale of the dust problem in Cape's South African mines following a mines inspector report of its crocidolite mine sites in and around Koegas, dated December 13, 1948, just two weeks before Riley arrived in the country to take up his new position.[36] Here was a good start, it seemed, to mapping lines of knowledge and control between London and South Africa.

To this Richard could add Jock McCulloch's boots-on-the-ground academic research on the asbestos industry in South Africa. At the very same time that Richard and Susannah were compiling their record, Jock was assembling characteristically fine-grained details of the toxic relationships between the South African government, the asbestos industry, and Cape itself (through both its South African operations and its UK headquarters) that helped sustain the appalling levels of health and welfare of asbestos mine workers and their communities.[37] From interviews conducted by Jock with Cape's senior management in South Africa, Richard learnt that they had always perceived the Cape group of companies they worked for as "British," which was reflected in the actively proprietorial approach taken by Cape headquarters in London to its operations in South Africa. It was London that signed off on investment decisions for local mines and mills, and it was London that was openly critical of disappointing outputs in Penge, and commendatory of impressive outputs in Koegas. London too was directly engaged in operational health and safety matters, such as deciding to introduce impermeable bags when shipping fiber.[38]

Laurie Flynn, with whom Richard's camaraderie was now developing into firm friendship, was another on whose sterling work Richard was able to draw. Flynn had been on the trail of asbestos corporate skulduggery for nearly two decades, using investigative journalism's stock in trade techniques of contacts, interviews, and cold calling to unearth a wealth of material that bore on the Cape case. It was through Laurie that Richard was introduced to the growing network of anti-asbestos activists and litigators in the United States. This was important not just because of the bank of asbestos general knowledge this network possessed. It was also opportune because some of it directly involved Cape UK, against whom several negligence suits had been filed in US courts by plaintiffs claiming their ARDs resulted from Cape-sourced asbestos products manufactured or sold in the United States.[39]

One of these cases, a class action filed in Texas in 1974,[40] hinged on the very same contention as Richard sought to make: that Cape's UK management and other employees knew very well the dangers of asbestos to human health and yet failed to take appropriate action. Among the boxes of files relating to the Texas case, Richard found two depositions that seemed to point clearly to precisely that circumstance. The first was given by Geoffrey Higham, Cape's managing director at the group's London headquarters. In it, Higham admitted to knowing that asbestos was dangerous from as early as 1931 (when the first asbestos regulations were introduced in the United Kingdom) and yet, in response to a follow up question about whether thereafter Cape "placed any kind of warning on the asbestos that you sold to the effect of its dangers," he said, "No, I don't believe we did."[41]

This was damning enough, thought Richard, but the second deposition, given by Richard Gaze, was even more shocking.

With a PhD in organic chemistry, Gaze was Cape's chief scientist and technical director with group-wide responsibility for any science-related aspects of the business, including keeping abreast of any medical research concerning the health effects of asbestos exposure and advising the board accordingly. He had joined Cape more than thirty years earlier in 1943, having learned that asbestos was hazardous during his interview for the job: "I was told by the person who interviewed me that certain precautions had to be taken in handling asbestos . . . [specifically] the dangers associated with breathing asbestos dust."[42] He made regular trips to South Africa and was very familiar with all Cape's installations there. He'd seen the conditions under which the miners and mill workers operated, and he'd spent time with the scientists at the PRU (Ian Webster, it will be recalled, believed Gaze to be one of those in the industry who understood the association between asbestos and ARDs).

In his 1975 deposition Gaze openly admitted learning shortly after taking up his position with Cape that breathing asbestos dust causes asbestosis and, thereafter, around 1960, accepting that mesothelioma was also caused by asbestos,[43] facts that he surely shared and discussed with Cape's senior management. Certainly, by 1963 they knew of these dangers, as evidenced by a letter dated August 30, 1963, from Cape's London-based group personnel manager addressed to Cape's senior executives around the world, including Gaze and Smither. The letter concerned a group instruction on ASBESTOSIS (the word is capitalized in the original), which had been recently approved by Cape's board of directors, detailing how this sensitive subject was to be handled: rather than urging that protective action be taken, the letter directed management "to educate employees" by "scotch[ing] all rumours and wild talk on the general subject of asbestosis."[44]

≈

There can be little doubt, therefore, that both Cape's board and its senior executives were fully aware of the threat asbestos posed to human health. More to the point, they also understood the responsibilities they bore to mitigate, if not eliminate, the threat. Warning labels on asbestos products may seem almost laughably inadequate to that end, but the very fact of their contemplation reflects an appreciation of the harmful nature of the raw material.

In England, at least, Cape was forced to act. Its Barking factory was closed in 1968, just before a new set of tougher asbestos regulations was introduced in 1969, significantly restricting permissible minimum sizes and levels of airborne dust particles in workplaces. This effectively banned the use of crocidolite and amosite (being the bulk of Cape's South African asbestos holdings) in the United Kingdom, on account of the very fine dust typically produced when manufacturing with amphibole asbestos forms. Yet even the fact that it took the imminency of legal prohibition to prompt decisive action was telling, given the horrifying levels of disease and death among the Barking workforce. Tony Mendelle, who was managing director of the Barking plant for twelve years before its closure, recalled in one television interview attending "about 110" funerals of workers during his time there. "I kept a black tie in my desk drawer, simply because going to funerals was a dismal part of management at that particular factory," he added, his clipped upper-class English accent at odds with his disconsolate demeanor. Three weeks after he gave the interview, he too was diagnosed with asbestosis.[45]

What these revelations offered to Richard was evidence of the state of awareness of those occupying Cape's UK headquarters regarding the dangers of asbestos and the dire levels of exposure endured by Cape employees (and others) in the United Kingdom and in South Africa. The fact that substantial mitigating actions had (eventually) been taken by Cape in the United Kingdom, but not in South Africa, had nothing to do with the need being greater in Britain or with ignorance of the working conditions and levels of illness in South Africa. As a matter of fact, both the poor working conditions in Cape's asbestos operation in South Africa and the severity of the health problems associated with those operations were well known to Cape's senior personnel in London. Rather, the reasoning behind Cape's behavior in South Africa boiled down to a willingness to live with blatant double standards.[46]

Just a couple of years before Richard took on the case, Cape had celebrated its centenary in 1993 with the publication of a modest little pamphlet of eight pages entitled "A Distinguished Past and a Confident Future."[47] In contrast to its much longer sixtieth anniversary booklet in 1953, this later one openly acknowledged the health hazards of asbestos, noting that "as the dangers associated with asbestos fibres came to be more fully recognised, further steps were taken to reduce the risks to the health of employees and to members of the public." The implication here was that this scientific enlightenment was happening in the late 1960s and early 1970s, which was misleading—not just because it can be strongly contested that recognition of the dangers of asbestos had been established at least thirty or even forty years before, but also because steps to reduce risks had been taken in the United Kingdom from the 1930s onward. When the publication then continues with "the company embarked on a massive programme of research to develop a range of asbestos-free products," as well as "safe techniques for stripping asbestos from buildings and other installations," it is, once more, talking about its *non*-South African operations.

Eventually, the text gets to Cape's businesses in South Africa, but in terms so gauche as to beggar belief:

> Having developed products which contained no asbestos the company decided to sell its mines in South Africa in 1979 and to use the proceeds to purchase additional factories and to exploit new technology for the manufacture of insulation materials and building products.

In other words, after acknowledging the imperative to protect employees and the public from the dangers of asbestos and after shutting its Barking factory in 1968 as a consequence, the company was nevertheless happy to maintain and even ramp up its mining and milling of asbestos in South Africa for another eleven years.[48] Far from a "distinguished past" thought Richard, yet still what confidence Cape held for its future. Perhaps here, in its self-assurance, was the key to getting behind the company's defenses of "we didn't know" and "not our responsibility"?

With this question in mind, Richard headed out for a run that evening to ponder and puff his way around a hilly, forest-like park near his home in Coulsdon, on London's southern outskirts. Often, he'd found, a solid dose of exercise would distract him just enough to generate a new perspective on especially knotty problems, while at the same time compensating somewhat for all those sedentary hours spent in offices and airplanes. It also "loosened a few coils," as Munoree puts it, allowing "the Richard beyond the case" to reappear, albeit, she adds with a sigh, "he'd likely soon turn the run or the match or whatever sport, into another competition."[49] The unintended as well as intended consequences of competitive sport, it must be said, were also apparent to Richard when I quizzed him on the topic:

> I did judo a couple of nights a week for several years but often came home with a bleeding mouth or nose, or broken toes. I did find it quite stress relieving, but my body was completely the wrong shape for that sport. Munoree was totally unsympathetic and used to tell me: "I don't know why you pay all that money to get beaten up when I could do it for free!"[50]

Putting to one side the fraught matter of mixing marriage and sport, on this occasion Richard returned from his run with an idea, or rather a possible lead.

He'd recently met Rachel Lubbe, who, as indicated earlier, would become the lead plaintiff in the initial case Richard filed against Cape in Britain's High Court in February 1997. Born in 1940, she'd spent the first nineteen years of her life in Prieska before meeting and marrying Schalk Lubbe and moving to Koegas. Schalk had a small farm there, though by then he was working in Cape's nearby crocidolite mine. Until 1984 the pair lived in Koegas, where Rachel worked occasionally as an administrative assistant in the mine offices. Even so, Rachel's exposure to asbestos dust had in fact been lifelong and almost entirely environmental—first in Prieska and then in Koegas—in her school, street, home, and office. She remembers vividly the puffs of dust rising from her husband's overalls when he came home each day and when she was washing them.[51] Rachel had been diagnosed with malignant mesothelioma in March 1996.

Through his now well-established connections with US asbestos litigators, Richard was aware that Schalk had been deposed in another US asbestos case involving Cape, this one in Jones County, Mississippi.[52] During his time at the mine, from 1958 until its closure in 1980, Schalk had risen through the ranks to become mine secretary in 1972, representing all the mine's administrative staff. It was in this former capacity that he'd been asked to provide evidence. Richard's run-inspired idea was to scour the nearly 400 pages of Schalk's two depositions for indications of Cape's double standards and the reasons for how and why the company seemed so comfortable maintaining them. Working in tandem with Susannah, who helped summarize Schalk's depositions, Richard uncovered some key findings.

Cape's London directors, Schalk said, visited "on a regular basis . . . every three to six months," and sometimes with Ronald Dent (Cape's chairman), Gaze, and Higham all visiting at the same time.[53] Dent, Schalk recalled, "was very much concerned about sales and the control of asbestos dust in the whole process of production . . . because of the bad publicity we received in the South African press, and the number of cases of people who died of asbestosis cum mesothelioma." Pointedly, Schalk then added, "whether he was doing something to alleviate the problem is a different question."[54] It turned out, according to Schalk, that while the Koegas mine seldom if ever complied with South Africa's dust control limits then in place (no matter that compared with other countries, those limits were "very, very soft"), such "bad news" results were suppressed under a prevailing "don't ask, don't tell" understanding among management. "It was also common knowledge that if we had to adhere to the requirements and instructions, we would have closed the mine within days."[55]

When, as sometimes happened, dissenters did raise their concerns about working conditions, they were ostracized and eventually dismissed by head office in London. This fate, noted Schalk, befell A. C. M. Cornish-Bowden, then chair of CASAP's board—his fellow-directors (Schalk suggested either or both Louis Kuyper and Justin MacKeurtan) "spoiled his name" leading to "a coup d'état"[56]—as well as A. P. Bonzaaier, the medical officer at the Koegas mine. Bonzaaier's impassioned warnings to visiting directors from Cape UK that, for example, "you must remember, you are killing people on these mines," were simply not tolerated. "He was eventually fired . . . by Mr Kuyper," declared Schalk in his deposition.[57]

A final, pervasive red flag that Richard and Susannah gleaned from Schalk's testimony was his reference to the role that racism played in exacerbating the impact of Cape's chronically poor levels of dust control at its work sites. Alongside the entrenched distinctions in medical screening and treatment between white employees and black or coloured employees, Schalk (who was a white Afrikaner) noted that a few years before the Koegas mine was shut down, "showering facilities" were finally introduced on site. But only "for white employees," he stressed, "where they undressed and put on their working gear before they went on duty. And when they came back, they left it there and then they went home." All other mine workers carried home the layers of asbestos dust crusted on their bodies and impregnated in their clothes to share with their families.[58]

≈

Adding all this to their wall-mounted web of Cape's operations, lines of control, and levels of awareness of the dangers of asbestos, Richard could see grounds for a strong case of liability. Strong enough, he hoped, as he filed the case in London's Royal Courts of Justice on Saint Valentine's Day 1997, to convince the court to allow the case to proceed in the United Kingdom, by dismissing the inevitable objections from Cape that the case belonged in South Africa. It was with these issues in mind that he couched the plaintiffs' argument as simply and as directly as possible: "by reason of such knowledge [of] the dangerous nature of asbestos, the Defendant company [Cape UK] was under a duty of care to those living or working in the vicinity of the mines, mills or factories." To which point Richard and counsel added the long list of medical and scientific reports available to Cape since the publication of the UK chief inspector of factories' damning report in 1899, as well as all the evidence of its awareness of them that he and Susannah had so painstakingly compiled.[59]

The time also seemed right. Everyone in Britain was by then well aware of the dangers of asbestos. A widely-publicized report on the health impacts of asbestos commissioned by the UK government in 1985 had shocked nearly everyone with predictions of a growing wave of asbestos-related deaths in the decades ahead due to the long latency of ARDs.[60] More recently, in 1995, one of the authors of that earlier report had published updated figures showing deaths from mesothelioma alone would likely be running at 2,700 to 3,300 per year by 2020.[61] Newspapers contained stories of families and communities devastated by asbestos, alongside polemics criticizing companies for doing too little too late to repair the damage they caused.[62] On television and radio, victims could be seen and heard fighting for their every breath and struggling to come to terms with what had happened to them.[63] Insofar as public sentiment is ever a factor in cases before the courts, it was then titling in favor of Richard's case against Cape.

But in the end, none of this was enough. Mr. Michel Kallipetis QC, the presiding judge, never engaged with the merits of the duty of care argument: "That is not the question with which I am concerned," he declared; rather "I have to decide which jurisdiction has the most natural and closest connection with the causes of action."[64] And on that point, he was persuaded by Cape's preliminary argument that South Africa was indeed the proper forum for any such claim to be heard. "If there is a duty . . . upon the English company," Kallipetis declared, "it seems to me that that can easily be litigated in South Africa."[65] Further, there is "no pressing circumstance which would justify me . . . deciding that the interests of justice . . . require that the action be heard in this [UK] jurisdiction rather than in . . . South Africa."[66] Accordingly, on January 12, 1998, Mr. Kallipetis granted Cape's application to stay (or halt) the proceedings in the United Kingdom.

Richard was certainly disappointed, deflated even, but not resigned, as he knew he would appeal. Reflecting a "glass half full" perspective commonly found in plaintiff lawyers, he says of that time, "We would never have taken on these cases had we not been prepared for a long haul."[67] After all, his clients had been waiting decades for any sort of justice and while, in truth, they bore more hope than expectation that the present case could deliver it, Richard really believed that justice would, eventually, prevail. Still, there was no denying that his clients' stakes were high, as illustrated by the fact that Rachel Lubbe had died on June 29, 1997, barely one week before the hearing had begun, with her husband, Schalk, replacing her (as administrator of her estate) as lead plaintiff. She was fifty-seven years old.

CHAPTER 5

Apartheid Capitalism
—*Black Lives Mattered Less*—

I grew up during the Apartheid years, living in white areas, attending white-only schools and had all-white friends. I can still remember the white-only benches and the 6 p.m. curfew when Africans had to be off the streets. I am however not proud to say that I viewed the Africans' plight in South Africa with very little sympathy and thought. To that end I would say that my only excuse is that I was not aware of the facts. I think the word Richard used in this regard was "brainwashed" on the occasions we spoke of the political situation in South Africa.

—Suzanne Alderete

SUZANNE HAD BEEN RICHARD'S SECRETARY in London during the first eighteen months or so of the case. Richard remembers her as "genial" and "highly efficient," precisely as the job demanded, aside the skewed perspectives of her privileged upbringing as a white South African. But as time passed, Richard adds, "She became more and more engaged with the material we were dealing with, and you could see how it affected her."[1] Suzanne moved to the United States in the spring of 1996 and as a parting gift Richard gave her a copy of Laurie Flynn's *Studded with Diamonds and Paved with Gold: Miners, Mining Companies and Human Rights in South Africa.* She had in fact met Laurie with Richard some months before, when Laurie visited Leigh Day's offices to share stories and swap sources. She wrote the above quoted lines in a letter to Laurie by way of introduction and to say how profoundly moved she was by his book. "My reaction after reading your book," she continued, "was one of outrage and downright shame not only on my own behalf, but for the thousands of other white South Africans like myself, that just simply have no idea of the pain, suffering and humiliation that the African people have had to endure over the last 100 years or so."[2]

Suzanne wrote the letter in August 1996, just after South Africa's talismanic Truth and Reconciliation Commission (TRC) commenced its public hearings, among the many aims of which was to tear away the veils of ignorance and deceit that Apartheid ideology had peddled for so long.[3] Archbishop Desmond Tutu, who alongside Nelson Mandela inspired the establishment of the TRC and was its chairperson, was later to write: "Most of the white community [was] brainwashed by propaganda spewed forth by the government-controlled electronic media," such that they viewed members of the anti-Apartheid African National Congress (ANC) "as savages who wanted to overthrow a Christian, God-fearing government."[4]

≈

The past as well as present politics of South Africa permeated Richard's case against Cape like ink in water. Not only were the conditions of Apartheid government essential to Cape's perpetuation of its double standards regarding the health and welfare of its South African workers and their communities, but also, crucially, the objectives and capabilities of the new ANC government that had replaced it were important to Richard eventually winning—more than two years later—a final appeal before the House of Lords, permitting a trial to proceed in the United Kingdom. Little did he know how tortuous the path would be getting to that point.

Richard and his clients had not yet attracted the prominent public profile they were later to enjoy (after, that is, the handful of plaintiffs expanded to several thousand), but the matter had gained some traction in the media on account of Richard making a nuisance of himself. One piece on him and his work published in South Africa some six months after the case had been filed in England opens with, "The man sitting behind me at the Truth [and Reconciliation] Commission hearing asked so many difficult questions that, to detract from my ignorance, I asked him who he was."[5] Richard and the case were also on the minds of politicians and powerbrokers in the ANC. Two of those were the premiers of the two affected provinces—Ngoako Ramatlhodi of Limpopo Province and Manne Dipico of the Northern Cape Province—both of whom used to make regular trips to London to discuss the case's progress with Richard.

By then Leigh Day had moved its offices to the slightly more salubrious and much quieter premises of Priory House in St. John's Lane, which, despite a rather grand frontage (it adjoined the ancient and venerable St. John's Gate), was in fact a squat 1960s office block previously occupied by a meat-importation business for the nearby Smithfield Market. Still, it offered the firm more room and a tad more gravitas for the visiting premiers. Sarah Leigh, who was not directly involved in the case at that time, remembers bumping into Richard on the stairs one afternoon with "three very dapper gentlemen in three-piece suits." She said hello and shook their hands and then moved on. Later she rang Richard: "Who were they?" she asked, with not a little wonder at the political as well as legal waves being made by the young lawyer whom she and Martyn Day had hired just a few years earlier.[6]

The premiers were always accompanied on these trips by members of their respective offices. Often this included Tommy Ntsewa, chief of staff and legal adviser to Ngoako in Limpopo, and Thabo Makweya, a senior official in the National Union of Mineworkers of South Africa (NUM [SA]) working with Manne's Northern Cape government.[7] Both recall very clearly how important they and their bosses considered the Cape case to be, not merely for the asbestos-ravaged communities in their respective provinces but also for the nation as a whole. When I interviewed the two men separately in March 2023, both stressed that tackling the legacy of asbestos mining was a high priority for each of their then newly formed provincial governments. "Asbestos came to the top of the list very quickly," noted Thabo, "workplace health and safety always being a big concern for miners."[8] Tommy told me that "the Penge mine was a key issue—the first thing on my desk when I started working for Ngoako." How, he wondered, "are we, as a government, going to rehabilitate the abandoned mines sites and care for the people still dying quietly in the villages surrounding them?"[9]

Tommy Ntsewa puts you in mind of a mill pond—calm, deep, and reflective. He's frank and avuncular with a broad, gentle-featured face beneath a jaunty pork-pie hat pushed well back from his forehead in a manner that could mean laidback or world-weary, but in fact signals he's ready to do business. In low, modulated tones, his assessment of the South Africa of his youth is matter-of-fact: "You *had* to be political growing up in the 1970s and 1980s." Yet, as a law student he knew only the positives of asbestos in building materials and nothing of its negatives (the tentacles of brainwashing and deceit were far-reaching). Reading up on it, "I was shocked," he says. "Disease, death and little cleanup." Later, when visiting Penge after heavy rains, he recalls, "I could see asbestos-filled silt flowing out of the old mines into the river where people were drawing their drinking water." As he began his work with the Limpopo government in 1997, he saw Cape's former employees in Penge as "victims of Apartheid." We were "inheriting the vestiges of the regime," he says, "and had to work out how to deal with the consequences, including how to deal with the companies from that time."

Dismantling the mechanisms as well as the culture of institutionalized racial segregation was neither easy nor quick. The TRC's efforts to unpack the role that corporations played in Apartheid capitalism[10] led it to conclude that "business was central to the economy that sustained the South African state during the apartheid years . . . [and that] most businesses benefitted from operating in a racially structured context." That said, the TRC reserved its harshest criticism for "certain businesses, especially the mining industry, [that] were involved in helping to design and implement apartheid policies."[11] Put simply, South African mining corporations under white rule "exploited the cruel migrant labour system and made unabashed use of apartheid labour, and actively peddled its availability, as an advantage to international investor."[12] Among the several dimensions to such exploitation by the asbestos mining companies, the two most obvious were cheap labor and the inadequacy or even absence of laws governing occupational health and safety standards for black and coloured workers.

South Africa's Occupational Diseases in Mines and Works Act (ODMWA, 1973), for example, was nothing short of a study in overt racial discrimination with top-line benefits and protections provided only to "White persons," something less but still significant to "Coloured persons," and almost nothing for "Bantu persons."[13] So-called risk work could be undertaken by white and coloured workers only if they possessed a certificate of health fitness, while no such fitness requirement was made of Bantu workers.[14] White and coloured workers were subject to periodic medical examinations paid for by the state,[15] while Bantu workers had no such requirement. Any medical examinations that were conducted had to be arranged and paid for by their employer (which effectively meant they seldom, if ever, happened).[16]

Compensation payments for work-related injuries for white workers were commensurate with the nature and extent of the injury or disease and the employee's level of seniority (the average salary of a white mine worker at that time being roughly nine times that of a black mine worker).[17] Such payments also extended to spouses and dependents and were pensionable and transferable to spouses and dependents.[18] For Bantu workers, by contrast, there were one-off payments for only certain compensable diseases (notably, tuberculosis, silicosis, and pneumoconiosis), conditional on providing sufficient medical evidence, which was often lacking due to its prohibitive cost, ranging between rand (R)600 and R1,200 (approximately USD$750 to USD$1,500 at that time). No consideration was made for their spouses and dependents.[19] As the average annual wage of black mine workers in the mid-1970s was approximately R1,200,[20] these provisions effectively consigned a mine worker and their family to a life of penury once they became too ill to work.

Richard was painfully aware of how ruinous this regime was for families and whole communities of asbestos mine and mill workers, not least from reading Marianne Felix's vivid description of the plight of one ex–asbestos miner from Mafefe in Limpopo Province. After stopping work and being diagnosed with mesothelioma at the age of forty-four, Lucas Maalebogo Maenetja was awarded a one-off compensatory payment equivalent to four months' salary. "He was angry," says Marianne, telling her that "with disease in my body I have no hope. And my main worry is that I still want to educate my children."[21] Lucas died shortly thereafter, barely eleven months following his diagnosis.

Condemning such abhorrently racist laws and policies was easy after Apartheid officially ended in 1994. Removing and replacing them were more difficult tasks, not least because of the awkward circumstance that faces all revolutionary organizations that find themselves inheriting the powers and responsibilities of government. With a rationale to topple the previous political system and with skills and tactics honed to achieve that end, such groups must engage in some serious reorientation of purpose and practice when they succeed in replacing the *ancien régime*. The ANC was no exception in this regard.

This, according to Tommy Ntsewa, affected the Cape case in two ways. First, it meant that there still existed sufficient activist fervor for both federal and provincial governments to have "no hesitation supporting the litigation against Cape." Second, while there may have been some appetite for the case to be pursued in South Africa, the practical reality of the state being able to support likely thousands of impecunious litigants through legal aid funding or similar assistance was a very different story.[22] As it would later turn out, this second insight would prove to be critical in the case eventually being allowed to proceed in the United Kingdom.

≈

In the meantime, the two premiers were in no doubt as to the significance of the case. With regard to the Northern Cape: "We were very keen to support Leigh Day," Thabo Makweya says, gesturing as if to lift and push the firm along, "as it helped us raise the profile of the dangers of asbestos and the need for its removal from people's homes." As regards Limpopo: "We saw it as a big part of rehabilitating past injustices," says Tommy Ntsewa, while former Premier Ramatlhodi stresses that "we were dealing with the lives of entire communities in some instances, such as Mafefe,"[23] referring to an area west of Penge that contained many small amosite mines (or adits) and from where many laborers were recruited to work in Cape's Penge mine and mill.

Echoing a heartfelt sentiment I heard time and again from many involved in the story, Richard was held in the highest regard by officials in both governments, as a strategist as well as a lawyer. They were somewhat in awe of his dedication to helping find justice for the communities, to holding Cape accountable, and to be doing so on behalf of people living thousands of miles from his home. The Northern Cape's Premier Dipico, for example, wrote to Richard in the warmest terms: "Your steadfast belief and commitment to the cause of those affected by asbestos-related diseases in our country has inspired many."[24] Others, such as Leigh Day's Prieska office manager, Jack Adams, called Richard an "avenging angel," reflecting both the God-fearing nature of Jack's local community and Richard's fierce determination.[25] It was certainly true that strategy— whether terrestrial or celestial—was key to Richard's promoting the case within the political arena of South Africa and through the legal forum of the English courts.

Central to Judge Kallipetis's earlier decision of January 1998 in the proceedings granting a stay of the action in the United Kingdom was his conclusion that the litigation could and should be appropriately pursued in South African courts, precisely because that was where the relevant actions (that may or may not have been negligent) had taken place. The English courts, he asserted, were *forum non conveniens*, or *not* the appropriate forum. But this, maintained Richard and his legal team (barristers David Johnson QC and Graham Read[26]), was to misconceive the basic premise of their clients' argument. For it was their contention that the relevant negligent decisions and actions leading to the injuries suffered by the plaintiffs were taken by Cape management operating out of the company's London headquarters. Even if the consequences of such negligence occurred in South Africa, their roots were to be found in Britain. Thus, they held, the appropriate forum in which to try the case was the Royal Courts of Justice on the Strand in London.

The *forum non conveniens* argument, as used by defendants to ward off attempts by plaintiffs to try cases in jurisdictions unfavorable to the defendants, has a long history in English Law.[27] It was (and still is, in certain respects) an especially attractive device for transnational corporations whose activities, by definition, cross borders and jurisdictions. It is attractive because, typically, a defendant corporation wants to protect its major assets located in its "home" country, where the parent company is domiciled, from potential liability for wrongs occurring in "host" countries, where it or its associated companies operate. It is also an appealing device for those companies that want to avoid being held to account in any jurisdiction after it becomes clear that access to justice for claimants in local (host) state jurisdictions is often practically impossible.[28]

The conditions under which this defense is successfully claimed are enigmatic. Definitively expressed in English law by the House of Lords in the 1987 case of *Spiliada*—which, coincidentally, also involved a dangerous mineral (sulphur)—they boil down to two intersecting limbs.[29] The first requires that the defendant demonstrate that there exists "an available forum which is clearly and distinctly more appropriate than the English forum" for the trial to take place. Should that demand be satisfied, the second limb shifts the burden onto the plaintiff to show that despite the alternative available forum, there exist special circumstances "suitable for the ends of justice" that nevertheless require that the trial take place in the United Kingdom.[30]

That phrase "suitable for the ends of justice" is almost as elastic as it sounds, and the legal team Richard had assembled to take on the appeal all believed they would have a pretty good shot at arguing it in their favor, if it got to that. But in bringing their case to the Court of Appeal, scheduled for May 1998, the team was banking on denying Cape's argument based on the first limb of *Spiliada*. That is, they were intent on showing that South Africa was neither "clearly" nor "distinctly" a more suitable forum. Cape UK, they argued, had been directly responsible for the negligent actions that injured (or killed, in the cases of Rachel Lubbe and Matthys Nel) their clients, both before and after the company's restructure in 1948 creating its South African affiliate corporations. Consequently, the United Kingdom *was* the appropriate forum to bring an action against a UK company.

Counsel engaged to advance this line of argument comprised a new lead.[31] Initially, Richard had briefed Brian Leveson QC, a top criminal silk (senior counsel), to take on the appeal, but early one morning in March 1998, Brian rang Richard to tell him that, regrettably, he'd have to withdraw. By way of reparation, however, Brian took time to spell out what he thought was the best strategy to pursue before the Court of Appeal. Richard clearly remembers the phone call, not only because he was struggling to hear and be heard as he threaded his way through Smithfield Market (London's bustling wholesale meat market) on the way to work, but also because Leveson's suggested plan of action turned out to be a master stroke.

The United Kingdom's membership of the European Union (EU) added a twist to the jurisdictional question before the court that was a potential weak link in Cape's argument. Under the 1968 Brussels Convention,[32] the European Community (EC, precursor to the EU) had effectively blocked the use of *forum non conveniens* by any EU-based defendant (similar to Cape UK) as a defense to an action brought by any EU-based plaintiff. Whether actions brought by *non*-EU-based plaintiffs (such as the present South African claimants) were also covered under the Convention was still then a live question, the resolution of which would ultimately require a definitive ruling from the European Court of Justice (ECJ) in Luxembourg eight years later.[33] While the Brussels Convention point had already been raised at first instance before Judge Kallipetis,[34] Leveson underlined the potential strategic advantage of leading with this issue, rather than shying away from it, thereby exposing the bench to the prospect of having the matter referred to the ECJ. Leveson's insight was his strong suspicion that Court of Appeal judges were thoroughly disinclined to have matters transferred from their hands into those of their judicial brethren in Luxembourg. Richard was very taken by this approach and duly acted on it by instructing Barbara Dohmann QC, a commercial law silk with experience in Brussels Convention arguments, as the new lead counsel.

With this line of attack settled, Richard and his advocacy team returned to the same place where he had lost the trial. London's Royal Courts of Justice may look rather like a Disneyland castle—and indeed for many outsiders, its business may appear fantastically esoteric—but once inside, it is as humdrum, earnest, and hard-working as any respected professional institution.[35] It was into this bustling environment one bright May morning in 1998 that Richard Meeran, Susannah Read, Barbara Dohmann, and Graham Read strode through the enormous cathedral-like Great Central Hall to reach the Court of Appeal at the rear of the building.

After a brief recap of their strategy, they took their places behind the bar table with Cape's legal team to their right. There was a sense of do-or-die for both sets of lawyers, even if both were doing their professional best not to show it. Obviously, as the appellants, Richard's team was desperate to overturn the lower court's decision, despite intending to run the same basic line of argument (albeit tweaked) before the Court of Appeal. For their part, Cape's lawyers had already heard enough from the other side during the trial to know that they would be facing seriously credible arguments as to their client's negligence if the appeal was allowed and the case permitted to proceed before UK courts. Adding to Cape's anxiety was the especially damning asbestos decision in a recent UK High Court case of *Margereson* (as mentioned earlier in chapter 1), involving two mesothelioma victims who had, as young girls in the 1930s, played on asbestos dumps adjacent to a factory in Leeds, Yorkshire. While the factory was not owned by Cape, the case nonetheless demonstrated how persuasive English judges found arguments concerning environmental exposure to asbestos in establishing a corporation's negligence causing foreseeable injuries.[36]

Cape was represented by its long-time solicitors, Davies Arnold Cooper, who had chosen to brief counsel comprising Sir Sydney Kentridge QC as lead alongside Brian Doctor, and Richard Coleman as junior. Kentridge and Doctor were both South Africans, though they were practising at the English Bar. Kentridge was a legal titan in South Africa and the United Kingdom.[37] Distinguished and patrician in manner, he supplemented his long career in commercial law by notable anti-Apartheid cases, having represented Nelson Mandela in his 1956 treason trial and Steve Biko's family during the inquest into Biko's death in police custody in 1978. Backing up his accomplishments, Kentridge's mellifluous voice and assured delivery carried considerable authority, such that altogether, Richard candidly admits, "He was something of a hero of mine, even if now he was on the other side."[38] Brian Doctor was more prize fighter than Olympian in appearance as well as manner. Pugnacious and wily, he took his "zealous advocate" role very seriously for his corporate clientele, as he proved throughout the Cape litigation, doing his level best to rebut and undermine Richard and the plaintiffs' case at every turn. He well-earned the moniker "Sledgehammer" given to him by lawyers on the other side. Together with the up-and-coming Richard Coleman, the Cape team constituted formidable opposing counsel.

That said, their zeal sometimes got the better of them. For example, during one session before the Court of Appeal, Doctor handed up a document to Kentridge while the latter was in full flow on the question of whether and to what extent exposure to asbestos was the cause of the illnesses and deaths of the plaintiffs. Assuming it would support the point that lines of cause-and-effect are blurred, Kentridge began reading from the document. It was a statement made by the brother of the late Matthys Nel (whose wife was the fourth-named plaintiff in the case) attesting to the fact that while neither of their parents had ever worked at the asbestos mill in Prieska, the family had lived in the town for nearly twenty years in three homes at varying distances from the mill located near the town's center. Noting that the family's history was "tragic" (ravaged as it was by deaths from mesothelioma), Kentridge highlighted a passage in the statement describing "clouds of dust . . . being spewed out of the chimney of the mill," prevailing winds blowing the dust over the town, and "threads of blue asbestos fibre [being found] on the railway line."[39]

Both Richard and Graham Read recall how just about everyone in court was bewildered by this spectacle, as it seemed clearly to be making the plaintiffs' case for them—most especially in respect of the lethality of environmental exposure—rather than supporting Cape's defense. Indeed, at one point Lord Justice Evans interrupted Kentridge to reiterate the plaintiffs' main contention that "there cannot really be any argument as to the fact that these were the unfortunate victims of these lung diseases and that the cause of these diseases was exposure to asbestos."[40] Realizing that he had just underlined that very point, Kentridge shoved the Nel document back into Doctor's hands with an irritated harrumph and changed tack by arguing that one cannot be sure if the asbestos in question came from Cape's mines and mills or from "who-knows-where" in the surrounding "asbestos mountains," as that part of Northern Cape was commonly referred to.[41]

This embarrassing faux pas aside, it was in fact the ploy of Richard and his team to lead their appeal with the Brussels Convention's *forum non conveniens* argument that proved to be their sucker punch—not just because it was an aggravating distraction for Cape's lawyers,[42] but also because the bench immediately grasped its significance. All three judges—Lords Justices Evans, Millett, and Auld—engaged with Barbara Dohmann on the question of whether and if the Brussels Convention was relevant. The matter was neatly summed up in one brief exchange between the bar and the bench:

> JUDGE 3 (MILLETT LJ): With respect, if you win the appeal and we decide that the case should be tried here, there is no need to go to Europe [meaning the European Court of Justice (ECJ)] at all.
>
> SPEAKER 1 (DOHMANN): That is correct.
>
> JUDGE 3: Why should we delay this litigation by two years, going to Europe on a trip that may be completely unnecessary?[43]

While the court's reluctance to have the matter referred to the ECJ was pleasingly obvious, there nevertheless remained the task of winning the appeal. Dohmann and Read succeeded on that score by persuading the Court of Appeal that Judge Kallipetis in the High Court below "had failed to give any weight to the fact that the negligence alleged against the defendant company [Cape UK] is distinct from any allegations which might be made against the person or subsidiaries responsible for running their South African businesses from time to time."[44]

Cape's lawyers had repeated their argument made in the lower court that the matters at issue were the actions of Cape's subsidiaries in South Africa and whether they had met the occupational health and safety standards then set by South African law. In brief, they claimed that "the duty of care, if it existed, did not exist in England. If it had a locus, it must be where the [injured] person who falls within its ambit is situated."[45] But this was a mistake, as Lord Justice Evans made clear in a pivotal passage of the Appeal Court's judgment. "This submission confuses two separate questions," he noted. "First, what law governs the tort alleged in a particular case? Secondly, what was the location of the constituent elements of the tort?"[46] In answer to the first question, it was indeed arguable whether the applicable law was South African or English, but as the duty of care was allegedly owed by a parent company located in England (per the second question), it was reasonable to try the case under English law in English courts, even if other elements of the tort (breach, causation, or damage) may be governed by South African law. Such cross-jurisdictional features are, in fact, the essence of torts labeled "transnational." Or, as Lord Justice Evans chose to frame it, "There is nothing inherently wrong or unreasonable in bringing proceedings in England against an English defendant in respect of alleged negligence committed for the most part in this country, *even though* having its injurious effects abroad."[47]

≈

It is hard to overstate the significance of the Court of Appeal's judgment and the reasoning behind it, as the path was now clear for the substance of the case to be heard before the English courts. Delivered on July 30, 1998, it was a hugely satisfying outcome for Richard, Susannah, Barbara Dohmann, and Graham Read who were all in high spirits as they regrouped over dinner that evening in a posh restaurant in Holborn to celebrate. It meant that they could get down to the real business of the case of laying bare the dreadful and ongoing consequences of "the instructions and advice" provided by Cape UK that "showed a careless disregard for the foreseeable risks of injury to those who were closely affected by the asbestos operations in South Africa, taking account of the knowledge which they had or ought to have had of the health risks involved," as they had just argued before the Court of Appeal.[48]

Still, it was sobering to see how determined Cape and its lawyers had been to shirk any responsibility by arguing so strenuously before the Court of Appeal that (1) any claims of negligent behavior should be directed at its South African subsidiaries and that (2) no such negligence would be found because those subsidiary companies had abided by relevant South African laws. While Richard was confident that he could mount a good argument against their first point, the second point presented an obstacle.

The occupational health standards regarding asbestos in South Africa during the time Cape operated there had been pathetically inadequate—certainly, that is, compared to the standards set in the United Kingdom from 1931, when Britain introduced its first set of asbestos regulations, and more so after 1962, when they were strengthened. There existed no regulations governing asbestos mine site dust levels in South Africa until the enactment of the Mines and Works Act in 1956. Even then, however, they were regularly flouted, despite being far less stringent than those in the United Kingdom by permitting maximum dust levels more than ten times greater than in Britain. When looking for an explanation for such leniency, Richard was hardly surprised to learn that these amenable levels had in fact been "set" by the asbestos industry itself.[49]

What, therefore, was so galling about Cape's two-step line of argument was how disingenuous it was. The very reasons why South African standards were so low and late in coming were because of the concerted efforts by Cape and the rest of the asbestos industry in lobbying against any such regulation. Their attempts to suppress scientific evidence demonstrating how necessary such regulation was for protecting the health of their employees working in their asbestos mines, mills, and factories had been both systematic and largely successful. That the relevant government agencies at the time were so receptive to such lobbying and so willing to accept Cape's assurances that dust levels were being controlled (and then officially to report as much) showed how beholden they were to the industry and how complicit the government was in covering up the suffering and its causes.

"I am satisfied that with the variety of intensive measures now in existence, the risk of contracting asbestosis can, proportionally speaking, be said to be slight," announced Minister of Mines Carel de Wet, as he opened a new pneumoconiosis clinic in the Northern Cape in September 1967. "The industry is fully aware of, and fully accepts its responsibilities in this matter [of preventing asbestosis]," he continued, doing his best to sound convincing.[50] The minister's true concerns, however, were likely more economic than medical. For in the very same edition of the *Diamond Fields Advertiser* in which his reassuring words were reported, the paper ran a major story on the recent retrenchment of some 500 workers at Cape's Koegas mine. The move, the article explained, followed directly from the refusal by English dockers to offload a shipment from the mine because of health fears over handling blue asbestos. The warning signs were clearly there for anyone who cared to look for them.

Government-appointed inspectors of mines in South Africa had begun taking dust samples in asbestos mines in the early 1940s, mainly because there was no legal obligation on asbestos companies to engage their own "dust inspectors" until 1965. In evidence tendered in court by Cape, the company claimed, nevertheless, to have appointed a "ventilation officer" at Koegas and Prieska in 1954,[51] who, naturally, was in regular contact with the local mine inspectors in Bloemfontein and Kimberley. Over the next twenty years or so, Cape's own records show a litany of almost faultless report cards from Ministry of Mines' officials. In respect of Koegas and Prieska, "Conditions were found to be good and the dust hazard was not serious" (1940); "A high degree of dust control is maintained in surface mills" (1959); "The mine was satisfactorily ventilated and in a safe condition" (1964); "Underground working conditions at Koegas were excellent" (1970); "The mine was wet and clean and no dust was visible in the atmosphere" (1973); "The Koegas mill was clean and dust extraction and suppression arrangements were effective" (1974); "The plant and surrounding environment at Koegas were found in good condition and fibre and dust counts were satisfactory" (1977).[52]

The story was similar in Penge, even if a little less enthusiastically commendatory. Here again Cape (through its subsidiary

Egnep Pty Ltd) had employed a ventilation officer "at least since the early 1950s," who worked closely with the local mines' inspectorate to their mutual satisfaction, such that, in Cape's own estimation, "in general and on average the [dust] levels were largely within the limits determined and set by the authorities in South Africa." To which official reports added, "Conditions at Penge in Amosa are generally satisfactory," and, in reference to the Penge mill, "The machinery and fans work efficiently from a dust point of view and visible dust is limited."[53]

Cape was in fact content to defend any claims of negligence on the basis that it had complied with South African laws and regulations such as then existed, no matter how inferior they were to standards set elsewhere, including, notably, in its home jurisdiction of the United Kingdom. "Occupational health standards adopted in other countries did not apply to the mining and milling of asbestos in South Africa, and as such, cannot be compared," Cape's lawyers blithely claimed, then adding, by way of further explanation, "there are no other countries in the world mining amphibole asbestos (save for one operation in Australia)."[54]

The audacity of such reasoning astonished Richard. Surely, he thought, they can see that it misses the point of the alleged negligence in question being situated in the United Kingdom, not South Africa? And, further, that it skips over the stark reality that Cape already knew of the heightened dangers posed by amphibole asbestos being so strongly associated with mesothelioma.[55] If anything South Africa's "occupational health standards" should have been higher than those in other countries, not lower. But maybe not, he realized. Maybe this was precisely how Cape's lawyers intended to fight.

Mulling over the Appeal Court's ruling and, especially, the discomfiting understanding of Cape's intent, Richard spent many hours talking with Russell Levy, a close friend and colleague at Leigh Day.

Russell had joined the firm a couple of years after Richard and for much the same reasons. Both were and are natural rebels who have a healthy disregard for legal conservatism if it stands in the way of social justice and a huge appetite for legal reform if it helps clear the path. Both are outsiders—Russell is white but had been brought up in South Africa in a family of anti-Apartheid communists. Both are also smart and opinionated, albeit Russell is brasher and more assertive. They share the same biting sense of humor: "Richard is one of the least self-effacing people I know," Russell tells me with a grin when I ask him about Richard's intellectual modesty. To which accusation Richard replies, "It takes one to know one." They enjoyed sparring with each other on points of law and legal strategy over lunch or a beer on a regular basis, with Russell often "bringing Richard back down to Earth on some of his ideas." On this particular occasion, Russell's hard-nosed South African cynicism made light work of Cape's behavior. "Shocking," he said, "but what do you expect when they got away with it for so long?"[56] How and why Cape had "got away with it" was, of course, all down to the accommodating circumstances of South African politics.

≈

When Chris Wagner declared that in South Africa "asbestos was always about politics," he was entirely correct, even if somewhat unwittingly. He was being interviewed by Jock McCulloch at his (Wagner's) home in Weymouth, England in 1998, shortly before he died, and was referring to his profound regret "ever having worked on asbestos-related disease."[57] This was a truly astounding admission from the man widely credited with bringing the link between asbestos and mesothelioma to the world's attention in the famed *British Journal of Industrial Medicine* article written with Marchand and Sleggs in 1960. In truth, his life-long regret stemmed from the fact that politics had gotten so much in the way of his professional interests. "He was only interested in science," McCulloch notes. To be sure the country's politics had corrupted science, but under Apartheid it had also fostered social conditions from which the asbestos industry had profited enormously for more than thirty years, allowing economic incentives to subvert the health and welfare of hundreds of thousands of mine workers, their families, and the communities they lived in.

Sophie Kisting was (and still is) dedicated to studying the science of occupational health and, like Chris Wagner before her, worked at the National Centre for Occupational Health (NCOH; now NIOH) in Johannesburg.[58] Sophie, however, was not only acutely aware of the social and political settings in which her discipline operated. She also viewed them as essential features of her work rather than as cumbersome roadblocks. For her, the key to understanding and, importantly, addressing many occupational health and safety concerns was to see them in their wider contexts.

With a keen sense of social justice honed during her childhood in South West Africa (now Namibia), which was then also subject to Apartheid rule, Sophie never considered medicine and politics as separate entities. She recalls her time training as an intern in Cape Town's Somerset Hospital, for example, when helping to take blood and assisting seniors with medical assessments of political and other prisoners held on Robben Island, just a few miles off shore. "We all hoped in our youthful enthusiasm that one day it would be Nelson Mandela or Robert Sobukwe [the Island's most famous prisoners] we'd treat," she tells me with somewhat bashful pride.[59] While that never happened, Sophie was nonetheless a natural and powerful ally to Richard's present cause, not least because of her broad perspective on the causes of the "invisible epidemic" of ARDs, as she and her colleague Lundy Braun labeled it. "This epidemic," they argued, "was not simply the result of ignorance or the deliberate manipulation of information, rather [it was] shaped by industrial labor policies and practices and governmental legislation that took specific and changing forms during settler colonial rule and Apartheid in South Africa."[60]

Through her research at the University of Cape Town and her work as a medical adviser to the NUM, Sophie was coming face to face with the consequences of this epidemic in communities across Limpopo on an almost daily basis. She couldn't help asking herself what structural causes lay behind the epidemic's medical presentations and how they might help make the calamity more visible and those who allowed it to happen more accountable. One of her and Lundy Braun's most important revelations was the impact traditional employment practices of the asbestos industry had on the whole family. Ironically, the fact that work on the mines was available to men, women, and children was seen as great boon for families, absent—vitally—their knowledge of the extreme dangers they were submitting themselves to.

"With the family as the primary unit of labor in the Cape Asbestos Belt [stretching from Limpopo to the Northern Cape]," wrote Braun and Kisting,

> female and child labor was integral to the functioning and profitability of the industry and to the survival of families. Men did the heavy manual labor—drilling, blasting, and loading rick into

wheelbarrows and cocopans (steel wagon[s] that run on rails). Women and children hand-cobbed (separat[ing] asbestos from the host rock into clumps the size of an egg), sorted ore, sieved fiber, and weighed and packed loose asbestos into bags for transport.[61]

Richard was seeing the same wholesale exposure to asbestos dust in the files of former Cape employees and in interviews with claimants, as his potential client base started to grow exponentially. It was also during this time he first encountered health assessment certificates endorsed by the Medical Board of Occupational Diseases (MBOD). These had been issued to former mine and mill workers who had recently, albeit belatedly, been examined by MBOD doctors, and they were now bringing them along to show Richard. Notably, subsequent access to the full records held by the MBOD itself was to prove crucial in compiling evidence of the extent of ARDs among asbestos communities in settlement negotiations with Cape and its lawyers.

What was striking in these certificates was not just the almost metronomic repetition of symptoms as recorded by the MBOD, typically, "coughing up coloured phlegm, sharp needlelike chest pains, tiredness after every physical activity, shortness of breath,"[62] but also how consistent were claimants' descriptions of working conditions across the decades. One female bag sealer at the Penge mine told the interviewer: "I would be covered in dust at the end of each working day all over my body and clothes. No one could recognise us at the end of a shift." Also at Penge, a cobber described how she "had asbestos dust in her mouth, ears, and nose. It made her cough and sneeze," and another cobber said that he

breathed in the asbestos dust my entire shift as I was not given a mask to wear and I worked so closely with the asbestos. I handled rock and asbestos with my bare hands. . . . I also breathed in the dust that had settled on my work clothes as my work clothes were only washed once a week. I did this on my day off. This activity also exposed me to asbestos dust as I used to shake the dust out before washing my clothes.

Each of these claimants had worked for Cape during the 1960s and 1970s, and yet their descriptions seemed little different from the experiences of a fellow cobber who had worked at Cape's asbestos mill in Prieska between 1948 and 1949:

> I came into constant contact with asbestos as I used to handle it with my naked hands. We worked above ground under a covering. We would each receive a pile of asbestos rocks. We were seated on the floor and had to crush the rocks with a hammer and then sort the fibre from the rock. . . . I lived within an environment where asbestos dust was a matter of course and everything was constantly covered in blue dust.

All these workers were black or coloured. None were then aware of the damage asbestos causes. Each one was now sick. Their accounts span the very period throughout which medical and scientific evidence exposed the grave dangers asbestos posed to human health and yet Cape did so little to protect its employees. The testimonies of these Cape miners and mill workers make that much abundantly clear, no matter Cape's assertions to the contrary. The fact, what is more, that during this time the size of its workforce was also multiplying to an all-time high of 20,000, as South Africa's asbestos production reached its peak in the mid-1970s, starkly demonstrates just how far profit was preferred over people.

≈

As I stepped out of my motel room, a blast of hot air radiated off the concrete. It was my last day in Prieska and Jack Adams had come knocking at my door to take me once again to the "Red Block" on the edge of town. Stout and bald, with a smile even bigger than the outsized glasses that kept threatening to slip off his nose, Jack was formerly a security manager for copper and gold mines all over the Northern Cape, before taking on the running of Leigh Day's small Prieska office in 1999. Alarmingly punctual and well organized, he was now doing his best to manage me as I hurriedly stuffed notebooks, pens, and a camera into a bag and followed him to the car. During our week together, he and Cecil Skeffers had shown me umpteen sites where blue asbestos was still visibly present. But this time Jack wanted me to see how embedded it was in the daily lives of those who lived in Prieska's poorest neighborhood.

Emblematic of Apartheid's long legacy, this was and still is the town's black district, where small, red-bricked (hence the name) shacks are huddled along dirt streets with kids and dogs roaming freely in the almost complete absence of traffic. We stop randomly to ask an old lady sitting on her doorstep whether she'd let us look at her brickwork. She nods her consent, seeming to know Jack (or at least know of him), and she smiles shyly when I say hello. Accompanied by an excited gaggle of youngsters (her grandchildren, it turns out), Jack immediately points to numerous spots where iridescent sprigs of blue crocidolite, like the cut ends of electrical wire, protrude from the mortar between the bricks. The kids are laughing and pushing each other while the old lady simply shrugs.

Jack explains that the sand used in mixing the mortar back in the 1950s and 1960s, when these homes were built, came from the banks of the nearby Orange River. Plentiful and easily accessible, it was seen as a great advantage to house builders, even though the sand was contaminated by asbestos fibers that gently fell from the ever-present blue dust clouds hanging over the whole town in those days. Indeed, to the extent that the asbestos was noticed, it was seen as beneficial in adding strength and fire protection to the buildings.

Later that same day, I walked to the outskirts of Prieska to visit the town's now derelict swimming pool perched next to those same sandy banks of the river. Long, deep, and wide, and surrounded by the still visible remnants of landscaped grounds, it had been built around the same time as many of the houses in the Red Block and clearly, in its day, had been a rather splendid facility. I was especially interested in the old changing rooms adjacent to the pool. They were missing windows, doors, and a roof, and much of the paint work on the walls had been eroded over time exposing the bricks beneath. I spent a good twenty minutes going from room to room looking closely at the mortar and found no evidence of any asbestos. The pool had been for whites only.

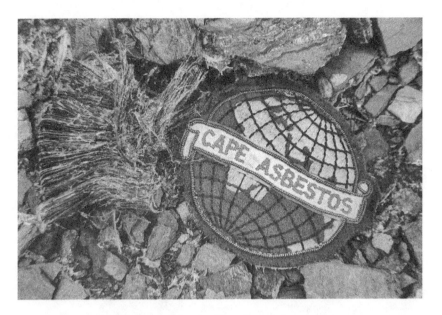

A clump of blue asbestos lying beside a Cape Asbestos company badge.

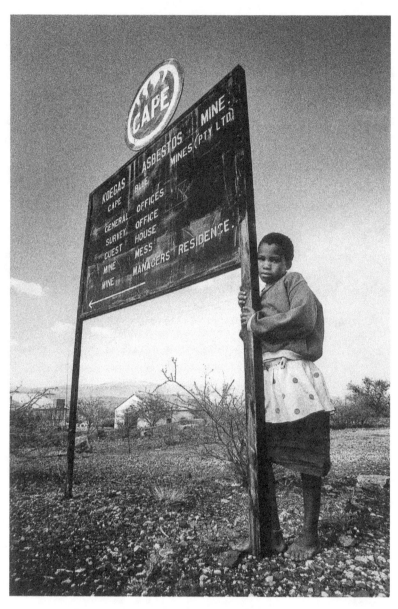

Young girl clutching a sign at the entrance to Cape's abandoned blue asbestos mine at Koegas.

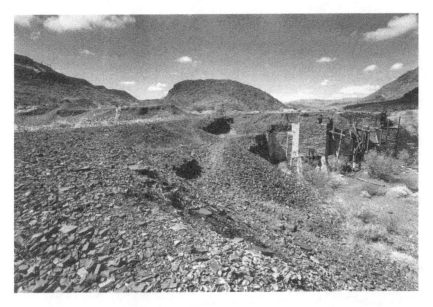

Unrehabilitated former blue asbestos mine (or adit), showing mine entrance surrounded by piles of tailings.

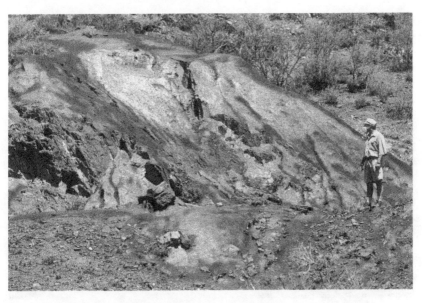

Man wearing a respirator mask standing in front of an unrehabilitated slag heap of blue asbestos tailings at a Koegas mine site.

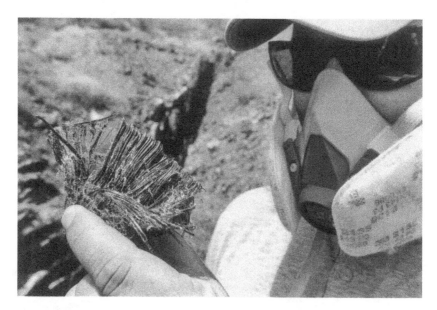

Blue asbestos fibers at an unrehabilitated mining site Westerberg, Koegas.

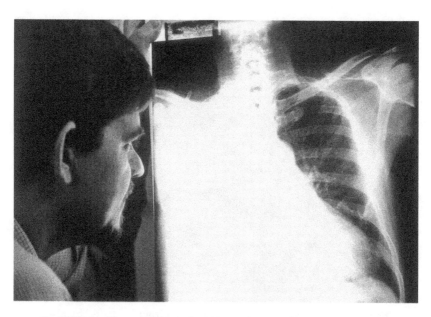

Dr. Wilhelm Pieterse of Prieska Hospital examining a chest x-ray of a patient suffering from an asbestos related disease.

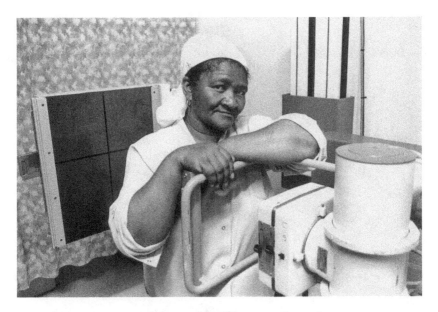

ANN VAN STADEN, fifty-one, asbestosis.
"My father worked in the time office at Koegas. I was still at school
when we used to play on the asbestos after the miners tipped the
'koekoepanne' [or 'cocopan'—a small trolley on rails used to transport asbestos ore]. I've worked at this hospital for 21 years and I've
seen many, many people die from asbestos dust. When you see them
gasping for breath you think: 'Lord, what will my hour be like?' I
never thought this same fate would befall me. My youngest daughter
also has a spot on her one lung. The doctor says it is the disease of
Prieska. I am unhappy with Cape because we never knew that this
was death."

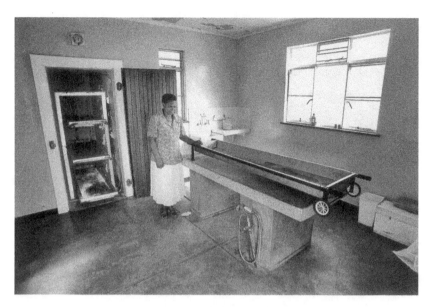

AUDREY VAN SCHALKWYK, fifty-four, asbestosis.
"I was 12 when I started helping my parents work asbestos at Koegas.
Now asbestos will be my end. For the past 23 years I've worked at
the hospital and I've seen many people end up in the mortuary.
Little did I know that I would also end up here because of asbestos.
My father died in 1993 because of the dust and my mother is also
suffering because of it. We are five children and three of us also
have it. I wish Cape can see how our people are suffering."

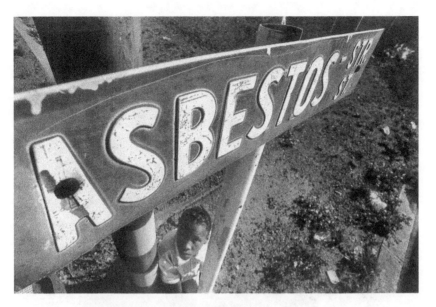

ASBESTOS STREET, Prieska South Africa.
During 1930 Cape Plc build a crushing mill in close proximity to residential and business areas in Prieska. The mill was in operation until approximately 1964. During this period residents of Prieska were exposed to asbestos fibers, either as employees or in their daily activities around the town.

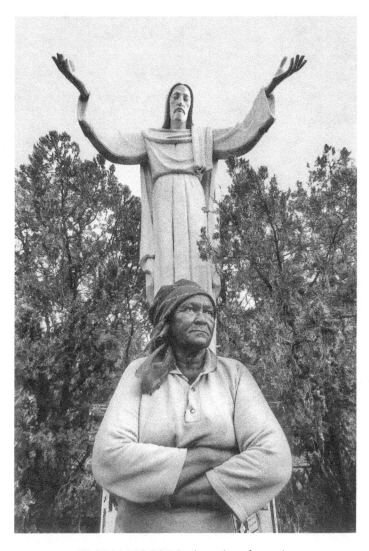

GLODIA MOGORO, sixty-six, asbestosis.
"I was 15 when I started to work for Cape, and now the doctor tells me I have asbestos on my lungs. They never told us about the dangers of asbestos. What can we do about it now? I have a constant pain in my chest and I am weak. We will probably never get anything from Cape."

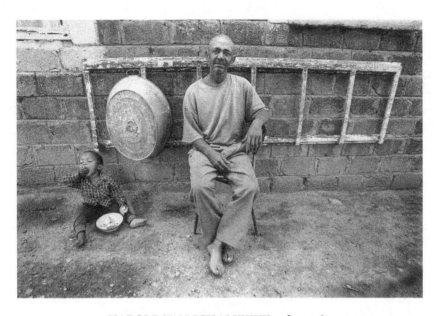

HAROLD VAN SCHALKWYK, asbestosis.
"I worked for Cape, and I am suffering because of them. If I die now who will look after my children? Both my parents died because of the dust."

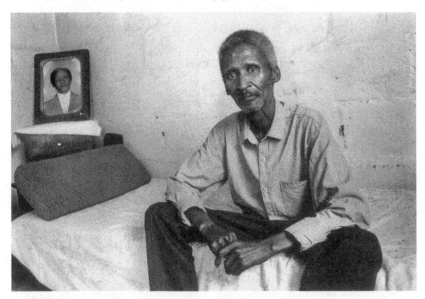

HENDRIK AFRIKA, fifty-six, asbestosis.
"I've made my peace with the fact that I am dying. I am unhappy with those people who took all those millions and who led us to our death. My mother died because of the dust. Today, they deny us. I'll never forgive them. I worked as a sample boy at the Prieska mill and they never warned us that it was dangerous work we were doing. They must give back what they took from the people."

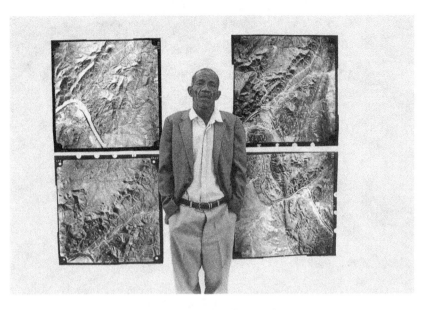

WILLEM OLYN, sixty-three, asbestosis.
"Cape exploited us and they make us suffer every day. Prieska is polluted. One day our children will suffer as a result of it. My father, my mother and my sister died because of mine dust. My wife also has asbestosis. The asbestos is eating me up and it is taking me to my grave. We are dying here."

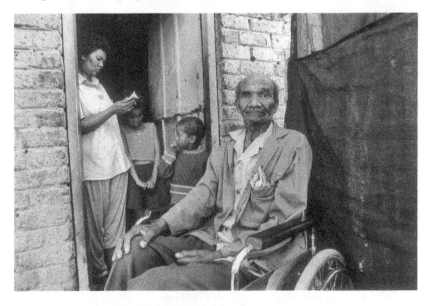

JAN VAN STADEN, seventy, asbestosis.
"I am ready to die. But there are five people depending on my pension and when I die they will have no income."

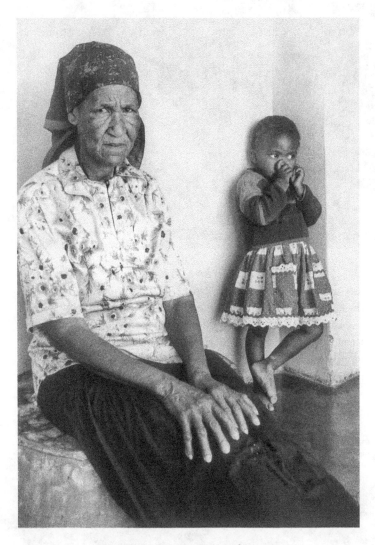

RAGEL OLYN, sixty-six, asbestosis.
"We worked hard for Cape and now we hear the dust was poisoning us. The dust was everywhere, in our houses, in our clothes and when you coughed the phlegm was full of dust. Now my health is poor, I cough and my chest pains. The dust has eaten holes in my lungs. Must I just accept it?"

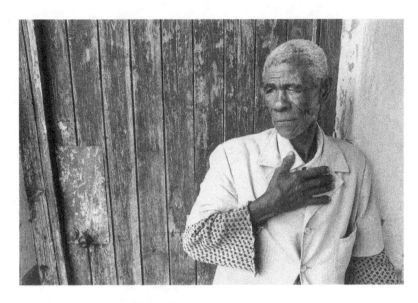

HENDRIK SAAIMAN, seventy.
"My whole family worked for Cape. I can't say if my father died of the asbestos dust, but he did complain about his chest and he had a bad cough. I was 12, or even younger, when I started to work at Koegas. We had to cope with the dust, it was how we earned a little money. It is only now that I hear that the dust affects your lungs, in those days we knew nothing."

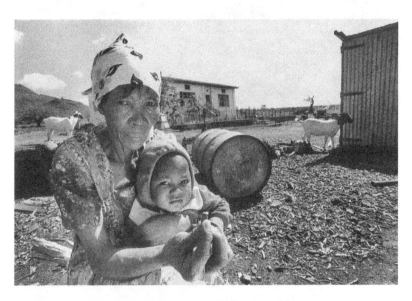

SARAH THYS, wife of a farm worker, Koegas.
"The asbestos lies blue in front of my house and we have to be careful, but the children still play with it especially this one."

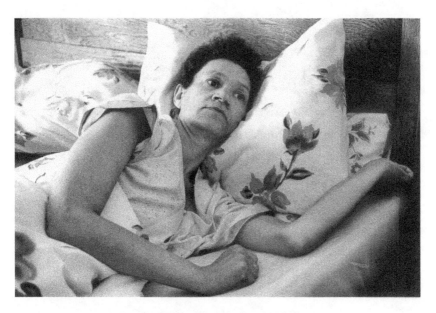

STEF JANSEN, forty-four, mesothelioma.
"I never worked at a mine but we stayed near a mine dump in
Prieska. Now I spend almost the whole day in bed. My movements
are very limited and I drink morphine every 4–6 hours for pain.
I am still young and the thought of dying is not nice. I have three
children and I cannot be a mother for them anymore. No member of
my family has reached the age of sixty because of the asbestos.
Why did they not warn us? They should at least not have brought the
mill into the town."

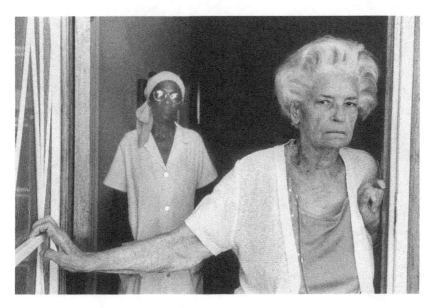

BETTIE JACOBS, sevety-five, mesothelioma.
"Because of the mill there was a lot of asbestos dust in Prieska.
I never worked at the mine but we walked past the mill when we
went to the river. The health inspector, Mr. Cilliers, used to take
dust samples from my porch, because the wind blew a lot of dust in
the direction of my house. According to the doctor, I've lived in
Prieska too long. Mietjie helps me in the house. She must help me to
dress, because I get too tired to do it myself. I don't hate Cape, but
I feel there is a lot they can do for the people."

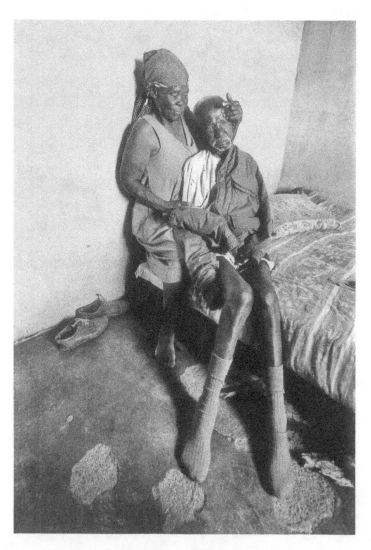

ISAK PRETORIOUS, sixty-five, mesothelioma.
"Give back what belongs to me. My health!"

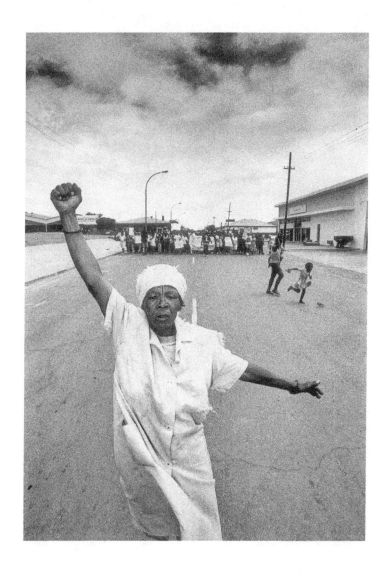

This page and opposite: Community protest action against delays in
the legal system in Britain.

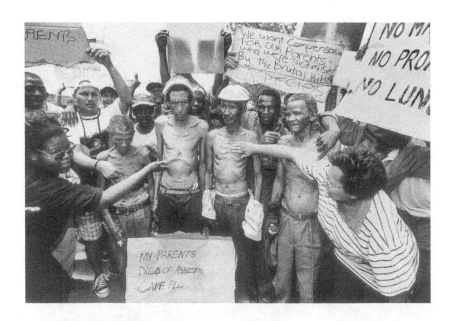

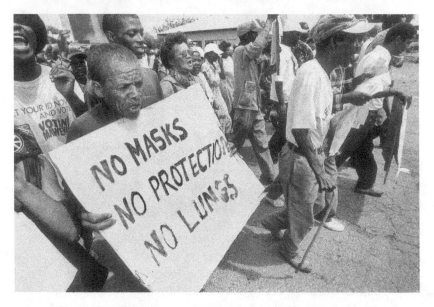

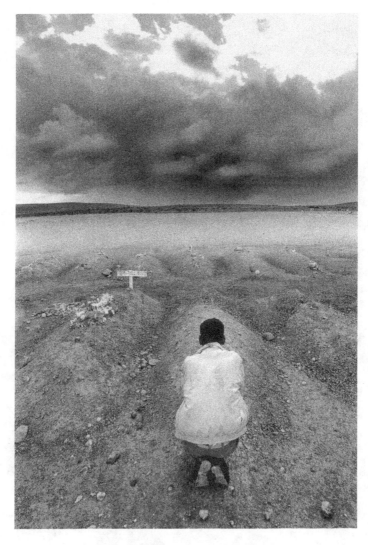

DIEDERICK OOR, born May 12, 1934;
died September 20, 1999.
"My dad used to work at Koegas. He suffered a lot before he died,
and that makes me sad. My mother died from the same asbestos
dust. Maybe my sister will also die from it. These things happen."

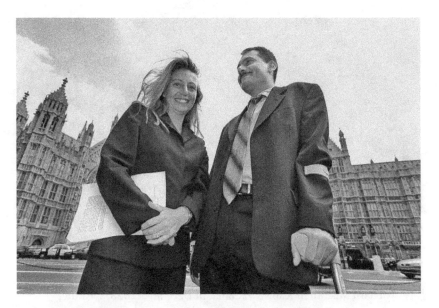

Susannah Read and Richard Meeran standing outside the House of Lords shortly after delivery of its historic judgment in *Lubbe v. Cape Plc*, July 20, 2000. A copy of the judgment is under Susannah's arm, and Richard is on crutches following another sporting mishap, this one resulting in a snapped achillies tendon. *Credit*: Andy Paradise

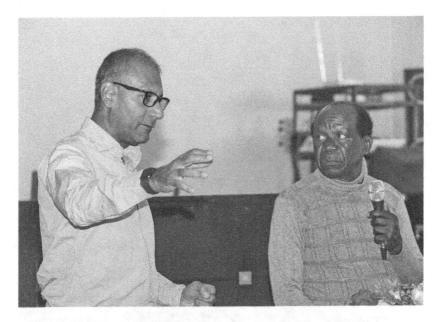

Richard Meeran in Kabwe, Zambia, in December 2023, speaking at a meeting of claimants in a class-action lawsuit against Anglo American Plc, concerning allegations of lead-poisoning of some 140,000 women and children. A community representative stands alongside. *Credit*: Leon Sadiki

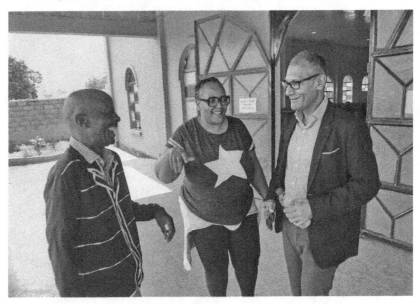

Zanele Mbuyisa (center) and Richard Meeran talking with a community representative in Kabwe, Zambia, in December 2023, following a meeting with claimants in the lawsuit against Anglo American. *Credit*: Leon Sadiki

CHAPTER 6

Corporate Cover-Up
—Fake News and Twisted Science—

HAVE YOU EVER WONDERED WHICH superhero you'd like to be or perhaps which new one you'd like to create? If either of these idle (or megalomaniacal) thoughts has crossed your mind, then I think it's a fair bet that you went for neither Asbestos Man nor Asbestos Lady—that is unless you happen to be one of the pair of enterprising Californian public relations specialists, whose enthusiastic pitch to Cape's North American subsidiary included initial mock ups of "The Asbestos Family Hero Album." "We see many possibilities for expansion into different public relations areas using the asbestos family idea," their cover letter gayly suggests. "Possible areas include coloring books, industrial films, advertising brochures, children's books and even fire prevention ads (such as Asbestos Man as a possible helper to Smoky [sic] the Bear)."[1]

The database for Marvel, an American media franchise, documents the existence of Asbestos Man since 1963 and Asbestos Lady since 1947 (with "The Torch" being their common arch foe), so the idea seemed to be to combine them and their future progeny in a fully-fledged superhero family. Whatever the motive and however deeply Cape entertained the notion, it could not have been lost on all concerned that, according to Marvel folklore, Asbestos Man was always depicted with a mask and oxygen tank because he was "a cancer survivor" and Asbestos Lady had died at the age of forty-five of "idiopathic mesothelioma."[2] Graver still, the pitch was made in August 1971, one year after the enactment of the US Clean Air Act, which classified asbestos as a hazardous pollutant, and two years before the US Environmental Protection Agency banned spray-on asbestos, thereby immediately halting its use, for example, for insulating and fireproofing the steel beams and elevator shafts of the World Trade Center beyond the fortieth floor of the North Tower.[3] Altogether it seemed—to say the least—a most inopportune time to be "glorifying asbestos," as Richard put it.[4]

Richard had happened upon the letter when riffling through a hoard of Cape documents in the basement of Jim Walker's law firm in Bloomington, Illinois. Richard had been introduced to Jim by Laurie Flynn (who was with him in the basement) on account of Jim's long history of pursuing negligence and personal injuries claims against US-based corporations supplying or manufacturing asbestos. It was a fire that had brought Richard and Laurie to Jim's door one still, frigid morning in December 2000, though not the one in the steakhouse Jim took them to that evening (welcome though that was), but rather a fire some years before that Cape claimed had destroyed a huge cache of its company records stored in a warehouse in London. The irony of such a fate befalling an asbestos company aside, the visitors hoped that in Jim's basement they might find some of the missing materials detailing Cape's state of knowledge of the health effects of asbestos—the "what, where, and when," as it were, of the company's awareness.

≈

Laurie's own research had already helped fill in some of the gaps. In the process of collecting material for his raw, uncompromising 1981 television documentary, *Dust to Dust*, on the extent of the Cape's cover-up of asbestos-related diseases and deaths in South Africa, Laurie had connected with Jim and other US attorneys involved in suing Big Asbestos. He'd assumed, rightly, that among the thousands of documents and testimonies tendered in court during those trials, there would be some bearing directly on the levels of awareness among Cape's senior management. After referring to medical literature in the 1960s, including Ian Webster's 1962 Pneumoconiosis Research Unit (PRU) report, and Cape's "experience with their own workers," Laurie was left in no doubt that Cape "knowingly exposed its workforce to high risk and whose former employees are dying in poverty." When, during filming, he asked Jim Walker what he considered to be the state of Cape's knowledge at the time, Walker paused for a moment before replying: "It's analogous to the situation of firing a gun into a crowd. You may not know which of them will be killed but you know for certain that some of them will be."[5]

The documentary contains a lengthy segment on the plight of former Kuruman asbestos miner James Ebang, his wife, and their children. Ebang had been suffering from asbestosis for some time and was recently diagnosed with mesothelioma. He was no longer able to work, could barely walk, and could not sleep lying down because he became feverish and often choked. He received R41 (USD$40 in 1982) in compensation from the government every three months, which bought a sack of mealie meal (maize) and a little coffee. The family often went hungry, and the children no longer attended school as their parents could not afford the fees. "When he dies I will have to bury him in a sack," said Ebang's wife. "I feel bitter and sad." The program's juxtaposition of the $500,000 damages payout Jim Walker secured for his asbestosis-suffering client from Cape's North American subsidiary underlines the appalling inequities of the Ebangs' treatment.[6]

Another of the revelatory documents unearthed by Laurie from Jim Walker's cache was the 1975 deposition of Cape's managing director, Geoffrey Higham, which we encountered earlier in chapter 4, in a US case involving Cape's asbestos products.[7] An engineer by trade, Higham had joined Cape in 1965 and rose to the top position in 1972. As the Cape group of companies' most senior executive, his understanding of the nature of the group's business was of critical importance both to its overall direction and how it navigated risks and opportunities. Yet, in the matter of managing the dangers posed by the Cape's core product, Higham seems to have been alarmingly deficient. In the deposition he started well when asked how long asbestos has been known to be a hazardous material "if not handled properly." "Since 1931," he replied, referring to the United Kingdom's asbestos regulations introduced that year.

But alarm bells began ringing with his woolly or contradictory responses after being pressed on what precautions were or should be taken to handle asbestos properly. "It boils down to the fact that wherever asbestos is used, and in whatever form, the dust that is emitted from it must be contained and limited to a very small amount," he said, adding that for Cape this means that "we set standards above [the minimum legal requirements] . . . our objective is that there shall be no dust emitted in our operations." Elsewhere in his deposition, however, Higham qualifies this objective by stating that "generally, we are aiming at 2 fibres per c.c. [cubic centimeter] standard," that being the maximum permissible quantity of airborne asbestos in UK workplaces in the mid-1970s. The fact that at the same time the maximum fiber count under South African regulations was set at 12 fibers per c.c. was not mentioned.[8] Nor was any reference made to the measurements taken by Cape itself at its South African sites, which, for the Penge mill, as Richard later discovered, averaged 24 to 70 fibers per milliliter between 1976 and 1979.* Bad though these Penge levels were, they were an improvement on the shocking levels of 630 to 800 fibers per milliliter recorded at the Prieska mill in 1948.[9]

Revisiting this testimonial, Richard found a new insight into Cape's managerial processes. Beyond confirming that Cape's directors had been fully aware of the health dangers of asbestos for nearly fifty years before closing its South African operations, Higham's candor also showed how UK-centric the company's managerial thinking was. Throughout his deposition Higham made no distinctions between Cape's UK and regional operations in terms of occupational health and safety. Rather, he repeatedly referred to "all operations," collectively. The standards against which the whole group was then being held, apparently, were those established in Cape's home jurisdiction of the United Kingdom, where legislation classified asbestos as hazardous and prescribed maximum airborne fiber counts in the workplace far more strictly than in South Africa.

Recalling that it was also in this deposition that Higham had admitted that prior to 1972 Cape had placed no health warnings of any kind on its products, Richard pondered on the implications of such frank confessions.[10] If the company neglected to warn others, notably its customers and clients, of the potentially harmful effects of asbestos that Cape itself was fully aware of, what hope, he thought, was there that the company would

---

* Note that per cubic centimeter and per milliliter are equivalent.

care to protect the health of those most exposed to the hazard—its workers, their families, and local populations? In light of evidence from his clients, and as repeated many times over with every additional claimant interview, the answer seemed obvious.

Despite purported intentions to the contrary, Cape had failed to take proper care of workers in its South African subsidiaries and surrounding communities. Furthermore, such failure resided as much with Cape's directors in London as it did with those on the boards of its companies in South Africa, not least because of the significant overlap between the two groups. In his first affidavit in the *Lubbe* case in June 1997, Richard had already listed no fewer than six individuals who held shared directorial roles in both Cape UK and one or more of its South African enterprises (namely, Cape Asbestos South Africa Property Limited [CASAP], Cape Blue Mines Limited, and Egnep Limited). Geoffrey Higham, Richard Gaze, and Rupert Riley were all on that list.[11]

The list also included Justin MacKeurtan, a South African who'd spent seventeen years on the board of Cape UK, alongside his directorships of CASAP and Cape Blue Mines between 1957 and his retirement in 1974. MacKeurtan had been deposed in a further US case involving Cape's asbestos products, this one in 1996 in Jones County, Mississippi, but in contrast to Higham, his deposition was notably more guarded and prickly. Perhaps this was because by then asbestos litigation was rampant (especially in the United States) and the depth of righteous indignation with which claimants pursued their cases was evident. Or perhaps it was due to MacKeurtan having been at the very forefront of Cape's resistance to what scientists and doctors were telling the industry about the dangers of asbestos. Either way, his words in the more than 400 pages of his deposition speak to a man on the defensive (or offensive defense), as evidenced in his lawyer's frequent objections to the questions being put to the deponent.[12]

MacKeurtan's sensitivity to questions regarding his knowledge of and attitude toward ARDs was especially marked, bordering on the absurd at times. He claimed, for example, that "we cared for our miners very much," yet in the next moment, admitted that he didn't know whether anyone in the company had ever warned the miners of "a possible relationship between asbestos and cancer," adding, "but I personally didn't."[13] When pressed time and again on the question of the link between asbestos and mesothelioma, he simply denied that such a link had ever been proven, even by the time he was being deposed in 1996. At another point, he detailed a bizarre conspiratorial tale about the recorded minutes of a pneumoconiosis conference in New York in 1964 (which he had not attended) having been "written *before* the conference had started," as discovered, he claimed, by "the British delegation [who] noticed a whole series of brown paper packets in the hall, in the corner," as they arrived at the venue.[14]

However, it was in terms of his engagement with scientists and medical specialists that MacKeurtan's testimony was most revealing. His profound skepticism of reports associating asbestos with any particular disease was fueled by his insistence that all dust is dangerous and by his zeal to find what he referred to as "the truth" about the health dangers posed by asbestos. This latter point, which he repeatedly made, was especially perverse, sinister even, as it reflected an intention hellbent on thwarting or interfering with the science of occupational health in ways that would benefit the asbestos industry. "I wanted to find out what the problem was and get to the truth," he says, by way of explaining his summary dismissal of Chris Wagner's 1960 study of thirty-three mesothelioma cases in the Northern Cape. "I don't believe it had been researched sufficiently. It was his opinion but was not proven. In my opinion, it was not proven."[15] These are certainly remarkable claims to make of what has become the world's most cited work in the field of occupational health, especially from someone with no medical or scientific qualifications and whose formal education ended at high school.[16] MacKeurtan was equally dismissive of Ian Webster's work at the PRU in Johannesburg. "Yes, he was always bringing up problems at these meetings," was his irritated response to a question about whether he recalled Webster making a statement about the relationship between asbestos and mesothelioma.[17]

No doubt MacKeurtan felt entitled to be "skeptical about some of the things that were said" on account of the twin facts that Cape had substantially funded the PRU (initially contributing some £25,000 to its asbestos research, according to MacKeurtan, and thereafter smaller annual sums),[18] and that he sat on the Engineering Sub-Committee of the national Asbestos Research Project. The former bought him influence in the scientific process itself, while the latter was pitched as an alternative—often oppositional—voice to scientific outputs. It was by way of this pincer movement that Richard could now see what MacKeurtan meant by seeking "the truth": it was "truth" on Cape's terms, or at least on terms that best suited the asbestos industry.

The Engineering Sub-Committee itself was emblematic of this manufacture of an alternative reality. It had been created as one of two subcommittees under the Asbestos Research Project, the other focusing on medical concerns, while the project itself had come into being in the most ignominious circumstances. Established shortly after Ian Webster had tabled his damning "Report of a Mesothelioma Survey" at a PRU meeting in May 1962, the project was designed as an industry fix for one of those "problems" that irked MacKeurtan.

Asbestos producers, as we saw earlier, were so panicked by this report's findings—most especially evidence suggesting that environmental exposure to asbestos dust was a principal reason for "the alarmingly high number of cases with mesothelioma" found in the area—that they took immediate steps to suppress and discredit the research. Indeed, when MacKeurtan first heard the results in a meeting with Webster, he was "outraged," throwing his hands in the air and lambasting a startled Webster with "How dare you!" after the scientist had delivered his conclusions.[19] Galvanized into action, the industry lobbied the minister of mines who duly responded in a letter to asbestos producers on August 1, 1962, urging *them* to conduct "intensive research into asbestosis and mesothelioma and the prevention of these diseases, with particular emphasis on dust prevention," and to advise him accordingly.[20]

Shortly thereafter, an executive committee for the newly formed Asbestos Research Project (the attention-grabbing word "mesothelioma" in the title of the survey it was replacing having been pointedly dropped) was established with a membership reflecting a very different research agenda to that pursued by Ian Webster and Chris Wagner. Of its fifteen members, six came from asbestos mining companies (including two from Cape— MacKeurtan and CASAP's mining director, Louis Kuyper), and four came from relevant government departments (Mines and the Miners' Medical Bureau). Another three were drawn from the government's chief scientific body, the Council for Scientific and Industrial Research (CSIR), the principal aim of which was (and still is) to support public and private projects through directed research that aligns with the country's socioeconomic priorities. The last two members of the committee were the only recognized medical specialists in asbestos research, and one of them was an adviser to the government's CSIR.

It was under the direction of this Executive Committee that the two sub-committees were formed, with the Engineering Sub-Committee holding its first meeting on October 23, 1962. It was obvious from the very outset that the Engineering Sub-Committee was intended not as complementary to the Medical Sub-Committee but as its competitor. With a membership drawn from the industry and government-stacked Executive Committee, the minutes of its first meeting made plain what the members considered to be their objective:[21]

> The problem facing us at present suggests that at this stage it is primarily an engineering problem, i.e. the elimination of the dust from the general atmosphere. The more detailed medical aspects are not of immediate importance, except in so far as long term prospects are concerned.

Such a brutally myopic analysis would surely have shocked those many victims of the "medical aspects" of asbestos, even if no one would disagree that dust had to be eliminated from *all* atmospheres, workplaces as well as "generally."

The minutes of this first meeting also revealed what was clearly the members' overriding concern—namely, what damage solving this engineering problem might do to their companies' profits. The asbestos industry, it warned, "cannot be too heavily loaded with the costs of dust elimination, which will cut heavily into profit margins." Much of the remainder of the meeting was thus taken up with outlining a scheme of damage control of the levels of compensation that it anticipated (correctly) would be demanded by a growing number of asbestos victims.

Shamelessly, it was suggested that "those persons who are exposed to asbestos . . . be classified into two groups: 1) compensable, and 2) non-compensable." The compensable group comprised mine and mill employees working in "dusty atmospheres" as well as other employees working in "non-dusty atmospheres who become accidentally exposed." While the non-compensable group comprised pretty much everyone else—including, notably, "the families of employees resident on the mines . . . who might become accidentally exposed to dust due to the pollution of the general atmosphere, contamination of roads, tailings used for general surfacing playing fields etc," *and* anyone who might handle asbestos products (stevedores, transport contractors, and factory workers, for example) "who are not employees of the mining companies."[22]

Richard had found this report buried in the NCOH archives, and after reading it, two things were clear to him. First, that no lawyer had sat on the Engineering Sub-Committee, nor had any lawyer cast their eye over this compensation scheme, for the scheme portrayed remarkable ignorance of the long-established "neighborhood principle" of foreseeability in the tort of negligence. That is, common law liability follows you if it is reasonably foreseeable that a person or class of persons is likely to be injured on account of your negligent behavior. Advising the minister to exclude environmentally exposed asbestos victims from any statutory compensation scheme, therefore, directly countermanded this cardinal legal principle. That said, it could be done, as statutes will nearly always displace tortious principles in common law jurisdictions such as South Africa, and indeed the proposed scheme became the basis for later legislation that provided compensation only to mining employees and, further, only to those engaged in designated "risk work."[23]

The second thing that jumped out at Richard was the fact that during those years in South African history such cruel, self-serving audacity was not seen for what it was but rather viewed as an appropriate and rational response to "the problem."[24] It was nothing short of a cover-up in plain sight.[25]

A central plank in Richard's argument against Cape was that in addition to it bearing liability for the ARDs of the mine and mill workers employed by its subsidiaries, Cape's liability extended to those with environmentally acquired ARDs, as they too were reasonably foreseeable casualties of the company's negligence, given the state of scientific knowledge at the time. Wagner's ground-breaking article with Sleggs and Marchand in 1960, alongside Webster's "Mesothelioma Survey" two years later, were not seen by the asbestos industry as chastening warnings of the human cost of its operations. No, they were seen as existential threats to the profitability of asbestos companies that had to be resisted as forcefully and cheaply as possible.

Correcting these grave, preventable injustices was in fact the key driver behind Richard's determination to sue Cape in the English courts. "Cape's business was a worldwide chain of production, orchestrated and controlled from London," he maintained, "starting in South Africa where the asbestos was mined and milled, transported to local ports, and loaded unto ships, then offloaded in the UK, Europe and the US, and ending with the manufacture of asbestos products in all of these places."[26] What sustained this production line was demand created by consumers in the West. And while widespread ARDs occurred along the entire chain for decades—sustained by the ability of Cape and the industry as a whole to conceal the risks of disease and to operate with impunity—it was mounting fears about the health of US and European consumers that led directly to the end of asbestos operations in South Africa. It was not concern for the well-being of South African miners and communities, including women and children, who had borne the brunt of the decimation. It was this cruel indifference and the apparent dispensability of human beings that galled Richard most of all, impelling him to seek justice for Cape's victims in the courts of the country in which the company was headquartered.

≈

Had Richard any doubts about the industry's stance in this regard, they would have been dispelled by the contents of a report of the Engineering Sub-Committee in 1965 that he found as he dug deeper into the files. Compiled by Cape's own (CASAP) mining director in South Africa, Louis Kuyper, the report documented the multiple stages in the mining and milling of asbestos when significant quantities of dust were created. Altogether, it listed nine such stages and no fewer than forty-three separate operations as "sources of dust liberated into the atmosphere." They included drilling and blasting; crushing ore, cobbing, milling, sorting, and bagging fiber; spillage during transport and disposal of waste. The "dust raised by winds and by persons or animals walking on dumps" was another issue, as was utilizing tailings to surface "playing fields, roads and school playgrounds" and the "use of second-hand bags, which once contained asbestos for 'sack' huts, bedding etc."[27]

Such frankness from the industry and Cape itself seemed to be as unwitting as it was ghastly, but it was nonetheless a combination pursued throughout the report. For example, when discussing how to tackle dust suppression, its authors concede "that it is usually impossible to make significant improvements to old mills"—to which problem the only solution offered is to "accept" that for a period, there will have to be "double standards" of dust control until the older mines can be replaced. It appears to have crossed no one's mind on the subcommittee that these old and dangerous mills should simply be shut down. Such blinkered thinking is all the more reprehensible given that at the very same time, two high-profile studies undertaken by leading researchers in the United States and the United Kingdom had both damningly concluded that there were no safe ways to mine, mill, transport, or manufacture asbestos, such is the lethality of exposure to its fibers.[28]

Most startling of all, however, were the report's conclusions in which the subcommittee first demanded that "sympathy and tolerance must be shown to producers who have been unremitting in their efforts to find answers to problems and in improving their plants" and then pleaded that "it is hoped that other [dust producing industries] will receive similar attention to that showered on the asbestos industry."[29]

Shaking his head in wonder at this warped sense of reality—that seemed not just to side-step medical and scientific evidence but to act as if it did not exist—Richard couldn't decide whether it was a result of myopic naivete or arrogant selfishness. Likely a bit of both, he thought. But in any event, it was not just the asbestos industry that was engaged in this elaborate stunt. Support was also coming from parts of the medical and scientific communities. This ignominious chapter in South Africa's history of occupational health research spotlighted the crux of the cover-up that Richard believed Cape had been actively involved in creating, that being the toxic intersection of profit motive and scientific endeavor. It was a "corruption of science," as Jock McCulloch labeled it, that sustained a pernicious industry and perpetuated the death and suffering of thousands of the country's poorest and most marginalized communities.[30]

≈

Of all the features of the asbestos industry's dreadful history to which Jock McCulloch devoted so much of his career as a social scientist investigating (and which ultimately cost him his life),[31] it was the producers' perversion of the truth that agitated him most. With dogged, level-headed precision, Jock had been pursuing these lines of duplicity and deception for many years in his native Australia (the only other source of mined crocidolite) and, especially, South Africa. The journey had led him to a profound, if baleful, conclusion about science and scientists when faced with realpolitik. "The discovery of an association between a disease and a chemical product is a political act," wrote Jock. "Its creator and the knowledge itself are immediately embroiled in an environment where the virtues of honesty and objectivity are largely irrelevant."[32] Richard's efforts to test Cape's levels of honesty and objectivity by suing it for negligence chimed well with Jock, who was happy to share his knowledge and thoughts.

Jock was not surprised that among Richard's initial claimants were white victims (Matthys Nel and later, Pauline Nel), as one of the most striking features of Jock's investigations of Cape's cover-up was the extent to which it hid critical information from its own employees, whatever their race, including senior staff. Like Richard, Jock had read the November 1996 deposition of Guy Wilson, a white, long-time Cape employee and CASAP's company secretary and board member, in the Jones County case against Cape in the United States.[33] Wilson had been adamant that during his employment he was never informed of the dangers of asbestos, nor was he aware of any company efforts to suppress medical research on asbestos or pressurize government officials.[34] Such responses may have beggared belief coming from such a senior officer in the company, but after Jock interviewed Wilson at the Wanderers' Club in Johannesburg in July 1996, he tended to believe that Wilson had been thoroughly (if somewhat gullibly) deceived. Wilson told Jock that he had visited Cape's mines and mills on a regular basis throughout the 1960s and 1970s, often accompanied by his wife and, during school holidays, his children. "It was an adventure driving to isolated communities along unmade roads," Jock recorded him saying, before adding that Wilson "now says that he would never have done so" had he known of the danger.[35]

On one of his own trips to South Africa in the late 1990s, Richard happened on a similarly perturbing story with a tragic ending. One evening in the bar of Johannesburg's Parktonian Hotel where he was staying, he met Schalk Burger, then a senior director in the South African Department of Mines and previously, in the 1970s, a mining engineer with one of Cape's subsidiaries (Cape Blue Mines) in Pomfret in the Northern Cape. Now in his sixties, Schalk was a shell of his former self. During his time with Cape, he'd often taken his daughter, Amanda, with him to the mines on weekends when she was aged between two and four years old. At the time of the meeting with Richard, Amanda was twenty-nine, with three kids, and had just been diagnosed with mesothelioma. "Schalk and his wife were caring for Amanda and the children after her husband had dumped her when she became ill," Richard recalls. "I remember him tearfully showing me photographs of her on his mobile phone. She died a couple of weeks later," he adds with a sigh. Determined to do something in response, Schalk joined the case against Cape as a claimant acting on behalf of his daughter's estate, but the bitter irony of what had killed her never left him or his wife.[36]

≈

As Cape's long-time technical and scientific director, Richard Gaze had responsibilities for keeping abreast of scientific literature and alerting management of any relevant health and safety issues arising therefrom. By his own admission, Gaze had been fully aware of the nature of asbestosis from the early 1940s and of mesothelioma from 1960. Furthermore, he must have seen evidence of these diseases on his frequent visits to the company's operations in South Africa.[37] Yet, such health warnings as Gaze did make were either insipidly ineffective (more pink than red flags) or brazenly ignored, in which case he seems to have run up a white flag. Either way, if fellow directors like Guy Wilson hadn't heard them, it was unsurprising that comparatively lowly miners and mill workers were equally in the dark.

Jock's view of Gaze tended toward him being cowed by his (nonscientific) bosses, such that Gaze was twisted into impossible positions when trying to straddle the often competing demands of scientific and business communities. In one instance, at a major scientific conference on asbestos in New York in 1964, Gaze proclaimed that it was very difficult to prove an association between asbestos and mesothelioma, citing, in support, the apparent absence of the disease in South Africa's amosite mines.[38] Yet in his presentation he failed even to mention Ian Webster's "Mesothelioma Survey," which had been conducted two years earlier and, as Jock put it, "effectively solved the very question Gaze subsequently claimed was so complex."[39] Why? Well, because Webster's study had been so thoroughly derided and suppressed by Cape's own words and actions, as delivered through the menacing South African Asbestos Producers Advisory Committee, that almost nobody knew about it. Gaze, therefore, could conveniently and safely ignore it.

Richard's opinion of Gaze was similarly critical, though he was inclined to add that Gaze had been browbeaten to a point where he lacked professional care or even competence. During his 1975 deposition, Gaze (who was then still employed by Cape) had stressed that "I am very conscious of safety questions. I regard it as being my duty to take these up at Board level in the companies on which I serve [namely, Egnep, CASAP, and Cape UK]." Further, he agreed that he felt "a sense of duty to see that safe practices are carried out by [Cape's] subsidiaries as a member of the board of . . . the parent company."[40] When asked directly about his actions regarding the promotion of safety at the mines and mills, however, Gaze's answers were underwhelming: "To my memory, I have never specifically advised the Board of Cape Industries [Cape UK] of a safety question." While he then qualified this by saying, "I would normally only expect to do this if I was not able to obtain satisfaction in my capacity as a director of the subsidiary company concerned,"[41] he seemed remarkably ignorant of what safety precautions existed in the South African firms. When asked: "Can you tell me whether or not your company [CASAP] has a safety department?" he responded: "You embarrass me, because I ought to know and I don't know."[42] Richard Gaze died of mesothelioma in 1982, aged sixty-five.[43]

≈

It was not just scientists employed or otherwise funded by Cape or other asbestos corporations that sided with the industry's preferred view of science. Its malign influence reached into the very heart of the medical establishment in South Africa. When the ever-vigilant and pioneering Christopher Sleggs began seeing significant numbers of lung cancer patients at the West End Hospital in Kimberley in the mid-1950s, all of whom were coming from the asbestos mining communities in the Northern Cape, he took note. In one of his earliest actions, he wrote to the director of the Institute of Medical Research in Johannesburg in October 1956, detailing a number of cases with new or peculiar symptoms that he was "convinced are not tuberculosis." He referred specifically to "a woman with proved mesothelioma" and to the recent death of a male patient "from progressive pleural thickening . . . which incarcerated both his lungs leading to heart failure." Sleggs signed off in an adamant tone: "I am convinced that there is an increased incidence of carcinoma of serous membranes in this district."[44] In terms of an early warning of what was to become an epidemic, this could hardly have been more emphatic. Nevertheless, there is evidence that certain pillars of the medical profession in South Africa paid little or no heed to the warning. Nor did they take any appropriate remedial action. In fact, quite the opposite.[45]

True, it was the CSIR that initiated Ian Webster's undertaking of the PRU mesothelioma field survey in the Northern Cape and Transvaal a few years later in 1960. But it then presided over the active suppression of the survey's interim results in 1962 and for decades thereafter accommodated the asbestos industry's self-interested efforts to query and compromise mesothelioma research by the PRU and later by the National Centre for Occupational Health (NCOH) and the National Research Institute for Occupational Diseases (NRIOD).[46] On this shameful legacy, two doctors, Neil White and Eric Bateman, reflect ruefully that "it is not a happy story nor one of which the medical and scientific communities or the public at large can feel proud!"[47]

Another august body, the South African Medical Research Council (SAMRC), was also accused of seriously impeding mesothelioma research undertaken by two NRIOD scientists, Leslie Irwig and Hannes Botha, at the behest (once again) of the South African Asbestos Producers' Advisory Committee (SAAPAC). First, the two men were "ordered" by A. J. Brink, president of the MRC and dean of the Faculty of Medicine at Stellenbosch University, not to deliver a paper detailing their findings on the mortality trends from ARDs in South Africa to an international environmental conference in New York in June 1978. Irwig, who was scheduled to deliver the paper, felt duty-bound to remove it from the conference program. Subsequently, SAMRC pressured

NRIOD not to publish the paper for several years. This time, however, the scandal attracted attention, most notably when Laurie Flynn reported it in his *New Scientist* article in 1982.[48] The responses to Flynn's investigative probing were instructive. Both Irwig and Botha "refused to discuss the affair" when Flynn interviewed them for the piece. After it was published, SAMRC's executive wrote an indignant response, diluting its responsibility by implicating others while not denying that it compelled Irwig to pull the paper or that the paper's eventual publication was delayed for years.[49]

Just as alarming was a long, cringeworthy letter Ian Webster, NRIOD's then director, wrote in response to Irwig, who had complained to him about the affair. Attempting, as he puts it, to record "the sequence of events" resulting in the paper's censorship, Webster's subjugation to the will of the asbestos industry leaps off the page. Slapped down by SAAPAC's "emphatic" demand that the paper not be presented, as well as fearful of SAAPAC secretary Fritz Baunach's likely rabid "attempt to refute the substance of the paper" if it had been presented, Webster is clearly a man under intense pressure. He finishes the letter in a pained tone: "I am as distressed as you over the asbestos industry's attitude to the work of the Institute and the publication of results. . . . I understand your feelings on this matter all too well and although I would have preferred to continue in my attempts to educate the industry, your suggestion of a meeting to define policy may not be all that untimely."[50]

While there is no evidence of such a meeting ever happening (still less a duly "educated" industry), the artful and highly effective maneuverings of SAAPAC—the *éminence grise* of the asbestos industry in South Africa—were abundantly clear to Richard, not only in the work of Laurie Flynn and Jock McCulloch, but also in additional files held by NIOH, toward which

Tony Davies guided him. Reflecting on how long Ian Webster had been bullied by the asbestos corporations (almost two decades), Richard returned to a key section of the introductory paragraph in the PRU's 1962 report on the "Mesothelioma Survey" conducted by Webster:

> The unfortunate publicity that was given to the survey in its early days has resulted in certain mining groups feeling that reference to a form of cancer has attached a stigma to the area in which they operate, and that such stigma could adversely affect, not only the future recruitment of personnel for their mines, but even the economy of the industry as a whole.
>
> While emphasising that this Unit [the PRU] realises its obligation to humanity, it is desired to point out that it will endeavour to continue what is regarded by us as necessary research as discretely as possible and with due consideration of all policies which may be involved.[51]

The coy reference to "certain mining groups" fooled no one. The sensitivity of both SAAPAC and Cape to the stigma of asbestos's carcinogenic properties bordered on manic, such that— evidently—the discretion it demanded of scientific research was preferred to the science community's "obligation to humanity." The perverted pomposity of such reasoning is quite simply breathtaking.

Yet, the industry's iron fist around the throat of asbestos research was to last decades, as evidenced by a letter Tony showed Richard, written by the honorary secretary of the Northern Cape branch of the Asbestos Producers Advisory Committee to one of Tony's predecessor directors of the PRU in November 1975. "Following this morning's discussions at the offices of Cape Asbestos (Pty) Ltd.," it said, "I am directed by my committee to confirm with you that an arrangement dating back to the days of the Asbestos Research Project still stands, viz that no studies dealing with asbestos exposed mining and milling personnel are to be published without prior consultation with the writer or, in case he is not available, with the offices of . . . Cape Asbestos (Pty) Ltd."[52]

There were also "good guys" in South Africa's medical profession at the time, from whose dedicated and clear-sighted work Richard was likewise to learn much about the degeneracy of the asbestos industry. Tony Davies and Marianne Felix were longtime servants in this category. Richard was now spending more time in South Africa and in their company at the NCOH when he was in Johannesburg. Tony was unflinching in his discussions with Richard about the asbestos industry's crude inveigling of scientific research and the medical profession's response, as the pair migrated their conversations between Tony's office and the cheap eateries in the streets nearby.

Tony had already introduced Richard to the ground-breaking observations made in the late 1940s by Gerrit Schepers, who had documented what he called the "simply deplorable" conditions of Cape's Penge mine, including the Dickensian and extensive practice of child labor used for the dustiest tasks (trampling asbestos fiber into sacks as it was poured over their heads from above) while being kept in order by a bullwhip-wielding supervisor. The fact that Schepers found that many of these children had developed clinically observable cardio-pulmonary problems by the age of twelve reflects that they were being employed at an even younger age.[53] Indeed subsequently, it was estimated that of the 7,500 claimants in the Cape case, 6 percent had been employed under the age of 7.[54]

The use of children in the workforce reflected one of two specific employment practices used throughout the sector that provided the asbestos corporations with yet another layer of disguise and cover-up. Such young employees were virgin asbestos workers (having little or no prior mine or mill-work exposure to dust) and therefore had no preexisting lung problems that might shorten their useful working life. Child workers were also cheap and nearly always employed casually, meaning they had no contractual rights and scant if any company records of their employment.[55] They could be expendable too, as illustrated by the common practice of using "chissa boys" when blasting open new rock. Their job was to light dynamite fuses and then scurry away as fast as their legs could carry them.[56]

The second accommodating employment practice was the almost immediate dismissal of any employee who showed signs of lung disease, which, especially in the early decades of the asbestos mining (1930s to 1950s), was often after just a few years or even a few months of employment. For the corporations, this meant not only that they could jettison suboptimal manual laborers, but also that dismissed sick employees would disappear from the workplace as they returned to their villages to cope as best they could. Typically, they did not cope very well, "dying quietly" without health care and often unable to work anymore.[57] But that, from the corporation's perspective, was not something it had to worry about, as they were now off the company's books and their occupationally acquired illnesses were not recorded against the company's name. Cape's use of migrant labor from neighboring Botswana, Lesotho, Mozambique, and Zimbabwe, as well as Malawi,[58] extended this invisibility cloak still farther, as such foreign workers were neither registered nor cared for under South African labor laws.[59]

It was in respect of this scurrilous practice that Tony Davies (and Jock McCulloch) directed Richard toward the work of G. B. Peacock, an assistant health officer with the government's Department of Native Affairs during the 1950s. After one inspection of asbestos mines and mills in Northern Transvaal, Peacock recorded how barefaced the producers were in their use of such expendable "turnstile" employees: "The practice of replacing the entire mill staff every few months (I inspected one mill that had six complete changes of staff in 12 months) as a method of controlling asbestosis and dodging responsibility for the provision of adequate dust proofing is felt to be very wrong." To which he added his observations on the dire circumstances that befall the discarded workers: "Previous experience amongst natives living under tribal conditions in the immediate vicinity of our biggest asbestos mines in Northern Transvaal [Penge], showed a large number of natives who had left the mines because their vital capacity had been so reduced that they could no longer perform any useful work."[60]

There were other noble medical researchers who resisted the industry's controlling efforts in their work on ARDs. Neil White and Eric Bateman cite "a number of insightful epidemiological studies" undertaken in the late 1970s and early 1980s "by concerned scientists, calling for better control of South Africa's asbestos hazard,"[61] as exceptions in their otherwise candid retrospective of "a medical scientific community that for a variety of reasons had minimal discernible impact on policy or practice that might have prevented mesothelioma."[62] There were also critical interventions by others in the field that undoubtedly advanced awareness of the dangers of asbestos, even if, at the same time, their commitment to the cause was compromised by pressures applied on them by the industry.

Richard was by now well acquainted with this peculiar professional ambivalence as graphically illustrated in Ian Webster's work, born of his susceptibility to industry pressure, and by W. J. Smither (Cape's chief medical officer), who seemed torn between being appalled by the dust-polluted conditions the company tolerated at its operations in Prieska and Penge, while being unwilling to support further research into the medical consequences of such heavy exposure.[63] Another vivid example was Chris Wagner's fleeing the country and his *volte face* on the seriousness of asbestos's causal relationship with mesothelioma after he, Sleggs, and Marchand had done so much to alert the world of this lethal association. Such action is difficult to comprehend in any way other than a craven surrender to the vexed demands of domineering asbestos corporations.[64]

The whole conspiratorial saga was neatly summed up by Jonny Myers in his paper on "Asbestos and Asbestos-Related Disease in South Africa" published in 1980, the year after Cape had left the country. Myers refers to the carelessness of science initially making crass assumptions about "safe" levels of asbestos exposure that in effect prolonged "experimentation" on human beings, as scientists waited out the time lag for the carcinogenic effects of asbestos to reveal themselves. He also notes that waiting for such "incontrovertible proof" of asbestos's lethality offered an epidemiological gap into which "industry leap[ed], seeking a further lease of life for asbestos production and manufacture, putting out positive propaganda for the duration of this time gap of uncertainty."[65]

Myers's summation is a fitting testimony to the causes and human consequences of Cape's heel on the neck of science and to the shroud that the company tried, but ultimately failed, to throw over them. The challenge now facing Richard was how best to show all this at trial, in an argument built around the company's negligence and the damage it caused to people's lives and livelihoods.

CHAPTER 7

Outrage

—*Thumb Prints on Lawsuits*—

LIKE INDIANA JONES WITH A law degree, Richard returned to the office from his latest trip to South Africa laden with tall tales and evidentiary treasure. But this time there was a problem.

He'd driven out to the Cape's abandoned mine offices at Koegas in the Northern Cape with local social development worker Cecil Skeffers, who'd told him that "lots of interesting stuff is just lying around out there." Cecil was right. The mine site was desolate. It comprised one main building, a small accommodation block, and a few outhouses—all windowless, half-roofed, and being slowly reclaimed by the bush. It was hot and dry under a blazing sun as they picked their way through crumbling piles of asbestos roofing tiles and mounds of discarded, foot-long blue asbestos mine cores (the tell-tale cobalt blue shimmering under the silky-smooth surface of nearly every cylinder) to the office's front door. Cecil gave it a shove, and it creaked open. He wasn't surprised. Small communities of itinerants often commandeered deserted mine buildings, breaking whatever locks there were and ignoring the forbidding skull and crossbones signs at the mine entrance warning: "Danger. Old Mining Area.

Caving Ground." What surprised them was what they found inside. Open filing cabinets full of employee records, time sheets, and payment schedules dating back decades and seemingly untouched since the day the last Cape officer turned off the lights and left the building in 1980.[1]

As the case was now evolving into a class action involving thousands of claimants and given Cape's recent disclosure of a fire that had destroyed many of the records it held in UK storage, this find was potentially very valuable. Richard and Cecil packaged up and carried off as many files as the trunk and rear seat of Cecil's truck could accommodate and headed back down the road to Prieska. By the time Richard had returned to London with his booty a week later, the novelty of their discovery had worn off. But not so for his colleagues at Leigh Day. "You found them *where*? A blue asbestos mine!" Everyone in the firm was used to dealing with piles of dog-eared documents and bulging files occasionally layered with office dust. But documents and files potentially harboring crocidolite fiber dust was an entirely different matter. The whole cache was quarantined and a sample sent off for analysis. It took a few days before the results were returned, showing no evidence of blue asbestos contamination. Richard (and Leigh Day staff) could breathe a sigh of relief.

After relating this episode to me, Richard confessed that this was one of several occasions when he wondered whether he should have curbed his enthusiasm, which had perhaps, at times, bordered on foolhardy. He was chastened that he hadn't thought of testing the Koegas files before bringing them into the office in London and that neither he nor Cecil had worn masks as they'd shuffled through the dirt and debris at the mine site.

I must admit to having had the same nagging doubts when, twenty-five years later, I wandered maskless through the very same mine site with Cecil and Jack Adams as my guides. The slowly degrading asbestos cement tiles were still strewn across the ground and a huge mound of drill cores (like discarded artillery shells) was still heaped round the back of the office building. The whites-only swimming pool for mine managers and their families in the adjacent executive compound was now knee-deep in sludge and the once carefully manicured bowling green was a desiccated rubbish tip, albeit still presided over by a rusting placard declaring: "No children allowed." Down the road at the mine's railhead, where asbestos ore had been stockpiled, excavated anteater burrows exposed ominously thick deposits of blue asbestos fiber beneath the meager attempts to rehabilitate the dump with a thin layer of topsoil following the mine's closure. It was here, too, that Shawn Louw, who seemingly still lived on the site, held up the tiny sole of a toddler's shoe for me to photograph as we weaved our way past broken bottles and jagged-edged cans of spam and around a dried up "water pit," which were the only remaining evidence of the dozens of miners' families who'd once lived and worked there.[2] Nothing, it seemed, had changed much, even if the scene was now more *Mad Max* than *Raiders of the Lost Ark*.

≈

With the Court of Appeal's July 1998 judgment behind them, Richard and colleagues were now able to focus on the next stage of the trial of compiling evidence of Cape's negligence and documenting its consequences. While initially their plan had been to focus such efforts on the handful of original plaintiffs (in the expectation that Cape would at some point recognize the need to settle not only these few claims but also those of the many thousands like them), Cape's evident determination to contest the litigation compelled Richard to expand the number of signed-up claimants. The trial door toward which the case was now heading had been opened after the plaintiffs' jurisdictional victory in the Court of Appeal, although Cape had predictably sought leave to appeal that decision before the House of Lords. Given the uncertainty that comes with venturing into new legal territory, as Richard was doing with this case, he was hugely relieved when the House of Lords refused Cape's petition on December 16, 1998.

In denying Cape leave to appeal, their Lordships had elected on the day to hold only a brief hearing between the parties and to decide the matter mostly "on the papers." Having not known in advance whether oral argument would be required, Richard, Graham Read, and Barbara Dohmann had met in conference two days earlier at Dohmann's chambers. In the end their preparations that day were not put to task, but what was said during their meeting turned out to be pivotal in what happened next. For with the appeal route on the question of jurisdiction cut off, Cape's lawyers resorted to an alternative line of legal attack, this time aiming at Richard himself, claiming that he was guilty of an "abuse of process" by misleading the Court of Appeal. It was a move as devious as it was nasty but, nevertheless, one that very nearly worked as it played out over the months that followed.

≈

In the meantime, however, there were other important matters to attend to.

Richard celebrated Christmas Day 1998 with a day off to be with his family and friends. "I'm a pragmatist when it comes to Christian traditions," he says. But it was the only down time he allowed himself over the holiday period, before gearing up for the new High Court trial. In fact, life had been even more hectic than usual over the past few months as a tide of plaintiffs came on board and more staff had to be recruited in Leigh Day's London office as well as in its newly established offices in South Africa (in Prieska and Burgersfort, near Penge) to handle the workload.[3] By January 18, 1999, Richard was able to issue a new writ against Cape on behalf of Hendrik Afrika and no fewer than 1,538 others, to sit alongside the existing *Lubbe* action. Hendrik had been chosen as the lead plaintiff of this second writ, in part because of the symbolic importance of his surname attached to such a case, but also because of the emblematic nature of his circumstances.

When still a child, Hendrik had worked for seven years at the Prieska mill as a sample boy (collecting clumps of fiber for grading) and as a result had contracted asbestosis years later as an adult. He'd lived his whole life in the town's Red Block, in a neat little house painted duck-egg blue, and so had also been environmentally exposed to crocidolite dust. By the time he signed up with Richard, Hendrik was in his mid-fifties, wasted to the point that his limbs looked preternaturally long. His fingers were clubbed (swollen at their tips and with downward curved nails) in a fashion characteristic of advanced asbestosis,[4] and he had sad, pleading eyes.[5] He was numbed to his fate, though less so his wife, Gwendoline, who excoriated those she saw as the culprits. "They did not tell us of the dangers and now that we are ill, they don't want to take responsibility," she protested. "I would like to ask Cape's directors and shareholders to come to see what is going on here and what they did to our people."[6]

By the late 1990s, the epidemic of ARDs was at its height after decades of incubation in the asbestos communities of Northern Cape and Northern Transvaal. Limp bodies, sunken chests, and the ragged gasps of lungs under attack were seen and heard everywhere in these towns and villages. "Prieska is a living graveyard," said Cecil Skeffers at the time.[7] Anger, too, was rife. Gwendoline Afrika's finger-pointing was mirrored in Mafefe, where many of Cape's former workers at its Penge mine and mill lived. Zack Mabiletja, a colorful, firebrand community leader in the town, whose many years working with Marianne Felix had raised his awareness of the trail of disease left by asbestos, was taking the fight into politics. In one memorandum addressed to the provincial premier, the British ambassador, and Cape Plc, Zack mixed passion with powerful rhetoric. He began in an elegiac tone:

> In the foothills and plains of the Strydpoort Mountains in the Northern Province, thousands of men, women, and children are afflicted by a plague called asbestosis. This debilitating disease is choking off the life of the community. It cuts short adults working lives, condemns families to poverty, and ends with a slow, painful and early death.

He then got to the nub of his contention:

> This plague is the legacy of Cape PLC's mining activities in the area over several decades. . . . Cape brought no benefits to the area. It paid slave wages, it used child labour and it showed a complete and utter disregard for the health of its employees and the African people of the area.
>
> When the tide of world opinion turned against asbestos, Cape simply abandoned its responsibilities in South Africa and left. . . .
>
> We call on Cape PLC to face up to its responsibilities, to admit it has done a terrible wrong and to make recompense to its victims.[8]

In addition to committing these words to paper, Zack also delivered them verbally. As he stood in the back of a bakkie (pickup truck), flanked by local dignitaries, and in front of a crowd gathered outside government offices in Polokwane, the provincial capital of Limpopo, his message was loud and clear to all who heard it.[9]

Asbestos activism is intrinsically political. Thirty-plus years ago, it was also revolutionary. Under Apartheid, stark racial boundaries corresponded with the asbestos-related disease burden carried by each racial group, such that when people talked politics in places like Polokwane and Prieska, the asbestos industry, and Cape specifically, were always on the agenda. Growing up in Prieska's Red Block in the 1980s, Andrew Phillips remembers that "all the ANC [African National Congress] big shots used to stay at our house when they came to town." His mother, Fildah Bosman (whom we met in chapter 2), was a keen Women's League activist who'd warn Andrew not to tell anyone about their visitors. "I was only a kid, but I could tell it was part of an underground war," he says, before adding that in any case it wasn't hard to hide the ANC apparatchiks amid the hordes of "friends, relatives, and homeless" his kind-hearted mother was constantly taking in.[10] Living in such a "mecca," as he calls it, seems to have rubbed off on Andrew, as he later formed his own political party and was duly elected Prieska's mayor in November 2021.

Civil society was a key player in resisting both Apartheid and the asbestos industry throughout the 1990s, as South Africa transitioned to democracy. So it was no surprise that leading activists in the two provinces became natural allies of Richard and the case against Cape as it began to take shape. For example, Shadrack Molokane ("the ultimate operator," as Richard labeled him) was an important and well-connected supporter of the litigation, as were other community representatives, including Zack Mabiletja, on whom Richard relied to get information about the case to the locals in and around Penge. Similarly, Cecil Skeffers was a vital cog in the litigation machine for the people in and around Prieska.

Cecil had been one of the founders of Concerned People against Asbestos (CPAA) a few years earlier, in 1996, which, in addition to advocacy, was trying to get as many people as possible through government compensation schemes by assisting them in obtaining the necessary medical documentation from the Medical Board of Occupational Diseases (MBOD).[11] That so many former asbestos workers had been previously denied compensation was something very familiar to Cecil, who had earlier worked with the ANC, helping people negotiate the labyrinthian and discriminatory workers' compensation schemes under Apartheid. "That sort of practical help was really necessary," says Cecil. "Without it, people had nothing—no job, no income, no life."[12]

For Cecil, as well as husband-and-wife team Jack and Joyce Adams (who were also among the founders of the CPAA), the prospect of adding a new offensive dimension to their work by assisting Richard in the case against Cape was both appealing and exciting. Jack and Joyce were by then working in Leigh Day's new office in Prieska, and together with Cecil and a growing troop of long-silenced residents of the town, they were gathering as many claimants as they could find. With the same happening in Limpopo through Shadrack and Zack, a slew of further writs was issued in the High Court in London between January and April 1999, altogether representing several thousand plaintiffs.[13]

While there was indeed no shortage of potential claimants, getting all of them signed up as plaintiffs and in such a short time (the additional writs had all been issued within six weeks of the *Afrika* writ), was an enormous task. Building a case of this size is incredibly hard work, as Angela Andrews and Steve Kahanovitz told me—and they should know, being stalwarts of South Africa's Legal Resources Centre (LRC), famed for taking on high-profile, public interest cases.[14] "It's mostly drudgery," they say of having to compile questionnaires, organize affidavits, take instructions from clients, and sift through mountains of details looking for common themes and illustrative features, though one does occasionally find a revelatory "gotcha" nugget. Richard had hooked up with the LRC, not least to draw on the organization's long experience in fighting human rights and social justice cases in South Africa under Apartheid and now under its new, ambitious post-Apartheid constitution. Angela and Steve were enthusiastic supporters of the litigation against Cape and were especially helpful to Richard in evaluating and documenting the capacity (or incapacity) of South Africa's legal system to host such extensive litigation at that time. This was a matter that would, once again, be raised by Cape in the UK courts over the coming months and years.

≈

The unavoidably hard work of conducting questionnaires, taking witness statements, and collecting medical records was continuing apace, with more than 2,000 additional claimants signed up throughout late 1998 and early 1999 (which figure eventually grew to some 7,500 plaintiffs at the end of the case).* More London-based Leigh Day lawyers were also being engaged for the task. One of these was Sapna Malik, a recent graduate

---

* Categorized as follows: approximately three-quarters of claimants came from Limpopo, one-quarter from the Northern Cape, and 137 from Cape's Benoni factory near Johannesburg. Some 75 percent reflected an element of occupational exposure, while nearly all claimants had evidence of environmental exposure. In addition, 78 percent of claimants were registered as living; the remainder were registered as claims on behalf of the estates of deceased persons. Richard Meeran provided me with these details (communication, June 7, 2024), which he said he drew from a joint witness statement made by Richard and Anthony Coombs (who we encounter in the next chapter) at the conclusion of the case's final settlement in June 2003.

with a burning passion to right wrongs, bucket loads of talent, and a sharp, resolute intellect to back it up. She may not strike you as an ambitious alpha lawyer because she is so affable and self-effacing, with a kind and graceful manner, but that resolve is most certainly there. The day I interviewed her (by then a partner at Leigh Day) in the firm's offices in May 2023, she had just been made co-director (with Richard) of its blue-ribbon international law practice.

Back in October 1998, however, as she trudged from one Limpopo village to another and persevered through one interview after another, such prospects were far from Sapna's thoughts. She had originally flown out to South Africa for four days, which had then turned into four weeks. "But it was precisely the sort of work I wanted to do," she stresses. That said, she was still shocked by what she encountered. Poverty, sickness, discrimination, ignorance, and illiteracy; whole communities decimated, first by the pollution of asbestos mining when it was there and then by unemployment (and the inability to work) after it left. It was a sobering experience for Sapna in other ways, too.

At the end of one long day, she was helping a middle-aged black woman place her thumb print on a document by way of her signature. "She was shaking as I gently guided her hand towards the paper," Sapna recounts. "I asked her was she OK, and she sheepishly replied that I was the first white person ever to touch her. I was stunned. Not just by the fact that I'd never been called 'white' before, but at the depth of the racial divide this woman had obviously lived through."[15]

Sapna, like Richard, has Indian heritage, was born and brought up in England, and is acutely aware of racial divisions. "It really left an impression on me," she says of the encounter with this woman, as indeed did the whole exhausting, eye-opening trip. Working with Richard was inspiring, if also a little alarming, not least when she found that his "obsessive nature was beginning to rub off on me. The rest of life simply got pushed to one side."

Zanele Mbuyisa was another inspirational character whom Sapna met on a subsequent visit to South Africa. "We were about the same age," says Sapna, "and she too was a recently qualified lawyer." With obvious delight, she added that she loved watching this "forceful, dedicated black woman" in action. Zanele had learned to be tough, having grown up in the sprawling township of Vosloorus, 30 kilometers east of Johannesburg, in a single-mother household with four other kids. Her mother had instilled in her the importance of education, which propelled Zanele through law school and then to the Wits Law Clinic (WLC) in Johannesburg, another prestigious and hard-bitten civil liberties organization, where, as she says, "I began my training in 'real' law."[16] It was from the WLC that Zanele was plucked to join a small band of lawyers and helpers at Leigh Day's Prieska office in 2000. "The Northern Cape was a shock," she recalls. "Poor, hot, and openly racist." She felt especially marooned in such a tiny town as Prieska.

One of her first tasks there was to take a detailed statement from a very sick woman. This was Zanele's first encounter with mesothelioma, and she remembers admiring the stoic dignity with which her interviewee bore the illness. She was dismayed to hear that the woman had died a week later, and then she was angry: "It made me even more determined to help." She duly threw herself into the job, fearing neither hard work nor venturing her frank opinion.

It was Zanele, for example, who immediately brought to Richard's attention the fact that the toilets in Leigh Day's Prieska office were racially segregated. An overlooked legacy of the former tenants (Old Mutual, a finance firm) to be sure, but acutely embarrassing nonetheless. She began ordering office stationery from Kimberley rather than buying it locally because of the sly discrimination she encountered in town ("They complained about my poor Afrikaans accent"). And it was Zanele who pushed for the increasingly regular community meetings with victims and litigants to be shifted from the "white" church hall in Prieska to the much bigger Omega Community Hall of the "coloured" church across town. By her own admission, Zanele is something of a rebel, so some of her sense of being a square-peg-in-a-round-hole likely came from her anti-establishment views as much as being a young black woman amid a population that, while mostly coloured, was traditionally governed by white men.

She was getting to know Richard—who was another novelty to the locals, she notes—as they traveled the countryside together. "I could see how odd they thought Richard was—not giving a fuck how big his opponents were." She loved that about him, and while they often disagreed, she is eternally grateful to him. "I learnt so much. I was allowed to believe in myself. As a black township girl, it was a huge confidence boost. And coming from an English boy!"

She's telling me all this twenty-five years later, sitting in a file-cluttered office in her own law firm in Johannesburg, where she continues to push for justice for the powerless against the powerful, whoever they might be. Enormously energetic, with her hair pulled back businesslike from her face and spryly attentive eyes behind huge square, black-framed glasses, she says what she admires most about Richard is his integrity: "When I first met him, he said that 'the clients are the most important; they must be treated with dignity.' I've never forgotten that."

"But my God, he was a scary driver," she suddenly blurts out after a long, thoughtful pause. Perpetually distracted by whatever conversation was going on in the car and frequently turning around to stress a point to those in the back seat, Richard had a number of close calls with the old roadside telegraph poles engulfed by colossal grass birds' nests, which are so distinctive on the long, straight roads of the Northern Cape.[17] "Often he'd forget to change gear, and we'd be stuck in third for miles," she recalls. The first time this happened, she and Jack Adams were so startled that they simultaneously whispered: "What is he doing?" to each other, before one of them coughed and gently suggested that Richard might consider moving up a gear or two.

Driving long distances was a big part of the job at that time, as they traveled between towns, villages, and old mine sites, collecting materials, assembling clients, and explaining the case at community meetings. Zanele learned to drive while she was stationed in Prieska—though *not* from Richard, she protests, despite then admitting that she "banged into everything" (reversing seems to have been a particular problem). Apparently, however, she was not alone in this respect, such that the Avis Car Hire at Kimberley Airport regarded Leigh Day's business as a distinct liability.

Against (or perhaps in support of) this reputation, I can attest to Jack's merciless driving when, more than two decades later, he piloted Cecil and me the 140 kilometers from Prieska to the abandoned Koegas mine. My notes for that day read, in part: "He pushed my wee hire car [coincidentally also from Avis at Kimberley Airport] to its limits, doing 160 kms per hour accompanied by an alarming groan coming from the car's back end as its less than aerodynamic design was found out. Even off-road, Jack kept his foot to the floor, seemingly pursuing the idea that flying above the rutted dirt track was better than staying in contact with it." Nonetheless, we arrived and returned safely.[18]

When, back in their day, Leigh Day folk arrived at their destinations—with or without driving incidents en route—they were always warmly welcomed. Word had got about, so their visits to places throughout the Northern Cape and Limpopo were attracting bigger and bigger crowds. "We knew there was a huge latent demand for something to be done about the 'forgotten epidemic' of ARDs," says Richard, "but we were still taken aback by how many they were and how 'forgotten' they felt." His case files were now bulging as he criss-crossed the country, which meant that the workload back in Leigh Day's London office was expanding exponentially. Throughout 1998 and 1999, and especially in 2000, more of the firm's existing workforce was assigned to the case, and a raft of paralegals was recruited to take on some of the administrative heavy lifting, often literally as well as figuratively, given the quantities of physical documentation the case was generating in those pre-electronic storage days.[19]

≈

The sort of paralegals a case like this attracts (beyond the prerequisite of a strong back) are nearly always driven by the social justice cause it represents. They're seldom attracted by financial reward, or by big-end-of-town clients, still less by prospects of wearing sharp suits or occupying a corner office. Typically appointed for short terms, paralegals engaged on such big class action, public interest cases can seem like a ragtag bunch of young idealists. But while (commendably) starry-eyed they may be, they are also often among the smartest, most dedicated, and hardest working of their graduating cohort. So it was with the crew that Leigh Day employed for the Cape case, but with an additional special ingredient of a dash of style and drama.

Dave Neita is hard to miss. He's waving theatrically at me as I pass through the gatehouse of Lincoln's Inn in London's legal district. A bear of a man with a handshake to match, he's wearing an expensive-looking coat, and his mane of dreadlocks, now tinged grey, is buffeted by the chilly spring breeze. He's a barrister (at Lincoln's Inn) and a renowned poet, performing in both callings with the same loud, passionate embrace that he credits to a strong, loving mother and a happy childhood in Jamaica.[20] He treats me with similar enthusiastic warmth as I fire questions about his time as a paralegal on the Cape case over tea in the Members Common Room tucked beneath the Inn's magnificent Great Hall.

Dave joined Leigh Day a few months after qualifying as a barrister. He'd met a colleague of Richard's, Olive Lewin, in a Jamaican coffee shop on Oxford Street where he regularly performed poetry. She'd told him about the case and that the firm was looking for recruits. "I loved the idea of the case and being a part of a legal team fighting injustice," he told me, "so I signed up."[21] He admits that the sheer quantity of "discovery" documentation was "mind-numbing"—finding it, collating it, and, most tiresome of all, copying it. Photocopying was the norm at the time, though Dave took a lead in trying out the then revolutionary alternative of scanning documents, in the hope that it might lessen the burden. Some forty to fifty paralegals in all were involved in the case, so it was a big enterprise, and the esprit de corps was terrific, but after a while it wasn't quite enough for Dave. He wrote a note to Richard one day, pleading with him that he (Richard) take him to South Africa on his next trip: "I have to meet these folk. I cannot just read about them anymore."

Richard relented, and soon Dave found himself packing his bags. "It was the best legal experience of my life," he exclaims. Used to "throwing myself into spaces," on this occasion Dave did more looking, listening, and learning. The human stories of suffering, racism, and classism that "had jumped out at me from the pages I'd read" were doubly compelling when he met the people behind them. Dave also came to appreciate the full scope of the "orchestra that Richard was conducting." "He was incredible," says Dave, a real "people's hero," he adds with a flourish.

The trip also provided Dave with material for his professional alter ego when he and Richard stayed in one guesthouse where the guard dogs had been specifically trained to attack only black people. His poem "Racist Dogs" is a rumination not only on the depravity of such a divided society but also on the cold comfort offered by the owner who told them that he'd lock up the dogs "while you two are staying here."[22]

Taking Dave into the heart of this maelstrom of tragedy and injustice turned out to be a stroke of genius on Richard's part, as the experience energized Dave's considerable capacity to broadcast, galvanize, and dramatize. "His enthusiasm never waned," says Richard, "nor did his conviction that we would win, even if I was not so sure," he adds. Back in London, Dave helped to whip up support for the case by any means that came to his fertile mind—in new material for his regular poem readings; organizing a concert in the church hall opposite Leigh Day's offices to raise money for a mobile medical scanner for the communities in Penge and Prieska; and another, cheeky fundraiser within the office, based on bids to shave off Richard's moustache (to the lasting advantage of both the claimants and Richard's face).[23]

≈

Funding the case was now more pressing that ever. Managing the explosion in client numbers, the multiplying workforce, the creation of new offices in Prieska and later Burgersfort, and the now frequent shuttling of lawyers and staff between London and Johannesburg (and beyond), not to mention the rocketing cost of hire car insurance—all had to be paid for. So, in October 1998, shortly after their success in the Court of Appeal, Richard applied to the United Kingdom's Legal Aid Board (LAB) to extend funding beyond the original handful of claimants to encompass several thousands more.

It was a laborious task, requiring completion of two separate forms (one asking for basic details, the other a means test) for each of the first batch of just over 1,500 claimants (with that number steadily rising to nearly 7,500 claimants over the coming years), but ultimately almost all were successful.[24] Naturally, the claimants easily passed the means test. Crucially, they also qualified *despite* being foreign nationals (on the basis that their suit was against a UK company). "It was a lucky break," admits Richard, as the small window of a few years during which the United Kingdom permitted non-citizen, legal aid applicants was closed in 2000. Predictably, however, not everyone appreciated the claimants' (and Leigh Day's) luck. Scandalized accounts appeared in the British media falsely declaring that "South Africans cost [UK] taxpayers £9 million in legal aid" (in the end the figure was £2.5 million). Ruth Lea, the head of the United Kingdom's Institute of Directors, was reported saying that such legally aided cases involving foreign workers were "absurd" and setting "a very dangerous precedent," that could force British companies to "re-register overseas."[25]

Media and corporate beat-ups aside, securing funding (effectively guaranteeing LAB's coverage of the baseline costs of all *unsuccessful* claimants in the legal proceedings to follow) was essential for the case to proceed, even if, as Richard reflects, it only covered about half of Leigh Day's actual costs. The whole process had turned out to be a huge challenge, especially for the first five claimants, whose applications were initially rejected and granted only on appeal to the Legal Aid Appeal Committee. Thereafter, an extension of legal aid needed to be obtained at every new stage in the proceedings. "It was by no means a rubber-stamping exercise," he notes matter-of-factly, "but it took care of cash flow—the day-to-day expenses of the case—and that was critical."[26] The firm's partners had, after all, taken on the

case knowing that it would cost them financially (albeit, hope-
fully, not ruinously so); it was the principle of righting a grave
injustice that had drawn them in at first, and that remained their
abiding rationale for pursuing it.

≈

The size of the case, its sensitive subject matter, and the win
they had secured in the Court of Appeal in July 1998, followed
by the House of Lords' refusal of Cape's petition to appeal five
months later, had attracted serious media attention. Richard
was being interviewed and quoted in all the United Kingdom's
broadsheet newspapers, he was appearing on TV news chan-
nels and in documentary programs, and his name and reputation as a formidable maverick were now well known in legal
circles.[27] Richard was a savvy media operator, being proactive
(not just reactive) in his relations with activists and journalists.

One of his most effective, and certainly striking, ploys to generate publicity for the case arose from a chance encounter in a
bar in Kimberley with a young South African photographer
named Hein du Plessis. Richard was so moved by du Plessis's
ability to capture the dignity of his mainly elderly subjects in the
sample photographs he showed him that Richard commissioned
him on the spot to record the lives and struggles of asbestos victims in the Northern Cape. Shot in black and white, the resulting
images (many of which adorn this book) still have an immediate impact on anyone who sees them. Raw, sad, angry, and
bathed in pathos, they show bodies and lives disfigured by disease that the subjects in the photographs by then knew was
preventable, but had not been not prevented any more than the
danger had been disclosed to them. Richard organized a series
of public exhibitions of the collection (with invitations to the media), entitled *Cape Dust*, at venues throughout London, including

above Westminster Hall in the Houses of Parliament, the Royal Festival Hall, and the Stephen Lawrence Gallery. Later, as another fundraiser, he auctioned copies of the photographs in the same church hall opposite Leigh Day's offices as Dave Neita had previously used for his concert.[28]

Beyond his own efforts, Richard now found himself and the case being hoisted onto the broad and uncompromising shoulders of the global anti-asbestos movement. Aligned by the twin objectives of banning asbestos worldwide and bringing governments and corporations to account for the damage caused by its mining and manufacture, this loosely connected network of organizations, affected individuals, and sympathizers was as passionate as it was widespread. Laurie Kazan-Allen, one of its leading campaigners, became an important driving force behind the promotion of the Cape case. A tireless and self-effacing activist, Laurie was then editor of *British Asbestos Newsletter*, a scholar, author, and an extremely well-connected operator.[29] "Her support meant a lot to me," says Richard, "and her willingness to get involved alongside her great pot-stirring skills helped push the case to audiences in the United Kingdom and overseas."[30]

The well-publicized nature of the case and the sheer numbers of victims involved raised two critically important challenges for Richard. First, there was the tricky question of how to manage the expectations of the claimants, as individuals and collectively. While Richard was keen to incorporate as many victims as possible in the action, the very fact that he was acting as their lawyer in litigation against Cape in British courts naturally invited comparisons to be made with other asbestos cases or claims pursued in the United Kingdom. That British asbestos victims of corporate neglect were being awarded comparatively enormous five- and six-figure payouts (while awards in the United States were even larger, often ten times as much)[31] conjured similar expectations in the minds of many South Africans.

Richard, therefore, had to draw on every last ounce of his diplomacy and communication skills to convey accurate but also intelligible messages to his audiences about the nature of the litigation, its progress, and likely outcomes. It was, to be sure, a delicate exercise combining clarification of legal peculiarities, crystal ball–gazing, and candid realism. As though teaching a "Law 101" class, he had to explain that the legal system focuses on process rather than outcome, thereby sometimes producing outcomes that are unjust, or at least not as fair as people had hoped or expected. And while he seemed to walk this tightrope with some aplomb—"sitting above the people, but also part of them," as Dave Neita puts it—he was forever cautioning that winning the case was far from certain, let alone securing substantial sums in compensation.

However candid the message, it didn't stem the flood of interest in the case, as victims and their families warmed to the idea that, at the very least, it provided an opportunity to bring Cape to account. In Prieska, the venue for the crowds who came to hear Richard had to be moved (at Zanele's prompting) from the prim and proper "white" church hall to the bigger sprawl of the Omega Community Hall, which was the main venue for meetings of the coloured and black communities in town, but even there, as Jack Adams put it, "there was no room to swing a cat." Meetings always began with a prayer and when discussions became heated—which over the coming years of frustration they occasionally were—a peacekeeper would intervene, sometimes in Baptist song, to break the tension.

The gatherings were even larger in Limpopo, held outdoors, with people perched on every available vantage point. They also tended to be more political and unruly. The National Union of

Miners' presence and influence were more pronounced there than in the Northern Cape, but in both places the message was the same. People wanted atonement for what had been done to them, and in the liberated air of the new, post-Apartheid South Africa, they were demanding it. Managing these great expectations made of Richard by his clients was somewhat unnerving, but at least it was founded on a belief, however inflated, in his ability to deliver.

The second major challenge facing Richard was very different and far more threatening. Ever since the House of Lords had denied Cape leave to appeal in December 1998, Cape's lawyers had been formulating a direct attack on Richard's legal competence or, more precisely, on his professional conduct. On the face of it, their intention was to reopen the jurisdictional question by arguing that there had been an "abuse of process" on the part of the plaintiffs' lawyers in their conduct before the Court of Appeal during its hearings the previous July. What, however, they were really trying to do was to find another way to avoid facing a trial that focused on the question of Cape's negligence. Either way, on February 5, 1999, barely two weeks after Richard had filed the *Afrika* writ (alleging negligence), Cape's lawyers issued two new summonses in the High Court, one claiming an abuse of process and the other, flowing from the first, seeking a stay of both the *Lubbe* and *Afrika* actions as well as any new proceedings against Cape that Richard was then in the process of filing.

Of the first claim, Cape alleged that Richard had misled the Court of Appeal in 1998 by not expressly indicating that the original five plaintiffs in the *Lubbe* case would be joined by many (perhaps thousands of) others, if and when the question of jurisdiction was settled in their favor. Following the Court of Appeal's pronouncement that jurisdiction did indeed reside in the United Kingdom courts and Leigh Day's subsequent assembly of thousands more claimants, Cape's lawyers now argued that such expanded numbers of plaintiffs were neither anticipated nor flagged and that therefore the Court of Appeal had been misled. This abuse of process argument was in fact *ad hominem* in that it was directed solely at Richard's actions and intentions.[32]

The second summons issued by Cape sought to apply or re-apply for a stay of both the *Afrika* and *Lubbe* actions on the very same ground (*forum non conveniens*) as had been denied by the Court of Appeal eight months earlier in *Lubbe*. It was obvious, therefore, that Cape was banking on the introduction of the new abuse point as a game-changer in its otherwise rehashed juris-dictional argument that the United Kingdom was *not* an appro-priate forum in which to try these cases. Whatever the reasoning, it was a low blow, especially as there seemed little doubt that everyone involved in the case, including Cape's lawyers, had all assumed that the first five plaintiffs were just the tip of the ice-berg of potential claimants. It was a "gloves-off" moment to question Richard's professional integrity in this way, and it showed how hard (or desperate) Cape and its lawyers were pre-pared to fight the case.

Further evidence of the heavy-handed tactics the other side were minded to employ in besmirching Richard's character was provided a couple of weeks later when news reached him about some scurrilous activities of Cape's South African attorneys, Webber Wentzel Bowens (WWB). Lawyers from the firm had targeted community leaders in Prieska—Obert Mahlo, chair-person of the CPAA, and Christa Smith, a counselor with a prominent social services non-profit organization, as well as Cecil Skeffers (the three, coincidentally, representing the black, white, and coloured communities, respectively)—asking each of them what Leigh Day was doing in the town.[33] The WWB lawyers said they were only "looking for basic information" about the claimants engaging with Leigh Day, what sort of health checks had they undergone, and whether they (Obert, Christa, and Cecil) were claimants themselves. But they made it clear they were happy to pay for the information and—in respect of Cecil—also advised him that "Cape Plc was prepared to make a settlement offer of ZAR 100 million [£10 million at the time]."[34]

Underhanded though such approaches were, they seemed more aggressively ham-fisted than seriously menacing, Christa Smith noted in her subsequent affidavit that "the impression I got was that he [the WWB attorney] was on a fishing expedition as he was battling to get co-operation from people in the community."[35] Like the other two, Christa stonewalled her interlocutor, bluntly telling him that her husband had died just weeks before from mesothelioma at the age of fifty, having lived and worked in Prieska (and played in the mill's asbestos dumps as a kid) all his life.[36] There is no record of whether the WWB lawyer retreated shamefaced.

The story was the same in Limpopo. Zack Mabiletja recalls being contacted by a WWB lawyer who invited him to Johannesburg, booked him into a hotel room, and then promised him an all-expenses-paid trip to London if he would agree to testify against Richard. Presumably WWB wanted Zack to implicate Richard in Cape's abuse of process argument, along the lines of Zack having witnessed Richard's intentions to mount a multi-party action from the outset of the litigation (and thereby misleading the Court of Appeal in July 1998). But WWB overplayed its hand and the gambit failed. Not only did Zack find the lawyers' behavior odd, he found it intimidating. "I had an uneasy feeling about it all," he told me when I asked him about the episode. After meeting with the WWB lawyers that evening and telling them that he wasn't interested, he'd returned to his hotel room. "But I couldn't sleep. I left the hotel in a hurry at 5 a.m. the next morning to escape back to Limpopo." It's not hard to understand Zack's apprehension and antipathy. The fact that he had been, in his own words, "politicized by the asbestos problem" and that so many of his friends and colleagues had died of ARDs after working for years in Cape's mines, underlined both how inept was WWB's approach and Zack's resolve not to cooperate.[37]

There is little doubt that these overtures by WWB lawyers—no matter how spectacularly unsuccessful—were nonetheless attempting to tap into an old vein of support for Cape in both communities that, they hoped, harbored doubts about the merits of the current litigation against it. Cape had been the principal employer in Prieska and around Penge for decades, so evidently there were some (many, even) who at that time had much invested in the company's continuing prosperity.[38] The depth of such feeling was made clear by Matthys van Rooyen, who had practiced medicine alongside André Pickard in Prieska throughout the 1950s and 1960s. He described a prevailing skepticism in those early years whenever he and André warned of the danger asbestos posed to the community's health. "People saw *us* as dangers," he intoned. "You must remember . . . everything they own[ed] in the world was invested in Prieska. . . . They thought [we] would be trying to take away their livelihood." The most brutal responses came, unsurprisingly, from Cape executives, whose threatening and dismissive manner was summed up by one especially acerbic comment directed at Matthys's concerns: "With our directors in London earning a million a year, do you think they would listen to you?"[39]

By 1999, however, with Cape long gone and whatever economic benefits it had brought to these asbestos communities long forgotten, there were in fact very few Cape supporters or litigation skeptics to be found. Sure, both Zack (in Penge) and Christa (in Prieska) encountered some resistance to their advocacy activities, but it was mostly the petty power politics of local bureaucrats, jealous of the attention their protests were attracting.[40]

On one occasion, for instance, Prieska's mayor, Lillian Valacia, whose sympathies apparently lay with Cape, tried to sideline Richard and Zanele in a town hall meeting with community representatives when she started speaking in Afrikaans—which she knew neither Richard nor Zanele could understand—even though she could speak English perfectly well. After hearing the rough translation of one especially distasteful proposal (that whereas all white claimants' grants would be processed in Prieska, the next of kin of deceased black claimants' estates would have to travel 240 kilometers to Kimberly for processing), Richard interrupted her suggesting that perhaps the national media would be interested to hear about such blatant discrimination. She switched immediately to English and dropped the proposal.[41] Another time, again in Prieska, council members accused Christa of fomenting disquiet among the town's residents by encouraging them to listen to what Richard had to say. Indignant, Christa dismissed their complaints with a withering, "Well, the graveyard is full of people who laid down their lives because of asbestos!"[42]

And so it is. (Notably, the cemetery was one of the first places Cecil brought me to see when I visited Prieska.) Back then, as Richard and his team were shuttling back and forth across the country processing a rising tide of claimants, all they were encountering was outrage, anger, and fear expressed by the living, the dying, and the loved ones of those already dead and buried.

CHAPTER 8

Offensive Lawyers
—Clean Hands and Dirty Tricks—

HE HAD COME AND GONE IN A FLASH. Like any other in the steady stream of couriers dropping off documents and parcels at Leigh Day's reception desk in its Priory House offices in London, he'd chirped, "This is for you," as he handed over a manila envelope, turned on his heel, and left. It was February 1999, and with the Cape case feverishly ramping up business, the foyer was a hive of activity. But this delivery was different. It was a leak, orchestrated, apparently, by someone close to Cape who was appalled by how far the company was prepared to go in fighting the case against it. Hand-written in block letters, it was simply addressed: "PRIVATE—THE PARTNER DEALING WITH CAPE PLC." Inside was a sheaf of about thirty pages comprising two euphemistically entitled "audits" by a public relations firm engaged by Cape. One was a media audit and the other a political and communications audit. Both were recent, dated January 20 and 27, 1999, respectively. Together, they outlined a strategy for what amounted to a reputational hit job on Leigh Day.[1]

The principal purpose of this offensive was to devise a public relations vehicle that would divert attention away from questions

about Cape's responsibilities for the plight of thousands of its former employees, their families, and local communities in South
Africa and toward questions of whether British taxpayers should
be footing the legal aid bill for foreigners to sue a British company in UK courts. The public relations firm, Media Strategy,
was unashamedly explicit about this diverting tactic, which, it
suggested brightly, would "give Cape a good chance of turning
the spotlight away from the responsibilities of multi-nationals to
their former third world employees."

Neither was it bashful about encouraging the right-wing media (such as the *Daily Mail*) to paint the litigants as unworthy
of such assistance from the British taxpayer, precisely because
they were non-white and poor, as well as foreigners:

> The political ironies are so delicious for a paper like the Mail
> (a Labour Lord Chancellor having to choose between black
> workers and multi-nationals) that the details of the claims are
> likely to be of secondary interest. Cape cannot avoid being part of
> any story, but the taxpayer and the politics will be the headline
> issue rather than any alleged lack of safety procedures in a Trans-
> vaal mine 30 years ago.[2]

That the strategy necessarily involved targeting Leigh Day
as the orchestrator of the supposed wastage of public funds
and therefore deserving of condemnation, censure, and financial sanction was, it seems, especially attractive in providing
Cape with the opportunity to avenge all the trouble the firm
had caused Cape over the past three years or so. "A substantial
story about an 'ambulance chasing' law firm will be uncomfortable for Leigh Day," wrote Media Strategy (alluding to Leigh
Day's ongoing litigation against tobacco corporations as well as
the Cape case), especially, it noted, as any reduction or cancella-
tion of legal aid funding would "exert further pressure" on the

firm. Managing to combine displays of profound ignorance and callous disregard for the destitution of so many of the plaintiffs, the authors then added: "The spurious nature of many of the claims . . . will help to undermine Leigh Day's credibility. Is Leigh Day really going to apply for legal aid for someone identified only by the name of a village?"[3]

It was a prime example of a manifesto of supercilious bastardry, backed up by a forensically detailed plan of which politicians, government officials, and media outlets to target in delivering its objectives.

Davies Arnold Cooper (DAC), Cape's UK solicitors, were party to this affair, having been identified by Media Strategy as correspondents in documentation detailing Leigh Day's efforts to obtain legal aid for its clients. The firm had an exceptionally close relationship with Cape, having acted for the company for decades. "It seemed more like a family relationship rather than one based purely on business," Richard says. Such fealty meant that any perceived attack on Cape such as the present litigation was seemingly felt personally by its lawyers, who reacted accordingly. With Brian Doctor as counsel throughout the entirety of the case, Cape's legal team was tightknit and at least as passionate about protecting its corporate client as Leigh Day and its counsel were about procuring justice for their clients by calling Cape to account. It was these shared levels of commitment to their clients' respective campaigns that made their court battles so bitter and barbed the longer the case carried on.

≈

Graham Read from Devereux Chambers had acted as counsel for Richard in his earlier *Thor Chemicals* and *Connelly* cases,[4] both of which were forerunners to *Lubbe v. Cape* in tackling questions of corporate liability under UK law for damage caused by corporate actions overseas. Though a junior barrister at the time, Graham's constant presence throughout the Cape litigation was immensely important. Next to Richard, his knowledge of the legal dimensions of the case was unmatched, and even his understanding of the metastasizing complexities of its factual details was extensive, given the time he was spending with Richard and Susannah Read (no relation to Graham, incidentally). As the matter progressed, Graham found himself increasingly wedded to its outcome personally, as well as professionally. Though he desperately wanted to win the case on its legal merits, he was nonetheless focused on the needs and wishes of claimants. "The key thing," he told me, "was to get compensation for the victims, however the case turned out in the courts."[5]

Graham had previously crossed swords with Brian Doctor (who'd represented Rio Tinto Zinc in the *Connelly* case), so they were known to each other. But the two were very different as barristers and as personalities. While Doctor was bull-doggishly aggressive in court, Graham was more cordially cerebral. Graham is also extremely affable. A wry observer of the human condition, he punctuates conversations with witty asides, his face creasing and his whole upper body gently bobbing up and down as he chuckles in delight. With a hint of teddy bear in appearance, he shuffles along, often in a flurry of papers and thoughts he is forever bringing to order. Habitually, when his brain is duly motoring through the gears, he slowly forces his fingers through his hair, fashioning an unruly mohawk from the crest of which he seems to conjure some thought or order-imposing structure. He has, above all, a canny legal mind, especially adept at detecting strategic roadblocks and land mines laid by the other side—skills that he and Richard were often to draw on in the coming months.

Graham's take on Cape's abuse of process argument was characteristically empathetic and emphatic. The ruthless manner of the other side's targeting of Richard, seeking to attack his integrity and thereby tarnish both his professional reputation and that of Leigh Day, was exaggerated and cynical in Graham's view, especially when it was being used principally as a vehicle to undermine the first Court of Appeal's judgment in favor of the plaintiffs permitting them to argue their case before the UK courts. "I felt for him," Graham says of Richard. "What he went through at that time was incredible—being pilloried in the press and by the profession." Graham knew the abuse arguments were a mere forensic ploy, built on foundations of sand at best. "So what!" was his clipped response when I asked him about Cape's claims that Richard had always known that the final number of claimants was likely to be hundreds or thousands.

"So what," indeed, for it had been understood from the very outset by all parties—the litigants, their lawyers, and the judges before whom they appeared—that the well of claimants from which the first five plaintiffs had been drawn was very deep. Most particularly, neither Cape nor any of its lawyers had previously aired any concerns about numbers. They, better than anyone, knew how deep the well ran, yet their arguments thus far had focused primarily on jurisdiction and secondarily, on rebutting allegations of negligence. Indeed, rather than showing concern, they had been keen to highlight the prospect of additional claimants. During the first Court of Appeal hearing on July 28, 1998, for example, Brian Doctor expressly acknowledged the likelihood that behind the initial case of five plaintiffs lay many more. He was, in fact, adamant in stressing the "enormous ramifications" of such a circumstance. Noting that "for the parties themselves in this case, the individual claims are not that great,"

Doctor then added, "but your Lordships would know that the case is seen as something of a test case and that, as far as the defendant is concerned, there may well be other claimants of this sort."[6] What is more, Justice Buckley in the High Court, before whom Cape first ran the abuse of process argument in July 1999, also underlined this general acceptance among parties of the numbers involved, saying, "I am quite satisfied that everyone realised there *could* be many more claimants."[7]

Nonetheless, the fact that the numbers of plaintiffs did expand—specifically in the form of the *Afrika* writ of 1,539 claimants—was a significant development in Justice Buckley's view, such that while he "stop[ped] short of finding an abuse of process" by Richard, his Honour determined that Richard "did not tell the whole story" and was therefore "misleading." "I conclude," he continued, "that it had for some considerable time been Leigh Day's intention to bring a multi-party action."[8]

Such a conclusion was good enough for Brian Doctor's purposes. It didn't matter that he'd failed in his vigorous contention that an abuse of process (a more serious offense) had occurred when, as he put it, "Mr Meeran carefully selected the five Lubbe claimants for the purpose of the forum debate which Mr Meeran knew would arise . . . when in fact it was always a case on jurisdiction for many more potential claimants." Why not? Well, because Doctor's spotlighting the new circumstance of suits involving thousands, rather than merely a handful of plaintiffs, successfully persuaded Justice Buckley that "the number of claimants and whether the case is likely to run as a group action is [*sic*] highly material" to the question of which jurisdiction (South Africa or the United Kingdom) was most appropriate to try the case. And given, in Justice Buckley's opinion, that "almost everything" in the case took place in South Africa, he sided with Cape. His ruling on July 30, 1999, declared that the most appropriate forum was South Africa and, as such, duly granted stays on both the *Afrika* group action and the *Lubbe* case being pursued in UK courts.[9]

It was a sensational turnaround. In one fell swoop the claimants' victory before the Court of Appeal exactly one year earlier was undone. In a manner that felt to Richard like a beat up, a straw man concocted by Cape's lawyers, the trial door opened earlier by the Court of Appeal—affording the claimants the opportunity to argue the heart of the case, namely, that the damage and suffering they endured was caused by Cape's negligence—was once again slammed shut. It was a war of attrition, being waged by Cape and its lawyers, frantic as they were to avoid getting sucked into a legal argument on whether Cape owed the *Lubbe* claimants a duty of care and the potentially dire consequences the company would face should it lose that argument. I asked Graham Read whether at the time it felt a bit like Cape was fighting "Custer's Last Stand"? "More like Napoleon's Battle of Borodino," he countered, alluding to Cape's seeming preparedness to sacrifice so much—reputation, company finances, and even dignity—to duck responsibility.

One significant blow that Cape's lawyers managed to land on the plaintiffs' case came from their otherwise fruitless efforts to gather implicating information in South Africa on Richard's intentions and actions signing up new clients. As mentioned in the previous chapter, Obert Mahlo, Christa Smith, Cecil Skeffers, Zack Mabiletja, and Deon Smith had all resisted or rebuffed overtures made to them by WWB, Cape's South African lawyers. But in Tony Davies they found an old-school Christian charity and a willingness to help that dispelled any initial wariness Tony might have felt when approached by Nic Alp from WWB. "I was naive," Tony confesses, "though at the time I was just being frank!"[10] The approach seemed innocent enough: they "ask[ed] for assistance," he later stated in an affidavit, "to acquire background knowledge about a complex matter of which they said they knew little."[11] And in fact, background knowledge is what Tony provided them.

In February 1999, Tony had written a report detailing the incidents of occupational lung disease and pulmonary tuberculosis among former miners in Limpopo, many of whom had worked in Cape's mine at Penge. The report's intended audiences included Department of Health officials and other researchers, as well as the miners themselves and their communities, to be used as a means of helping them gain access to statutory compensation. But Tony believed it might also help educate WWB and Cape, so he provided them with a copy.

> As there was a mass of evidence, mostly adverse from Cape's point of view, I thought it would speed up the process. I thought the documentation which I gave to Cape's lawyers was to be used to provide them with badly needed background . . . demonstrat[ing] that there were hundreds of cases who could potentially claim if any were entitled to do so. . . . I was trying to be helpful in supplying them with material I thought might help Cape understand why they should settle these people's claims.[12]

The report was built on years of research during which Tony had interviewed and examined several thousand former mineworkers, so he knew what he was talking about. Yet still, Tony admits that his "initial suspicion [of the approach from WWB's lawyers] was that they might end up twisting my words in the time-honored legal manner." Which, in the end, is precisely what happened.

A passage in the report referred to Tony's "association" with Richard and Leigh Day having lasted some three years, during which time the firm had been preparing a case against Cape and was "currently involved in registering larger numbers of former employees of the company who have been certified by the MBOD [Medical Board of Occupational Diseases]." While the report went on to specify the help that Tony (and Marianne Felix) provided in identifying the five initial plaintiffs in the *Lubbe* action, taking care to distinguish that case from Leigh Day's "current" registration of many more, it was the disclosure of the three-year association with Richard that Cape's lawyers latched onto. Such a lengthy collaboration, they claimed, might be read as indicative of Richard's prior intention to orchestrate a class action, no matter that the initial *Lubbe* writ comprised just five claimants. Twisted though this logic is, it worked. Justice Buckley cited it approvingly in reaching his conclusion that Leigh Day had long harbored the intention to bring a multi-party action and to that extent had misled the Court of Appeal.[13]

Tony (and Richard) could see how mistaken this was. As Tony noted in his affidavit that since he was "writing [the report] in February 1999, it is of course true that the registration of further cases had begun, but it is wrong to conclude that the registration of large numbers of cases began three years ago." No matter the soundness of such reasoning, it went unheeded. Tony was stunned and embittered.

> As a professional medical doctor I am truly horrified by the way my report written . . . long after the events Cape now seeks to rely on, for a specific non-legal audience, has been "picked over" and distorted by Cape's lawyers, particularly as I only gave the document in order to help convince Cape that they ought to consider compensation for these ill people. I am afraid it reaffirms my worst suspicions of lawyers generally.[14]

There was one lawyer, however, to whom he humbly apologized for his naivete—Richard. But as Richard recalls the episode,

"I held no grudge and told him not to worry as it was par for the course in highly contentious cases like this one." The two remained firm friends until Tony's death in March 2024 at the age of ninety-two.

The abuse of process argument based on the contention that Leigh Day (and specifically Richard) had failed to provide full and frank disclosure of the prospect, or even just likelihood, of many more claimants joining the case, had now become a major problem. One that could very well sink the whole ship, as Buckley J in the High Court had just shown, taking down with it all cases and all claimants on board, as well as the lawyers trying to pilot it through the rough seas of the law. Yet, frustratingly, it was not a problem that had been unforeseen by Richard and Graham Read.

Following their victory in the Court of Appeal in July 1998, Richard and his team were faced with two strategic challenges. First, while initially it had been Richard's intention to limit the case to just the original handful of plaintiffs (in the belief that winning on their behalf would compel Cape to settle in respect of the many thousands of similar claimants waiting in the wings and thereby foreclosing any further litigation), an awkward set of circumstances forced him abruptly to change tack toward a mass sign up of clients. Some months earlier, Richard had confronted a Johannesburg personal injuries attorney named Malcolm Lyons, who wanted to take on some of the Cape asbestos claimants as his clients. After the enormous quantities of time and effort Richard had already invested in the case, he was loath to let Lyons sail in over the top of him. It was an acrimonious confrontation, as Richard made clear to Lyons both the history and the current delicate positioning of the case, albeit, in the end, they "reached a general and in principle understanding . . . [to] work together on further cases should *Lubbe* succeed."[15]

Yet, despite this agreement, shortly after delivery of the Court of Appeal judgment, Deon Smith in Prieska called Richard in London late one Friday evening, tipping him off to the fact that Malcolm Lyons's law firm partner, Karen Vermaak, was in town eager to solicit clients, with a church hall meeting scheduled to take place on the coming Monday. Immediately jumping on the next plane to Johannesburg, together with Leigh Day colleagues Frank Patterson and Sapna Malik, Richard managed to get to Prieska in time to intercept Vermaak. As they flew south, Richard realized that with other lawyers circling Cape's victims, Leigh Day's hand had now effectively been forced. He and the firm were in danger of losing control of the case if they stuck to their mere handful of claimants. He therefore decided that they now had no choice but to shift to a wholesale signing up of clients to prevent Lyons and Vermaak taking advantage of all Leigh Day's work, even if it was, as Richard later candidly admits, "a move I am least proud of because it was based on our desire to maintain control of the litigation and protect our commercial interests."[16]

Be that as it may, Richard, Sapna, and Frank were astonished by the sheer numbers of people eager to sign up with them. An initial meeting of potential claimants in Prieska's white church hall was large enough, but as they were leaving it they found Cecil Skeffers waiting outside "to ask whether we would be willing to address the coloured and black communities at the Omega Hall the following day," as Richard relates it. "We said, 'Yes, of course,' only to find when we got there, hundreds of people inside and outside the hall, all holding their MBOD certificates. It was completely overwhelming."[17]

Predictably, these events put paid to any prospect of Richard and Lyons ever working together.

This mischief concerning claimants was followed some months later by another, this time in the United Kingdom. Richard learned that Anthony Coombs, a solicitor with John Pickering & Partners, a Manchester firm specializing in asbestos injuries, who was working in conjunction with Malcolm Lyons, had just issued writs in England against Cape, on behalf of some 100 of its former employees without any prior consultation with Richard or Leigh Day. Following a heated telephone exchange with Coombs—"I don't think he fully appreciated the complexity of the case or how perilously poised it was at that point," Richard recalls—they agreed, uneasily, to collaborate by combining their cases.[18]

The second strategic challenge facing Richard and his team at that time was the pressing need to prepare their response to Cape's petitioning the House of Lords in August 1998, for leave to appeal the Court of Appeal's decision against Cape.

The two endeavors were not unrelated. Cape's application for leave to appeal to the Lords was based on the sole ground that the Court of Appeal had erred in its interpretation of the conditions upon which the shield of *forum non conveniens* can be successfully deployed by a defendant (which conditions, according to the Court of Appeal, Cape had failed to fulfill).[19] No mention was made of the matter of numbers of claimants. Still, Richard wondered whether in response to Cape's leave application, he and his legal team should nonetheless expressly state that the numbers of claimants had increased. To that end, Richard sought specific advice from leading counsel, Barbara Dohmann, who, together with Graham Read, had been retained as counsel by Leigh Day. Both Richard and Graham were (and remain) clear about the advice that was given, not least because it accorded precisely with their own views. However, frustratingly, legal privilege prevented them then, and prevents them now, from disclosing its contents.

What was and can be said is that leading counsel "was aware of the contents of [relevant] affidavits and of the likelihood of further claimants should the appeal succeed." And further, as Richard swore in an affidavit at the time, "Prior to the leave application before the House of Lords, we [Leigh Day] sought and acted upon advice from leading and junior counsel [who] were aware that we had at that stage taken further instructions from approximately 1500 future claimants."[20] To this it can be added that after the House of Lords' judgment in 2000, the Office for Supervision of Solicitors—then the disciplinary wing of the profession's regulatory body—dropped its investigation into the conduct of Richard and Leigh Day in relation to the matter as a direct result of a written explanation from Graham of the advice that Barbara Dohmann and he had given Richard prior to the House of Lords' hearing.

Notably, as mentioned earlier, Cape's lawyers were also seemingly nonplussed by the prospect of further claimants being added to the case against the company. They were certainly well aware that Leigh Day was taking instructions from hundreds more clients. Anne Ware from DAC, for example, in correspondence with Leigh Day, had expressly referred to a *You* magazine article published in South Africa in November 1998 likening the huge number of potential claimants to "a volcano waiting to erupt."[21] Yet, she and her colleagues had not (and did not) raise the matter in their petition to the House of Lords. Of course, the real reason why Cape's legal team had omitted to do so was "because they wanted to keep the argument in reserve as ammunition to support an 'abuse' argument in the stay application that they intended to make when further claims were issued."[22]

Indeed, if anyone was being economical with the truth it was Cape's lawyers. It was only after the Lords had denied them leave to appeal and after Leigh Day and Pickering Partners had issued further writs, that Cape's lawyers raised the abuse of process point by reapplying to the High Court for the case to be stayed. And despite such a subterfuge and the spurious nature of their abuse argument, the ploy had worked in helping turn Justice Buckley toward their side. Graham had had a hunch that it might when, on the penultimate day of the seven-day hearing in the High Court in July 1999, he could see that Brian Doctor was getting some purchase with the judge on the abuse point. That evening, Graham and the whole Leigh Day team were having dinner at the chic Café du Marché off Charterhouse Street, hosted by John Hendy QC, a labor and personal injury specialist and new lead counsel for the plaintiffs. It was a typically generous gesture of Hendy's, Graham recalls, "but throughout the meal I couldn't help wondering whether we might be better off finessing our counterattack for the following day."[23]

Though Justice Buckley had found against them, Richard and Graham could still see a platform on which to build their appeal. Buried in the very last paragraph of his judgment, after determining that South Africa was the most appropriate forum to try the case, the judge noted that "even if the claimants here succeed in establishing a duty of care on the defendant on the basis of decisions taken or policies laid down by it in England, almost everything else about the case occurred in South Africa."[24] But that alternate condition, Richard maintained, was in fact the point upon which the whole case pivoted. Namely, that Cape's UK-based decisions and policies *had been* instrumental in creating and perpetuating the circumstances in which the claimants had suffered damage, thereby demonstrating not only that there existed a duty of care on Cape UK's part, but also that it had failed to uphold it.[25] As, for these reasons, the United Kingdom was *an* appropriate forum, the matter reduced to a question of whether there were any additional considerations that might displace the *prima facie* conclusion that South Africa was the more appropriate forum. It was here that the second limb of the *Spiliada* test (regarding *forum non conveniens*) came into play, by asking the so-called ends of justice question. That is, are there compelling reasons to believe that a fair and just outcome would *not* be achieved in South Africa?

With the intention to fight on this particular question of jurisdiction, Richard lodged his appeal in August 1999 and duly instructed Barbara Dohmann QC once again to lead the case before the Court of Appeal, hoping to repeat the success they had with her in the first Court of Appeal case. Also, Graham Read was again briefed as junior counsel, alongside Kate Gallafent, a budding employment and civil liberties lawyer who'd recently joined Barbara Dohmann at Blackstone Chambers. No matter their intended line of argument, nobody on the team was under any illusion that Cape and its lawyers would once again hammer the abuse point. To that end Richard also later engaged Robert Owen QC, a professional conduct expert, when it became clear that the court was, like Justice Buckley in the court below, latching onto the abuse allegation.

However, before getting to the second Court of Appeal hearings scheduled for October 1999, they faced another setback. The initial bench appointed to hear the appeal included Lord Justice Evans, who had sat on the first Court of Appeal case. From Leigh Day's point of view, this was a good thing, not only because Evans was very familiar with the case, but also, of course, because, along with Lord Justices Millett and Auld, he had decided in favor of the plaintiffs. But these were precisely the reasons why Cape's lawyers did not want Evans LJ sitting on the bench for the second appeal, and they were on the look-out for anything that might help ensure he didn't.

There is nothing inherently problematic about an appellate judge sitting on second appeal involving the same litigants as well as many (though not all) of the same legal arguments. Indeed, there may be good cause for them to do so as they are, obviously, already familiar with the details of the case. Cape's lawyers, therefore, appeared to have little to go on—until, that is, an opportunity was handed to them on a plate, and by Richard's legal team, no less. Misguidedly, in retrospect, Richard had agreed to John Hendy QC (who was still lead counsel at the time, having led the plaintiffs' case before the High Court the month before), writing to the Civil Appeals Office suggesting that Lord Justice Evans be appointed to the bench for the second Court of Appeal hearings. This correspondence was duly disclosed to DAC (the foreknowledge of which alone, Richard now admits, should have set alarm bells ringing), who immediately seized on the information to challenge Evans's appointment on the grounds of conflict of interest, or his being "tainted by apparent bias," as DAC's David McIntosh alleged.[26]

Cape's lawyers' quick-fire application for recusal in early August caught Richard's legal team on the hop as his "go-to" counsel were all on summer holidays—Graham Read was in Cornwall on a family expedition to see a total eclipse of the sun ("a bad omen," he now says)—and unavailable at short notice.[27] Whether for that reason or the fact that the three-judge panel appointed to hear the application was so clearly unimpressed by Leigh Day and counsel writing to the Civil Appeals Office with such a request, the court granted the application and Lord Justice Evans was forced to remove himself from the case.[28] It was a wounding hit on Leigh Day's reputation as well as on the prospects of its forthcoming appeal.

Though seemingly more technical than substantive at the time, Evans LJ's recusal turned out to be a pivotal moment in the case. Richard and his team were never to know, of course, what Evans LJ would have made of the arguments presented in the second appeal, given that they remained substantially the same as in the first appeal, save the additional claimants and the allegation that Richard had misled the previous courts as to the group nature of the action. But there is no doubting the fact that the three new judges on the second appeal (Pill, Aldous, and Tuckey LLJ) saw these new circumstances as critical in finding unanimously against the claimants in their judgment of November 29, 1999, and reaffirming the stay granted by Justice Buckley in July. Their decision was, in other words, diametrically opposite to that handed down by their brethren in the first Court of Appeal case sixteen months earlier.

During the Court of Appeal hearings, Cape's lawyers had doubled down on the abuse argument, adding barely disguised invective to their accusations that Richard had misled the courts during the first stage of the litigation. Brian Doctor not only asserted that "the judgment of the [first] Court of Appeal in *Lubbe* is now seen to have been procured by material non-disclosure and abuse of process," but also, and with astonishing chutzpah, speciously blamed Leigh Day for "the two-year delay occasioned by the hearings in *Lubbe* [having] seriously prejudiced the group claimants themselves and their estates."[29]

The oral exchanges between the two sets of counsel across the four days of hearings were decidedly heated, leading Tuckey LJ to lament that in his judgment "the abuse argument has generated considerable acrimony between the lawyers which has led to allegations and counter-allegations which one would not expect to see in litigation of this kind." For Kate Gallafent, it was a baptism by fire for a newly admitted barrister: "I just wanted to hide behind the box files" piled on the table in front of her, Graham Read remembers her saying, half-jokingly, after one singularly vitriolic session.[30] There were also rumors that privately, the other side's lawyers were referring to Richard as "The Prince of Darkness," which Richard will tell you he took as something of a badge of honor, despite its unpleasant overtones.

Beneath the thick-skinned bravado, however, these attacks on his professional integrity stung, especially as they had clearly swayed both Buckley J in the High Court and now the Appeal bench toward Cape's side. One evening, in the middle of the Court of Appeal hearings, Munoree, Richard's wife, arrived home to find him slumped on the stairs, chin cupped in his hands, staring vacantly into the middle distance. "He looked beaten down and exhausted. I was worried," she recounts. Even when Nadia, their six-year-old daughter, broke through his torpor bounding across the hall, plonking herself onto her father's knee, and launching immediately into an impassioned tirade about a grave injustice she'd suffered that day in the school playground, a shadow still hung over him. The support as well as responsibilities of one's family are crucial in times like this, and Munoree's wise counsel that "you are on the right side of history" certainly buoyed him, but there was no denying he was struggling.[31]

≈

The full extent of the case's unraveling became clear when Richard read the Court of Appeal's reasoning. Lord Justice Pill, writing the lead judgment, set the admonishing tone:

> Lubbe plaintiffs cannot in my judgment complain if the issue as to which forum is appropriate is now assessed in the light of the large number of claims which it was always hoped would follow upon their action and which were commenced very soon after the earlier application for a stay was finally refused.

Aldous LJ's criticism was more directed, calling out Leigh Day's failure to inform both the initial Court of Appeal and the House of Lords of the prospect of the subsequent filing of additional claimants in a group action as little short of deceitful:

They [Leigh Day] believed that the chances of a stay being granted on *Spiliada* grounds was substantially less if a claim by five South African claimants was being considered by the court, than if the court realised that a group action was the desired result. They therefore sought to obtain that advantage, but to do so they had to mislead the court as to the factual background.

Tuckey LJ added, for good measure, that such maneuvering had "achieved nothing and was a waste of time . . . [which] would not have happened if Mr Meeran had disclosed his intentions from the outset."[32]

The placement of Richard's perceived delinquencies at the center of the court's reasoning was undeniable, but it could have been avoided, or substantially excused, if his own senior counsel, Barbara Dohmann, had been more forthcoming. At the very least, she could have stated that in her view the matter of numbers was irrelevant to the question of jurisdiction, that it was unnecessary to have drawn the matter to the attention of the House of Lords, and, critically, that Leigh Day and Richard had followed her advice on these points. She was a leading silk (and Chair of the Commercial Bar Association at the time), so her standing by Leigh Day and Richard, rather than leaving them to face the rap, would have made a real difference to the attitude of the court, and was, surely, the right thing to do in the circumstances. As it was, neither Richard's sworn testimony that he had sought and received such advice in unambiguous terms from Dohmann, nor Robert Owen's express reference to that fact and to Richard's affidavit during oral hearings, held sway with the bench. Lord Justice Aldous's caustic response to Owen's argument was to ask: "This is the Nuremberg defence, is it?"[33]

Barbara Dohmann did, however, spring something of a surprise by proffering to the bench an interesting anecdote regarding the first Court of Appeal's awareness of the potential for many more claimants to emerge should the *Lubbe* appeal succeed. She had recently attended a reception at which Lord Millett (one of the judges on the first Court of Appeal) was present. Dohmann had intimated to his Lordship that a complaint had been raised in the present (second) Court of Appeal hearing, that the bench on which he had sat had been misled. "Lord Millet laughed," noted Dohmann. "He said that it was obvious that there would be further claimants 'in spades' if the appeal was allowed."[34] This revelation underlined what was, in fact, already broadly accepted by all parties. As Tony Davies had so eloquently observed, "Anybody who did not expect . . . other cases would arise . . . would have to be very stupid indeed" (incidentally demonstrating that despite his contempt for lawyers generally, he and Lord Millett were at one on this point).[35] But the anecdote did little to address the decisive question of *why* Richard had felt no need to disclose to the House of Lords in December 1998 the fact that he had taken instructions from some 1,500 additional claimants, upon which point Dohmann remained silent.

The second Court of Appeal's judgment of November 29, 1999, duly found that "South Africa was clearly the more appropriate forum, . . . [as] there would inevitably be a number of legal and factual disputes relating to liability for any injury and the amount of any damages which would be better investigated and decided in South Africa." Crucially, in reaching this conclusion, the court held that "the institution of the group action was a sufficient change of circumstances to allow the court to reconsider its previous decision in Lubbe. The group action should be stayed on forum grounds and that meant that the Lubbe action should be stayed as well."[36]

In terms of the litigation's eventual nine-year span, this result was about as low as the case would get. No matter the heartening sight of Action for South Africa campaigners and others protesting outside the court in the pouring rain after the judgment was handed down, there was no escaping the fact they'd lost their appeal in emphatic terms. As lawyers, they had faced withering attacks on their professional integrity in court, precipitating, immediately thereafter, a formal investigation by the Office for Supervision of Solicitors into Richard's alleged misconduct.[37] Richard was angry. Believing the accusations against him to be grossly unfair and the resulting judgment wrong, he let rip with stony-faced invective in debrief meetings (astonishing because it was so at odds with his habitual poise). Yet, as things then stood, should there remain any appetite to bring the case to trial, the venue would have to be South Africa, a venue where Cape had effectively no assets or presence and where it knew the claimants' inability to pay for legal representation meant that neither Leigh Day nor any local law firm would be willing or able to take them on.

So it was with a grating sense of foreboding that a week later Richard carried all this news to South Africa to convey it as best he could to the claimants and their families. There was disappointment, of course, "but they'd become so used to the highs and lows of the case that they took it in their stride," Richard recalls. "They knew us so well by then . . . and they trusted us," he adds, admitting how gratifying, but also onerous, it was to carry such a weight.[38]

While he was with the communities, Richard was able to offer some hope that the case might still proceed in the United

Kingdom. After all, the litigation "scoreline" before the Court of Appeal was now 1–1, each side having won once before two differently composed benches of the court on what was essentially the same question of jurisdiction. Cape, of course, had also been denied leave to appeal to the House of Lords after losing before the first Court of Appeal. But now the opportunity presented itself to Richard and the claimants to see if, after their loss before the second Court of Appeal, they might fare any better before the House of Lords.*

Richard felt that one aspect of the second Court of Appeal's reasoning was notably weak and therefore open to being challenged on appeal to Law Lords. Alongside the contention that the substantially increased numbers of claimants tipped the scales in favor of South Africa as the most appropriate forum, the three appellate judges had rejected any arguments of the inherent injustice this would likely create, given the grave limitations the South African legal system was then laboring under. "The court," they said, "would not refuse a stay on grounds that legal aid was not available in South Africa or that the South African courts were not able to deal properly with the actions. Contingency fees were then lawful in South Africa and the court could not conclude that legal representation would not become available in South Africa."[39] Richard was adamant that the Court of Appeal was wrong on these points. "We had presented strong— we thought compelling—evidence of the near impossibility of bringing the case before the South African courts, and yet the court simply dismissed it," he says. So "we believed that there were solid grounds for an appeal and we were determined to fight on," he adds.[40]

---

* For dates and details of the aggregate litigation scoreline, see the Litigation Timeline at the front of the book.

Before the second Court of Appeal, counsel for the plaintiffs had indeed argued vigorously that the unavailability of legal aid was fatal to the prospects of a just outcome for the claimants in South Africa. Richard had also made clear in an earlier affidavit that while contingency fee arrangements were, in theory, an option in South Africa, the reality was very different.[41] He had obtained supporting testimony from a raft of leading South African attorneys detailing the significant practical difficulties encountered in pursing public interest litigation in the country at that time, including, notably, the unavailability of litigation insurance in South Africa, without which claimants would be exposed to unconscionable financial jeopardy should their case fail.[42]

Cape's South African lawyers, WWB, were also all too aware of the near impossibility of taking on such a large case in South Africa. This much was made clear in yet another theatrically inept artifice they attempted to execute in conjunction with the most unlikely of partners.

The Centre for Applied Legal Studies (CALS) at Wits University in Johannesburg was (and still is) one of South Africa's foremost institutions of human rights expertise and advocacy, whose director at that time was David Unterhalter. In September 1999, a couple of weeks before the second Court of Appeal hearings were due to commence in London, Stuart McCafferty and Nick Alp from WWB approached Unterhalter with an extraordinary proposition. If Cape provided sufficient funding, they suggested, would CALS consider representing the claimants in litigation *against* Cape in the South African courts? That such an arrangement would certainly flirt with ethical impropriety was obvious. But so too was its intent—namely, to try to generate evidence to undermine Leigh Day's contention that present circumstances in South Africa were such that adequate representation for the claimants would not be possible, resulting in an outcome that would likely be substantively unjust. McCafferty and Alp proffered a ballpark figure of R2.5 million (approximately $420,000 at that time) to fund the case, which after some thought Unterhalter believed to be about half of the likely cost. In any event, Unterhalter declined.

When, two months later and immediately before the Court of Appeal handed down its judgment in November 1999, Richard got wind of this bizarre overture (Unterhalter sent him copies of the correspondence), he wrote to DAC registering his concerns but also, he admits, to goad both DAC and WWB over their cack-handedness. "The suggestion that Cape should fund the claimants' litigation," he wrote, "must surely reflect an appreciation by your client (prior to the Court of Appeal hearing) that contingency fees in South Africa are not a realistic option for this case and that a very significant source of funding would be required in order for this litigation to proceed in South Africa." As nothing came of the proposal—Unterhalter was, evidently, "less than enthusiastic" about it—the matter was dropped. Some months later, though, Richard and Unterhalter did meet up to share a beer and a laugh over the strange affair.[43]

Establishing that legal aid was unavailable in South Africa had also been a saga of intrigue and behind-the-scenes machinations. Shortly after the second Court of Appeal's hearings had commenced, Richard was able to furnish the court with a letter from the South African Legal Aid Board (SALAB) stipulating that legal aid was no longer able to fund personal injuries litigation in South Africa. But soliciting the letter had not been easy.

Mohamed Navsa was then the chair of the SALAB, so Richard decided that approaching him directly would be the quickest and surest way of getting a frank appraisal of the state of legal aid in South Africa at that time. As Navsa was also a High Court

judge, Richard rolled up to his judicial chambers in Johannesburg one morning, hoping to see him. Richard explained the purpose of his visit to Navsa's clerk who told him that unfortunately
the judge was very busy that day. "I'll wait," said Richard, mus-
tering all the grim-faced determination he could manage,
whereupon the clerk returned a few minutes later to tell him that
in fact the judge was able to see him right away. After introducing himself, Richard came straight to the point. Navsa conceded
that the country's legal aid scheme was indeed financially crip-
pled but then added, astonishingly, that he was not prepared to
say so publicly, concerned as he was to protect the reputation of
the country's legal system as a whole. Richard was flabbergasted
by such an excuse, which would put in serious jeopardy the prospects of getting any sort of meaningful result for thousands of
Navsa's fellow countrymen and women.

After the meeting, Richard returned to Munoree's mother's
home in Pietermaritzburg where he was staying and spent most
of that night at her kitchen table, writing an intemperate ten-
page letter explaining what he thought of Navsa's reasoning and
its likely consequences. Ignoring the time-honored wisdom of
sleeping on it, he immediately fired off his diatribe by fax to
Navsa, copying it to all the other members of the Legal Aid Board
(which included the Minister of Justice and the Chief Justice of
the Constitutional Court). Navsa was livid, and the stoush was
only finally settled a week later, following an intense bout of lobbying that Richard recalls being one of the most surreal experiences in the whole case.

Chaperoned by the well-connected force of nature that is environmental activist Liziwe McDaid, Richard spent an afternoon inside the South African parliamentary buildings in Cape
Town, "marching" (as he remembers it) into people's offices re-
questing audiences and hanging around debating chambers'

doors waiting for sessions to end so they could nab ministers, politicians, and influential bureaucrats to explain to them the legal aid/Navsa dilemma. Their efforts paid off when they wrangled a promise out of Deon Rudman, the Director General of Justice, that he would speak to his boss, the Minister of Justice, Penuell Maduna, about the affair. Rudman kept his promise and Minister Maduna stepped in ordering that the SALAB write to Richard, declaring that "with effect from 1 November 1999, legal aid will not be granted in respect of the institution of actions for damages for personal injuries."[44] It was a significant victory for Richard—or so it appeared at the time—as the letter provided the Court of Appeal in London with seemingly compelling evidence of the incapacity and therefore unsuitability of South African courts to entertain such a case with so many indigent plaintiffs.[45]

There was, to be sure, no sharing a beer and a laugh with Mohamed Navsa following this outcome—even years later Navsa was still bitter over being so thoroughly side-stepped[46]—but Richard had found an important ally in the Minister of Justice. With a doctorate in constitutional law, Maduna was smart, urbane, and ambitious. As a politician, he could see the significance of the case in its broader context: the big numbers of victims in small mining communities; the wealth of a British company built on Apartheid exploitation; and the path-breaking nature of the case. It was legacy litigation coming hard on the heels of South Africa's new-found freedom and rebirth. As a lawyer, he understood how important it was to Richard's planned appeal to the House of Lords that they burnish the argument that South African courts were not then well placed to deliver a just outcome, should the trial be blocked in the United Kingdom. Above all, Maduna knew that the prospects of a sizeable financial settlement for the victims and their communities were far greater before the English courts than anything available to the claimants before South African courts or under the country's workers' compensation schemes.

As discussions between his office and Leigh Day continued, the minister dispatched Enver Daniels, the Chief State Law Adviser, to London in early March 2000 to discuss what was needed and what the South African government was prepared or able to deliver. It was to prove a decisive move. Based on the briefing Daniels gave him after he returned from London, Maduna was able to persuade his colleagues in the cabinet to endorse the South African government seeking leave to intervene in the forthcoming appeal hearing before the House of Lords.

≈

By the middle of May 2000, when preparations for the appeal to the House of Lords were well under way, the legal team hit yet another problem arising from the allegations of abuse of process directed at Richard. Even though no finding of any abuse had been made by the Court of Appeal, Anthony Coombs apparently believed that the matter created a conflict of interest between Leigh Day and the claimants' counsel. Coombs thus wanted to brief separate counsel for the claimants' writs he'd filed alongside those of Richard.

Richard had already briefed the redoubtable Dan Brennan QC and Michael Beloff QC as joint lead counsel (with Graham Read and Nicholas Kahn as juniors) when, on the eve of the statement of facts being lodged with the court, Coombs informed them that he had approached Keir Starmer, then a rising star from Doughty Street Chambers, to appear on his clients' behalf. Splitting the unified front of claimants in this way was seen by

Richard and his team as not only unnecessary, but also potentially fatal for the chances of the appeal's success for all claimants.

In response, Graham Read wrote to Coombs a long and considered letter setting out why he thought no such conflict existed, and Dan Brennan[47] had a quiet word with Keir Starmer pointing out the case's complexities and vexed history, of which matters Starmer was evidently not fully aware. The pincer movement succeeded, and Starmer withdrew, leaving the legal team as originally briefed to appear for all claimants.[48]

The episode had been an aggravating headache that was especially disagreeable so close to the scheduled hearing before their Lordships in mid-June 2000, but with it now out of the way, Richard and counsel could focus entirely on fine-tuning their argument. The thrust of it was the contention that the "ends of justice" would not be served if the trial were to proceed in South Africa (the second limb of the *Spiliada* test on *forum non conveniens*), with the Brussels Convention point that EU law may preclude any EU-based defendant from claiming *forum non conveniens* as an alternative, fall-back position.

Essentially, therefore, their lead argument was a repeat of the one they had advanced in the second Court of Appeal case to no avail. Under the circumstances, Richard was keenly aware of the need to reframe and reinvigorate the argument in such a way as to persuade the House of Lords to allow their appeal and extricate the case from a personal attack on him by elevating it to the level appropriate in a matter of such public importance. To that end, the dark cloud of the second Court of Appeal decision also provided a silver lining. By introducing the competing public interest factor in the "ends of justice" assessment of which was the most appropriate forum, the Court of Appeal provided a substantial foothold for the claimants to seek leave to appeal to the

House of Lords[49]—namely, the opportunity to put to the House of Lords that the Court of Appeal had been wrong in its assessment that the public interest in South Africa hearing the case was greater than the public interest of it being heard in the United Kingdom.[50] The key to demonstrating that the Court of Appeal had erred on this point lay in providing evidence that the South Africans themselves (including the South African government) did *not* see the public interest being served by having the case heard in their courts rather than in English courts.

News, therefore, of the South African government's intention to intervene by elaborating on the severe financial stringency facing the country was very welcome for Richard: "It is important for the House of Lords to have the information from the South African government on this," he told the South African press when they interviewed him about the case's prospects.[51] And he was right, for that information turned out to be pivotal. During the hearings it became increasingly clear that their Lordships were sympathetic to the public interest and ends of justice arguments as led by Dan Brennan, such that at one point, Michael Beloff (who had been enlisted specifically to lead on the fall-back Brussels Convention point) commented to Richard, sotto voce, "This is going rather well," as the need for his submissions steadily diminished.[52]

In their judgment, handed down on July 20, 2000, the Law Lords placed considerable emphasis on the fact that "written submissions on behalf of the Republic of South Africa contain no hint that public funds might, exceptionally, be made available to fund [the litigation]." Added to which, they were persuaded by the preponderance of written testimony from distinguished South African lawyers confirming that taking on the case on a contingency fee basis was not a viable prospect. No "firm of South African attorneys with expertise in this field had the means or would undertake the risk of conducting these proceedings on [such] a . . . basis," they noted.[53] Such authoritative and unambiguous evidence coming from the South African establishment was therefore critical in the eyes of the House of Lords and led directly to it finding in favor of the claimants. Not only did the Lords overturn the Court of Appeal decision, they lambasted their brethren for failing to "take account of the evidence."[54] Such unstinting criticism of the second Court of Appeal was especially gratifying for Richard, who maintained that its determination that legal representation "would become available in South Africa,"[55] was simply "bizarre" given the preponderance of evidence to the contrary.

It was, by any measure, a momentous decision by the House of Lords, with all five judges allowing the appeal to have the case heard in England.[56] A vindication of Richard's skill and determination to turn a "good idea, but doomed to fail" as he'd been told at the outset, into a good idea that succeeded. Against the odds, the cardinal principle of clearing a legal path toward justice for Cape's victims had triumphed over the determination of Cape and its lawyers to block the path with as many obstacles as they could marshal. "If these proceedings were stayed in favour of the more appropriate forum in South Africa," noted the redoubtable Lord Bingham, who wrote the lead judgment,

> the probability is that the plaintiffs would have no means of obtaining the professional representation and the expert evidence which would be essential if these claims were to be justly decided. This would amount to a denial of justice. In the special and unusual circumstances of these proceedings, lack of the means, in South Africa, to prosecute these claims to a conclusion provides a compelling ground, at the second stage of the *Spiliada* test, for refusing to stay the proceedings here.[57]

For the claimants, it was a slam-dunk decision, finally and definitively opening the door to suing Cape in UK courts. And it was made all the more emphatic by their Lordships ordering that the "defendant [Cape] must bear the costs of the proceedings before Buckley J and the second Court of Appeal."[58]

≈

The favorable hearings before the House of Lords in June 2000 were a very different experience for Richard and his legal team than those they had endured before the Court of Appeal barely seven months earlier. In part this was due to an unexpected moment of melodrama played out at the end of the first day before the Lords. Prior to commencement it had been tacitly agreed between the opposing legal teams that claimants' counsel would occupy the first day with their submissions, Cape's counsel taking the second day to make theirs. With mischief aforethought, however, Dan Brennan finished the claimants' submissions with forty minutes or so left in the first day. Clearly flustered and somewhat unprepared, Brian Doctor for Cape was "sent in to bat" for what—in test cricketing circles—is universally regarded as a difficult and dangerous short spell at the end of long day.

The experience was also agreeably different because the questions and interruptions coming from the five Law Lords were encouragingly positive for Richard and his team. They had given short shrift to Brian Doctor's abuse of process argument. "You are here now," Lord Hoffmann curtly told him, effectively rebuffing Doctor's main complaint that Richard had previously misled the House of Lords and the Court of Appeal.[59] The bench was clearly far more interested in questions of whether a South African forum would yield a just outcome in a suit against an English corporation, regardless of how many claimants had joined the case against it.[60]

In fact, there were now approximately 3,000 claimants spread across more than a dozen writs issued both by Leigh Day (accounting for roughly two-thirds of all claimants) and John Pickering and Partners (the rest). This total included an ever-increasing number of claims made on behalf of the estates of deceased people (around 400 at that time), which explained, in part, the sobering reality behind the fuzziness of the figures. "It was difficult to keep track of the number of deaths and consequently the number of deceased claims," Richard notes, which task only got harder as the case dragged on for another three years, by which time the numbers of claimants and deceased had both more than doubled.[61]

That the case would only be settled three years later was, however, not in the immediate contemplation of those on the claimants' side who attended the House of Lords on the day judgment was delivered. Audrey Van Schalkwyk (from Prieska), Shadrack Molokoane (from Mathabatha, Limpopo), and Jo Prince (from Benoni, where Cape's asbestos factory was located) were there representing the claimants, as were the two provincial premiers, Manne Dipico and Ngoako Ramatlhodi, together with Thabo Makweya, the Northern Cape's environment minister, plus, of course, all the lawyers. They were all delighted and relieved, as were the many thousands in South Africa, where the news was greeted "with shining eyes and delirious smiles," and cows were slaughtered in celebration in the former mining villages.[62] In London, there were also dozens of supporters (many wearing dust masks) and a bustling media throng waiting outside the court.

Ever alive to the possibilities of exploiting any positive publicity, Richard had devised a plan for a little theater once the judgment was made public, no matter that on that day he was in crutches following yet another sporting mishap (a snapped

Achilles, playing badminton). Together with Cape's lawyers, Richard and his team had received notice of the judgment in their favor barely thirty minutes beforehand, but it was enough for Richard's purposes. He took leave from his front row seat in the grand, red-liveried main chamber of the House of the Lords in the Palace of Westminster, just before the oral judgment was delivered. Thabo Makweya had been sitting beside Richard immediately before his sudden departure. "Where is he going?" Thabo wondered to himself, but soon forgot about it once proceedings began. It was a brief event—just a summary of the court's reasons and a simple statement of its conclusions—after which Thabo joined everyone else filing out of the room. "The first person I see outside is Richard, surrounded by reporters and TV crews," Thabo recalls. "He raced [hobbled?] up to me asking: 'What was the result?' I was stunned, momentarily dazed, until it clicked with me what he was doing. So I told him 'We won!' and he gave me a big hug. It was a great show," Thabo recounts, with a smile and a knowing nod of the head.[63]

Brian Doctor was conspicuously absent from the day's affairs. But as Richard retired to the SOS, a local pub in Smithfield,[64] later that afternoon for a celebratory drink or two (accompanied by the whole of the Leigh Day office, such was the importance of the victory), he had no doubt he'd be seeing more of Doctor and the rest of Cape's legal team over the coming months and years. It was only now, with the question of jurisdiction finally and definitively settled, that both sides could get down to the nitty gritty of arguing over the extent of Cape's negligence and how much it would cost the company to repair the damage.

CHAPTER 9

Redemption
—*Mending Broken Eggs*—

INDICATING THAT HE'D LIKE TO SPEAK, the man rose gingerly to his feet. He wished to respond to a remark made by an asbestos industry representative who'd sought to remind everyone of the many advantages asbestos brought to society. "You cannot make an omelet without breaking some eggs" was the astonishingly inappropriate metaphor the industry rep had chosen to make his point. Old before his time and in a halting voice no longer powered by fully functioning lungs, the new speaker's first words silenced the room. "I'm one of those broken eggs," he said. He then calmly spelled out that he was dying of an asbestos-related disease after having worked for years in Cape Town's notorious Athlone Power Station, which had only recently been stripped of the abundant and badly maintained asbestos insulation material used in its original construction in the 1970s.[1]

The setting for this piece of tragicomedy was an international asbestos conference being held in Johannesburg in late November 1998. Participants ranged from across the subject. Scientists, anti-asbestos activists, former employees, victims, lawyers, government officials, and industry and corporate representatives were all there, the aim being to bring as many stakeholders as possible together in the same room. Liziwe McDaid, who after chaperoning Richard through the halls of government had become such an enthusiastic and effective supporter of the case against Cape, was one of the chief organizers of the conference. Richard was also at the conference, but doesn't recall the "broken eggs" interaction, it being related to me by Liziwe.[2] "It was an important moment," she says, reflecting on how neatly it encapsulated the nature of pro- versus anti-asbestos movements. Collateral damage can *never* be acceptable to the latter when it constitutes death and disease in circumstances where the cause is understood and there exists the capacity to prevent it. If people from the asbestos communities had known that so many eggs would have to be broken, then they would have neither wanted nor needed the omelet.

≈

Following the House of Lords' judgment in July 2000, Richard's focus had begun to shift toward assessing the extent of the damage caused by Cape's negligence, which he was now very confident of persuasively establishing. If there was any silver lining to the dark cloud of protracted litigation over the past three and a half years, it was that considerable time and effort had been invested in compiling a compelling dossier of research on Cape's levels of awareness and responsibility.

That said, at this point the litigation could go one of two ways. Either the case proceeded to trial and the two sides would slug it out over whether and to what extent Cape had acted negligently and was therefore liable for damages. Or, realizing that the game was up, Cape might seek an out-of-court financial settlement. Either way, arguments and negotiations over corresponding levels of compensation for the claimants would be at the heart of proceedings. As near impossible as it is to mend a broken egg, so is the task of putting appropriate monetary figures on eviscerated lungs, devastated livelihoods, and lost loved ones. Furthermore, even if one can, there remained back then the elemental question of how much the company (and its insurers) could really afford.

Cape, as it transpired, chose to take both routes. Initially declaring it would "never surrender," as Brian Doctor tendentiously pronounced in court,[3] the company insisted that all claimants undertake new medical tests (to "verify" their health claims), as Cape would not accept the existing health records of a large majority of claimants held by South Africa's Medical Bureau for Occupational Diseases (MBOD). Despite the further delay, as well as the added expense and anxiety it caused the claimants, an initial sample of 650 new tests were conducted, with results that corresponded with those performed by the MBOD in around 85 percent of cases. Leigh Day argued that such correlation in this large sample was surely sufficient indication that the remaining cases would very likely have a similar "strike rate." Cape disagreed, and in an act boarding on malicious, it demanded that the health records of all the then more than 5,000 claimants undergo the time-consuming and expensive exercise of review. In the end, the strike rate remained at 85 percent.[4]

It was during this time in early June 2001, that the director of the MBOD, Lindiwe Ndelu, was forced to eject a pair of Cape's lawyers (Nic Alp from WWB and London barrister Charles Bourne) after she found them, uninvited, on MBOD premises and taking photographs without her or anyone else's permission. Apparently, the temptation for Cape to meddle in the affairs of science had not worn off even decades after its first forays in that direction under the guise of the South African Asbestos Producers' Advisory Committee. Perturbed by this incursion, Ndelu told Richard of the incident and also wrote to Mr. Justice Wright (who was, at the time, presiding over an interlocutory matter in the case in the High Court in London) complaining about the lawyers' behavior.[5]

Nevertheless, by the middle of 2001, Cape's circumstances betrayed some hints that it might be willing to settle. It had become clear that internally, the financial costs for Cape dragging out the litigation were beginning to sting. Graham Read recalls a rumor at the time about the exasperation of Cape's CEO declaring in a meeting that he had signed checks for the services of Charles Gibson—one of Cape's lawyers—for every day of the previous month."[6] More importantly still, the company was being shunted toward the negotiating table by the increasing external pressures bearing down on Cape's management and board.

Indeed, the rules of engagement had changed significantly. With the case no longer governed by narrow and dry legal argument over jurisdiction, broader concerns of public and political perception were now paramount. Societal awareness of the perils of asbestos was heightened and people's intolerance of corporate excuses was acute and scathing. Too many families and friends had been afflicted with ARDs, and litigation and compensation claims were now commonplace in the United Kingdom, as they were across all developed economies. A widely cited study published in the *Lancet* a few years earlier showed that in the twenty years between 1971 and 1991, the numbers of mesothelioma deaths in the United Kingdom had risen by more than 700 percent. A follow-up survey published in 1999 showed that across Europe during roughly the same period, Britain had by far the sharpest increase in the rate of mesothelioma deaths of any country surveyed.[7] The British media was also full of stories of lives devastated, corporations shirking responsibility, and the regulatory failures of governments. It was only in 1999, after mounting public pressure, that the importation, manufacture, and use of *all* types of asbestos were finally banned in the United Kingdom, chrysotile asbestos having continued to be in use following the bans imposed on crocidolite and amosite asbestos in 1985.[8]

There had been ample media coverage in the United Kingdom of the House of Lords' decision in July 2000, not just because of Richard's orchestrated theatrics on the day, but because the case reflected so many of these heartfelt concerns. The fact that the victims in the Cape case were mainly poor, black, and coloured Africans, rather than Britons, added to the outrage. Fran Abrams of the *Independent* reported that "Cape . . . could be forced to pay millions of pounds to . . . more than 3,000 South African miners and their families suffering from asbestos-related diseases [who] . . . were exposed to levels of asbestos dust up to 35 times the British legal limit." While David Pallister of the *Guardian* wrote that "the decision could have far-reaching consequences for British multinationals" operating overseas, before adding that "last year [Cape] made a pre-tax profit of £9.1m."[9]

But perhaps the most moving of all accounts of Cape's asbestos legacy came from a most unlikely source. Audrey Van Schalkwyk had worked for many years as a nurse in Prieska Hospital, where she had witnessed the rising tide of asbestos disease and death. Her parents had both worked for Cape—her father as a miner at Koegas and her mother as a "stamper" (operating a mechanical compressor) at the mill in Prieska. After school, she and her brother used to help their mother ram the asbestos fibers into hessian sacks. Her father had died of mesothelioma in 1993, and her mother was then succumbing to the same disease (she died eighteen months later in 2002). Audrey herself had recently been diagnosed with asbestosis. Richard had invited

Audrey to London to attend the delivery of the Law Lords' judgment and to participate in several preceding publicity events. Audrey is small, softly spoken and almost preternaturally poised, with gently contoured facial features and a shy smile. That said, she maintains strong eye contact in conversation, showing, one soon realizes, a gutsy determination.

One of the events Richard had organized was a private briefing with fifty or so members of the UK Parliament's second chamber, the House of Lords (not to be confused with one of its constituent parts, the Appellate Committee of the House of Lords, to give the full title of the House of Lords sitting as a court).[10] Before this august body and in a wood-paneled committee room perched above the main chamber, Audrey had been asked to speak. "Just tell them your story," Richard urged her, "tell them about your family and life in Prieska."

She spoke for about twenty minutes without notes and without hesitation. She appeared calm, but, she now admits, she was terrified at the time, especially having to speak in English. "It felt good to get it out in the open," she says, "but I was shocked to see that some of the people there were crying." As she recounts this story to me, sitting in her tiny, impeccably tidy living room in Prieska twenty-three years later, I notice that she too has a tear in her eye. "It was very powerful," she says, composing herself.[11]

Having people like Audrey speak at events such as these was a coup. For while seasoned operators such as South African politicians and Richard himself were also performing in front of audiences, microphones, and cameras at the time, none had quite the authenticity of Audrey, precisely "because she was so obviously *non*-political," as Thabo Makweya stresses.[12] He, too, had been taken aback by the emotional reaction of the aristocratic members of the audience that day. A diehard communist then and now, who habitually refers to colleagues (and me) as "comrade," Thabo had grown up viewing "the white man as the devil," as he candidly puts it. "To see many of them so genuinely moved—showing real compassion for our plight—was a revelation." So much so, he adds, to my surprise, that it gave him real hope for the ongoing process of reconciliation back home in South Africa.

There was, however, still plenty of room for more "obviously political" rhetoric. Unflattering comparisons, for example, of Cape in South Africa with Union Carbide in India, where a gas chemical explosion at a plant owned by the American multinational in the central Indian city of Bhopal in 1984 killed between 2,000 and 20,000 people and maimed many tens of thousands more, grabbing headlines and putting pressure on the company. The comparison had been made many times, but on this latest occasion, Action for South Africa's (ACTSA's) director, Ben Jackson, twisted the knife by noting that "you could say Union Carbide was negligent, but not intentionally culpable," alluding to Cape's decades' long coverup of the dreadful health effects of asbestos.[13] *Time* magazine reported extensively on the "environmental calamity" caused by Cape's asbestos operations in the Northern Cape, and the BBC, building on its damning *Newsnight* exposé of Cape in 1998, was researching another documentary entitled "The Fatal Fibre," focusing on the avalanche of asbestos litigation and compensation claims that was now hitting the United Kingdom, as it had done more than a decade earlier in the United States.[14]

Cheryl Carolus, the South African High Commissioner to the United Kingdom at the time, and her deputy, George Johannes, were also instrumental in building and maintaining a high diplomatic profile for the issues raised by the case. George, a long-time anti-Apartheid activist and "lovely guy," says Richard, was an especially enthusiastic supporter, helping to facilitate and host a steady stream of functions and meetings in the High Commission's rather grand premises occupying the South East corner of Trafalgar Square in London. It was there that Leigh Day lawyers, local activists, national and international media, and visiting politicians, government officials, and trade unionists from South Africa were able to mingle and swap stories.

Designedly political publicity stunts also proliferated during this period. Of all of them, it was the targeting of corporate annual general meetings (AGMs) by supporters of the case against Cape that were most spectacular. The AGM of CGNU, a newly established insurance giant created by the merger of Norwich Union (a Cape shareholder) with CGU, was being held in the main auditorium of the Barbican on London's South Bank on May Day, 2001. Nearly all in attendance were expecting the usual stodgy fare of company highlights, financial reports, and future projections. But not quite all, for there were a few in the audience who were determined to spice up the menu. What happened next is best described by *Guardian* reporter Jonathan Freedland, who witnessed the scene:

> Lined up on stage, politburo-style, was the board of 16 directors. Facing them were CGNU's shareholders, representatives of big financial houses but also private individuals with just a share or two to their name. The chairman, Pehr Gyllenhammar, gave his annual report and then asked for questions from the floor.
>
> The first came from a representative of the South African National Union of Mineworkers, who reported that 60 people from his community back home had died from illnesses linked to asbestos. He wanted to ask about Norwich Union's 2% share in Cape Plc. . . . "I ask the chairman to give a one-minute silence for those who died before ever receiving justice," [he] said.

The chairman, peering down from his lofty perch on the platform, said there were lots of causes he sympathised with, but he couldn't give a minute's silence for all of them. Next question? A second representative of the South African miners. Gyllenhammar shifts in his seat and repeats his earlier statement. Next? The director of Action for South Africa steps forward to say he's heard enough words from CGNU and wants some real pressure on Cape. "We are getting on with our normal business," says the chairman stiffly. He wants another question and beckons a white man in a suit to come forward. Except he's an official of the GMB union and he, too, asks about asbestos. CGNU press officers are writhing in their seats with embarrassment: their day has been hijacked.[15]

Cape's own AGM a couple of weeks later was similarly hijacked when members of ACTSA stunned board members sitting on the dais by reading out a list of the 300 or so claimants who had died since the litigation against Cape had begun.[16]

≈

When, in the face of this mounting pressure, Cape finally came to the table with a firm offer to settle in October 2001, it did so true to its recalcitrant form. Through its lawyers, the company offered to settle the case for a low-ball sum *inclusive* of legal costs (which would have left as little as £1 million for distribution as compensation),[17] claiming that was all it could afford. Richard had always known that it might come to this—a miserly, even offensive, offer, accompanied by claims of penury in the style of "Sorry, but we're broke. That's all you're going to get!"

The art of negotiating a settlement in the shadow of litigation is always a delicate one, as Richard explains. The "settlement terms [had to] represent a pragmatic solution to the financial reality of Cape's position rather than reflecting any relation to the true value of the case."[18] And the reality at that time was that Cape was hemorrhaging badly. During the course of the litigation, its share price had plummeted from £1.50 to £0.11.[19] What is more, Richard had to be careful how hard he pushed back on the low-ball offer. He did not want to provoke Cape's complete collapse, the dire consequences of which were made abundantly clear by the actions of another British-based multinational asbestos company taken at that very same time. In October 2001, Turner and Newell filed for bankruptcy in both the United States and the United Kingdom, "leaving thousands of victims worldwide without redress."[20]

Nevertheless, push back hard he did. Richard knew he could do so for two good reasons. First, it was clear that Cape's coffers were not as threadbare as it claimed, after revealing in its 2001 annual report that it had set aside an £8.3 million litigation fighting fund.[21] Second, it was equally clear that Cape had no intention to compromise in any meaningful sense. In that same annual report, the company explained that with its fighting fund, it would "vigorously contest" any negligence or compensation claims made against it and that "no provision has been made for settling the claims."[22] Such bloody-mindedness raised Richard's litigator's hackles, making him all the more determined not to accept any derisory offer that effectively let Cape off with a slap on the wrist and no admission of wrongdoing. "There would be no repetition of Bhopal," Richard promised, referring specifically to the fact that Union Carbide had managed to evade liability under US law by successfully claiming the US courts were *forum non conveniens*. Thereby, the company had escaped properly compensating the many thousands of Indian victims of its negligence, all the while making shameless denials of responsibility.[23]

As matters stood with Cape, however, the outlook was grim. As negotiations dragged on through 2001, Cape claimed that its financial circumstances were worsening by the day, threatening the claimants with what it called a "lose-lose" situation if they didn't accept its offer to settle.[24] By this Cape meant that as it could not afford to make a higher offer, it would have no choice but to push the case to trial (already set down for March 2002). If Cape prevailed at trial, then the claimants would get nothing, and Cape would be "in the clear." But if Cape lost and was ordered to pay damages, the company would likely go into liquidation, leaving the claimants with almost no chance of receiving any payout at all. Indeed, Cape had "crashed into the red" the year before, with a pre-tax loss of £14.8 million, of which the £8.3 million provision for fighting the South African litigation was evidently a large part.[25] Not to base a settlement offer on *that* amount and thereby provide the now more than 6,000 claimants with some level of meaningful compensation—as the Leigh Day and John Pickering & Partners (JPP) lawyers proposed to Cape—seemed to be unconscionably mean as well as pig-headed. But Cape and its lawyers were unmoved.[26]

Then, unexpectedly, a possible alternative route presented itself. What if Cape was taken over and a new management team put in place? And what if the new team was more amenable to a settlement, allowing the company to survive and rebuild, rather than be so fixated on winning that it might drive itself into the ground? Well, following a series of secret meetings between Richard and a mercurial financier named Peter Gyllenhammar, these hypotheticals became reality.

Cape's precipitous share price drop had attracted the attention of distressed debt financiers looking for a bargain. One such "vulture fund" was Montpellier Finance. which had snapped up a 10 percent stake in Cape after its shares hit rock bottom immediately following the House of Lords' judgment in July 2000. The fund was headed by Peter Gyllenhammar (coincidentally the nephew of Pehr, chair of the CGNU), who, along with having a sharp eye for profit-making opportunities, also understood the detrimental impact on such opportunities of a corporation shirking its social responsibilities.[27]

Richard reached out to him in late summer 2001, and they arranged to meet in Montpellier's offices in Moorgate. Over a bottle of very good wine the pair broached the idea that ending the litigation with a more generous out-of-court settlement might be mutually beneficial. The claimants would receive acceptable compensation, and Cape would obtain closure on an open-ended liability by ending the "madness of Cape trying to defend itself when clearly people were dying from the asbestos [it had] mined."[28] The two parted that night with an in-principle agreement to investigate the possibility of a pre-agreed settlement of the case should Montpellier make a move to take control of Cape.

There followed a series of clandestine meetings over several weeks between Richard and Montpellier's managing director, Paul Sellars, during which they discussed the key elements of the prospective settlement and how it would fit into the broader strategy of Montpellier's takeover of Cape. Richard and Paul got to know each other well, especially as Paul warmed to the compelling moral argument that justice had to be done, after he made an epiphanic visit to the asbestos communities in South Africa and contemplated the chastening personal imperative of "being able to look my children in the eye," as he puts it.[29]

Still, Sellars was no pushover. For him, any settlement had to make business sense for it to have any chance of being accepted by Cape and its backers. The ensuing bargaining over money was long and hard as it boiled down to narrowing the gap between how much Cape would be able to afford (including borrowing) and how much the claimants were due. The key to reaching a compromise, as it turned out, lay in a meeting between Sellars,

Richard, and Premiers Manne Dipico and Ngoako Ramathlodi in Leigh Day's office in the autumn of 2001.

After listening to a summary of where matters stood at that point in the negotiations, the two provincial premiers decided to put pressure on Sellars to up his offer. Dipico and Ramathlodi both knew former President Nelson Mandela well, so they "suggested telephoning 'the old man' there and then, for him to speak to Paul."[30] Paul wasn't so keen on that idea and duly upped his offer to a point where an agreement was finally reached. Montpellier, it was decided, would stage a coup by purchasing a controlling stake in Cape, oust its senior management, and replace the board, all on the understanding that a settlement with the asbestos claimants would then be reached based on a pre-agreed "framework settlement . . . in the region of £20 million."

After agreeing to these terms, things moved quickly. Montpellier promptly launched a raid on Cape in early November 2001 by increasing its shareholding to a controlling threshold of 30 percent, installing Paul Sellars as Cape's new chair, and simultaneously submitting the framework settlement to court for approval and to stay the forthcoming trial in March 2002. The takeover and proposed settlement took Cape's senior executives and lawyers completely by surprise.

They were still in a state of shock when they met Paul Sellars in Brian Doctor's chambers in Fountain Court the next day. "They couldn't believe what had just happened," Richard remembers Sellars telling him. Doctor, together with Cape's DAC lawyers led by Fiona Gill, were so incensed that it blinded them to the new reality. They proceeded to lecture the new chair about what a bad move it was, before Sellars reminded them that *he* was now in control, not the old management, and that Doctor and DAC were to take instructions from him, not the other way around.[31]

Had Sellars needed any further persuading that Cape had to change the way it was approaching the case, it came shortly afterward during a round of golf. "I was playing in a foursome alongside my son when I got a call. 'I'll have to take this,'" Paul remembers saying, much to the annoyance of his son. "I was being asked to approve payment of a huge bill from Cape's QC [Brian Doctor] and whether to continue paying the lawyers to fight the case. 'This has to stop,' I thought. It convinced me more than ever that we needed to settle sooner rather than later."[32]

Negotiations on the fine-grained details of the settlement began immediately thereafter between Sellars and his new management team at Cape, together with their DAC lawyers on one side and the Leigh Day and JPP lawyers, led by Richard and Anthony Coombs respectively, on the other. Locked into separate meeting rooms in DAC's unlovely Fetter Lane offices in London,[33] convening every so often to haggle over specific settlement terms, the bargaining between the two sides was hard, relentless, and exhausting.

The enmity between the two sets of lawyers was still palpable, now laced with added spite following the subterfuge of the Montpellier takeover. Leigh Day's hand in the affair was sorely resented by DAC, but the rancor also spilled over to DAC's relationship with its client's new chairman. Paul Sellars, for example, kept referring to DAC lawyer David Smellie—whom Richard remembers adopting "a kind of macho commercial lawyer" stance throughout the negotiations—as his surname is spelled, no matter how many times Smellie pointed out that the correct pronunciation was "Smiley." It was childish to be sure, but after so long and in the face of so much antagonism, it did offer a soupçon of light relief.[34]

Meanwhile, the lawyers on the claimants' side of the negotiating table had their own practical problems to worry about.

Nominal titillations notwithstanding, Richard was driving the lawyers in his team to their very limits. "He was in the zone," Leigh Day colleague Sapna Malik recalls, so determined was he to get a result. "We'd work all day and then long into the night. And without food," she adds, as Richard would simply forget, blind to the fact that while he might survive on nervous energy alone, others with normal constitutions were failing badly. Food, of course, was ordered in once matters were brought to Richard's attention, but it hadn't helped that while the Leigh Day lawyers were flirting with hypoglycemia, they'd not failed to notice the steady stream of hearty victuals being shipped into the DAC lawyers' meeting room across the corridor.[35]

Out of all these goings-on, however, a result was achieved, and a settlement agreement was concluded by late December. At its core it comprised a total compensation package of £21 million which, despite being considerably less than the £100 million originally claimed by the victims,[36] seemed, according to Richard, "genuinely as much as Cape could afford" and obviously a vast improvement on its original offer. In addition, it was agreed that Cape, through its insurers, would pay £2.25 million toward the claimants' legal costs, which matter had been such a bone of contention in the first offer.[37]

With regard to the principal amount, an initial payment of £11 million would be made by June 30, 2002, with 10 yearly installments of £1 million to be made thereafter. Crucially, the total was to cover all present *and future* claimants, with half of the £21 million to be made available immediately to the plaintiffs in the present actions and the other half reserved for subsequent victims of Cape's asbestos legacy. In other words, anyone (i.e., not just the claimants in the present case) "who can show that they [or their deceased relative] suffered from asbestos-related disease as a result of working at, or living in the vicinity of, one of Cape's former mining, milling or manufacturing operations in South Africa" would be eligible to make a claim under the terms of the agreement.[38]

This was a huge gain in terms of aiding the asbestos-blighted communities in South Africa, as otherwise all those present and future victims not currently party to the litigation (likely many thousands) would miss out. In that respect, a settlement on terms like these was in many ways a better outcome in situations where large numbers are affected over long periods of time than was winning the case at trial because any consequent award of damages to the winning plaintiffs would be restricted to them alone. But the gain came at a price.

Together, Richard and Anthony Coombs had to undertake to foreclose their firms mounting any future litigation against Cape regarding its liability for asbestos-related injuries incurred in South Africa. It was a calculated concession and "a necessary compromise," Richard explains, to secure the payout while providing Cape with finality and a chance to rebuild its business without the threat of further waves of litigating claimants. The settlement agreement was duly signed by all parties on the morning of December 21, 2001, and it seemed as though an early Christmas present had arrived.

In the litigation's long road, this really did seem like a moment to savor. A victory of sorts. Premier Ngoako Ramatlhodi of Limpopo Province thought so: "When Cape left South Africa in 1979, it didn't once look back at the death and devastation it had knowingly created. But now finally, the local South African communities can have a sense that the global justice system didn't pass them by." While Richard shared elements of this spirit, there was also more than a hint of wariness in his voice. "I don't pretend that this is some kind of triumph," he announced to a slightly bemused media, "but I think it will constitute some sort of justice for the claimants. The company has been held to account and it's an important deterrent." When he then added, "It's not a victory but if you look at where we started a few years ago, when everyone told us we were wasting our time, then it's a good result," you get the sense of a man more relieved to have stopped banging his head against a wall, than one basking in conquestorial glory.[39]

≈

Philosophical skepticism aside, there were more pressing practical matters to attend to. A trust fund had to be established to administer the £21 million (symbolically named the Hendrik Afrika Trust [HAT]), with trustees to be appointed to its board. Richard hoped that Cyril Ramaphosa—then chairman of South Africa's Black Economic Empowerment Commission and formerly secretary-general of the National Union of Mineworkers (NUM)—would agree to be chair. "I remember ringing him to ask whether he would consider it, but before I even put the question to him, he said 'Yes'," Richard relates. "He knew what I was going to ask! I guess he already understood the power of politics far better than I did."[40]

Leigh Day also began planning how to administer the claims and payouts of the almost 7,500 claimants registered thus far as well as the many thousands that would follow them for at least 10 years. Preparations included making initial calculations according to a schedule of payouts for specific types of disease and levels of severity of illness, which was attached to the settlement agreement. It was a sobering task. For mesothelioma, claimants could expect to receive up to a maximum of about £5,250; for asbestosis about £3,250; for pleural thickening or pleural effusion about £1,600; and for pleural plaques a maximum of about £700.[41] (By comparison, the average yearly income in South Africa at that time was approximately £4,650.)[42] The practicalities of securely delivering payouts to the many claimants who were illiterate and/or without a bank account also had to be tackled.

A local office and a point person in-country were crucial. The existing Prieska office was the obvious choice for a venue, and Zanele Mbuyisa was sounded out about managing the day-to-day details of the operation. Sarah Leigh, who had semi-retired from the firm at this stage, was rather summarily ushered onto HAT's board after Richard rang her one morning and "more or less announced that I was a member," as Sarah recollects, with raised eyebrows. She was, in fact, happy to help and soon found herself with Richard and Zanele on an eye-opening six-week road trip around the asbestos communities in South Africa.

On one visit to Limpopo Province for an outdoor community meeting in Mafefe, Sarah recalls her amazement at witnessing the scale of the task at hand. "People were everywhere. Hanging out of trees, perched on street signs, standing in the back of bakkies, all wanting to hear what Richard had to say."[43] The meeting started with prayers for the souls of all the lawyers at Leigh Day ("gratefully received!" quips Sarah), before Richard took to the stage.

"He was brilliant and touching," she says, with a discernible ripple passing through the crowd when Richard told them that this time he had some good news. He talked about the settlement and the trust and then introduced Sarah as a highly respected and important lawyer and one of the trustees. "She will look after your money," he announced to polite applause. Stifling her embarrassment ("I'm *terrible* with money," Sarah confesses), she rose, said a few words, and quickly sat back down again.

It wasn't until they were all on the plane heading home to London that Zanele told her what the interpreter had really said when translating Richard's kind introduction, which was something like: "She's old and her work is done." Sarah chuckles when she tells me this. She also laughs when recounting how Zanele gently scolded her for stopping to give people lifts when they were driving up to Limpopo from Johannesburg. "Apparently I wasn't supposed to do that in South Africa." But for all her self-effacing bonhomie, Sarah was, and still is, a formidable intellect backed by a strong vein of compassion and a fierce commitment to righting wrongs.

These preparatory arrangements were all well and good, but there remained the daunting obstacles of two further preconditions of the settlement. First was navigating the tricky matter of securing political approval for the provision in the settlement that released Cape from any future liability for environmental damages arising from its former asbestos operations. This task hinged on convincing the ANC that such a hefty concession was both unavoidable and desirable. Richard had been trying for some time to secure an audience with the party's power brokers when out of the blue he got a call from someone in the ANC secretariat. The matter had come up, he was told, during the ANC's annual summit then being held in Pretoria, and senior party officials and relevant ministers would like to hear from the lawyer himself about the deal. "Would he care to come to Pretoria to explain?" they asked him. "Immediately," they added.

Fortunately—or so it seemed—Richard was in Prieska at the time, so at least he was on the same continent. Time was too tight to hire a small plane to fly up to Kimberley (from where he'd catch a commercial flight to Pretoria), so he'd have to get there by road. But road trips (as we know) have a habit of tempting fate when it comes to Richard and Leigh Day lawyers. And so it proved this time.

The long-suffering staff from Avis were, once again, willing to let Richard hire a vehicle for this latest expedition. However, whether by accident or design, they claimed that all they had available at such short notice was a clapped-out, thirteen-seater minibus. It's 150 miles from Prieska to Kimberley, along an almost dead straight road through parched, desolate bush, with only one small town along the way. A peculiar mix of boredom and the death-defying speed of local drivers are usually the main concerns. But sufficient fuel is also essential, which fact, unfortunately, had not fully impressed itself on Richard before he left, as he'd forgotten to check how much was in the tank. And so, after some ninety miles, the minibus came to a slow, ignominious halt.

Plan B had Richard standing on the roadside dressed in a suit and tie with a briefcase in one hand and the thumb of the other gesturing at the few vehicles passing by. Due, perhaps, to the incongruity of his appearance, he was having no luck until a farmer stopped to offer him a lift in the back of his truck, "if you don't mind sharing it with the goats," the farmer explained, "'cause that's all the room I have." The goats, it seems, were rather taken by Richard's attire as "they nonchalantly nibbled at my suit and trampled my briefcase," he later tells me. As accommodating as this scene was, the goat-farmer's progress was too slow (ANC officials were keeping tabs on Richard's progress by cell phone), so it was decided that he would be intercepted en route by a driver of a late-model Mercedes dispatched by the Northern Cape premier, Manne Dipico, to ferry him the rest of the way. Richard barely had time to thank the stunned farmer as he detached himself from the goats and clambered into the purring Merc and sped off into the distance. "We tore along the highway and screeched into Kimberley airport just before the plane took off, but I made it to Pretoria."[44]

Once there, Richard managed to persuade the ANC and thereafter the South African cabinet to sign off on the agreement. It had not been easy to convince them, but his case was helped greatly by support from Justice Minister Maduna, alongside Premier Dipico and his Limpopo counterpart, Ngoako Ramatlhodi, who both saw the short-term benefits the settlement would bring both to their local communities and to their own political prestige.[45]

The second precondition of the settlement was more formidable, not least because it was so completely beyond Richard's capacity to do anything about it. Cape's financial backers had to agree to lend the company the money, and for that to happen, they had to be convinced that Cape was sufficiently well placed to carry such a heavy financial burden.

In town hall meetings in Prieska, Burgersfort, and Mafefe, Richard was at pains to get this point across, however frustrating it was for the communities to hear it. The irony that claimants like seventy-two-year-old Gideon Mkhonto, a former mine worker at Penge battling ARD, now found "himself worrying about the financial health of the company that made him sick," was not lost on either the claimants or their lawyers.[46] Such worries, as it transpired, were well placed. Despite all other efforts, the settlement initially faltered when Cape failed to make the first payment to the HAT on the scheduled date of June 30, 2002, and then foundered entirely in August that same year when Cape's bankers (Barclays Bank and the Royal Bank of Scotland) declined to make the necessary loans, on the grounds that they were not convinced of the future financial viability of the company with a £21 million liability sitting on its books.

"It was a devastating blow to claimants who at that point in time had expected to begin receiving their compensation payments," Richard recalls.[47] After the highs of the House of Lords' judgment in July 2000 and the in-principle agreement over settlement terms that followed it, this was (another) huge dip in the roller-coaster journey of the case. It also, once again, presented Richard with the unenviable task of explaining to the claimants why it happened and what would happen next. Pointing out that one of the reasons for Cape's precarious financial position was the enormous costs it had incurred defending the case was fair and accurate, but it did little to relieve the bitterness of people's disappointment.

With litigation recommencing almost immediately, it seemed like the whole adversarial show was back on the road. Montpellier sold its stake in the company, and Paul Sellars (who "felt bad" about the failure of the settlement)[48] was replaced as chair by Martin May, who was not at all inclined to settle the case for anything more than a bargain basement price. Cape's lawyers, emboldened by the settlement's collapse, also reverted to type in backing their client as aggressively as possible.

Richard's first meeting with Martin May was as dispiriting as it was in stark contrast to his relationship with Paul Sellars. "His first offer was ridiculous—£1 or £2 million, I think," says Richard, "but I knew they had more to give than that, so I flatly refused, telling him we'd accept nothing less than £8 million." Sometime later, May upped the offer to £4 million, but Richard stuck to his guns, insisting on £8 million. May was aghast: "That's not the way you bargain," he blustered, as if this was haggling over pottery in a bazaar, but Richard was unmoved, suspecting that Cape may well be under pressure from its own bankers to reach a settlement.

Finally, after more strained meetings with Cape and its lawyers, the company offered £7.5 million, which both Richard and Anthony Coombs accepted as it seemed clear to them that the company would not agree to pay more. Included in this figure was £1 million from Cape's insurers, General Accident South Africa (GASA), being the same amount it had agreed to under the doomed first settlement.[49] In addition, GASA agreed to £2.75 million for legal costs, being an increase of £500,000 on the previous offer under the first settlement.[50]

The claimants' total of £7.5 million was a let-down compared to what had been agreed to in the first settlement, but Richard and Anthony were able to supplement it with a further £3.2 million drawn from another settlement then being negotiated in parallel litigation in South Africa. This second case was against Gencor, another asbestos company, for which many of the Cape claimants in Limpopo Province had also worked at some time.[51] Their employment overlap was the justification behind the Gencor settlement's contribution to the Cape settlement, albeit, as we shall see, hard fought and fractious. At any rate, together, these two amounts brought the total sum of £10.7 million available for payouts to the Cape claimants. It was in fact a sum similar to what the claimants would have received under the earlier Cape settlement (recalling that the £21 million then was to have been divided evenly between existing claimants in one group and all future claimants in another).[52]

The most obvious forfeiture in the new settlement was the abandonment of the trust arrangement for managing future claimants. It was a serious loss. Everyone involved (most especially Richard, who'd been told time and again by folk like Tony Davies) knew that the ARD epidemic was a slow-burn affair, with the certainty that many thousands more cases would arise in the coming years and decades. But as Richard and Anthony's primary duties were owed to their existing clients, they were obliged to focus on their needs first, and so the trust was duly dissolved.[53]

Another difference between the two settlements was potentially advantageous. Cape's indemnity against any future claims for environmental damage and rehabilitation, which Richard had negotiated (reluctantly and at the cost of frayed nerves and a good suit) with the South African Cabinet as part of the first settlement, was dropped from the second one. Theoretically, therefore, Cape would be open to future claims for historical environmental damage by the South African government (though to date, no such legal claims have been made).

At the same time, however, Cape insisted on retaining its indemnity against any subsequent claims by existing claimants. And further, as part of Gencor's agreement to chip in £3.2 million to the Cape claimants' compensation pot, those claimants who'd worked for both companies were also obliged to waive any right to subsequent claims against Gencor or its subsidiaries.[54]

The contribution from Gencor was clearly important but securing it had been difficult and fraught. For while Richard Meeran and Richard Spoor—the South African lawyer who had initiated the action against Gencor in late 2001—were nominally on the same side as they shared some hundreds of claimants, their agendas were different. The Cape litigation was effectively finished and a settlement within reach, whereas the Gencor claimants were still in the middle of negotiations. Spoor wanted to delay any separate consideration of compensation for those claimants who had also been employed by Cape until he'd secured a settlement for all the claimants against Gencor. This made no sense to Meeran, as that would inevitably delay any payouts those overlapping claimants might receive.

Spoor's case was also precariously poised at this time, as Gencor was threatening to unbundle (i.e., divest) its assets *without* making any provision for the asbestos victims as prospective creditors.[55] Richard and Anthony Coombs joined Richard Spoor in seeking an injunction against Gencor doing so unless and until a settlement for all asbestos victims of its operations was established. Gencor duly complied, and an Asbestos Relief Trust

(ART) was created. However, Richard Spoor was reluctant to see any part of the monies in the trust carved out for the dual Cape/Gencor claimants. Rather, he wanted to have these claimants, like all the others, go through the process of claiming from the ART.

The resulting stand-off was tense to say the least, with each Richard accusing the other of scuppering their respective cases.[56] Ultimately, the impasse was broken by Gefco (the Gencor subsidiary for which a significant proportion of the Cape claimants had worked) agreeing to pay the agreed-on £3.2m for the benefit of those Cape claimants who had worked for it. Thereupon, tying up the matter, the terms of the ART were amended expressly to exclude the Cape claimants.

The Gencor negotiations were a bruising affair, tinged with distrust over the origins of a damning article that appeared in South Africa's *Mail & Guardian* in May 2002, concerning the then still extant December 2001 settlement for the Cape claimants. It was a scurrilous piece, strewn with factual errors upon which its authors mounted sensationalist accusations that Leigh Day was poised to take the "lion's share" of the £21 million for itself, that many claimants would be getting nothing at all, and that the firm had done nothing to communicate any of this to the communities involved. It was rank bad journalism, made suspiciously worse by the inclusion of a lengthy hagiographic section on Richard Spoor's case against Gencor.[57]

A week later, after a flurry of outraged correspondence from Richard Meeran (supported by UK legal aid officials) threatening a libel suit, the newspaper published a long, and, it must be said, groveling apology, admitting making "untrue statements," including "suggest[ions] that Leigh Day had acted unethically and irresponsibly," and "regret[ting] the false and inappropriate language used in the article and apologis[ing] unreservedly to

Leigh Day & Co and their clients for the offence and distress caused."[58]

Despite the lawyerly rancor, a settlement with Gencor had been reached, and everything looked set to be signed alongside the new Cape settlement agreement. But there remained one final episode of serendipitous melodrama before that could happen. Upon being notified of the details of the new settlements, the United Kingdom's Legal Services Commission (LSC) realized that the new arrangements included an additional £500,000 allocated to Leigh Day and JPP for legal costs. Ever mindful of the need to save taxpayers' money, the LSC duly reduced its previous commitment to bear £3 million of the claimants' legal costs to cover only £2.5 million of their costs.[59]

Having run the case on a pro bono basis since October 2001 (when the LSC had formally withdrawn all legal aid support), and having already racked up costs far in excess of anything it was going to recover from the case, Leigh Day could ill-afford yet another hit to its bottom line. One option might have been to raid the claimants' compensation pot for some or all of the £500,000, but that prospect was so distinctly unpalatable that it forced Richard down an altogether different but still desperate path.

It was early February 2003, and Richard was sitting in his office in London with both the provincial premiers, Dipico and Ramatlhodi, discussing how matters were progressing. The £500,000 dilemma had been mentioned, whereupon Richard had one of those hare-brained ideas his colleagues were so used to see him float. "Why don't I phone Cape's insurers and ask for an extra £500,000," he said out loud. The two premiers didn't quite know where he was going with this, but they nevertheless nodded encouragingly just to see what might happen.

Through a series of mergers and name changes GASA, Cape's South African insurers, was now part of insurance giant Aviva, the CEO of which was Pehr Gyllenhammar.[60] There and then, Richard phoned Gyllenhammar's Zurich office, and "surprisingly, I got straight through to him." Richard put his case as best he could and managed to squeeze the full £500,000 out of the insurers. "I think I shamed him into it," Richard recounts, "when I placed the call on speakerphone and told Pehr who else was sitting in my office." It might be added that as Pehr Gyllenhammar had been chairing CGNU's AGM in the Barbican eighteen months earlier when it was hijacked by anti-asbestos activists and community leaders from South Africa, he was already very well aware of the reputational pitfalls of displaying signs of hard-hearted resistance to the claimants' case.

≈

On Thursday, March 13, 2003, the two settlements with Cape and with Gencor were finally signed.[61] Gencor's unbundling proceeded as planned, while Cape's shareholders and (crucially) its bankers approved the deal. In the weeks that followed, detailed letters—in English, Afrikaans, and Sotho—explaining the terms of the settlements "as clearly as possible" were distributed to all the claimants, often by hand, at huge community meetings. Sarah Leigh recalls the lines of people queuing up to receive their letters, "many clutching their *dompas'* [passbooks] from their working days" as proof of identity. "Some could hardly walk," she recalls, while others were supported by friends and relatives as they shuffled forward.[62] Claimants were given until May 20, 2003, to register any objections, but "not a single client did object, nor did anyone object thereafter," Richard notes.[63]

South African banks were invited to bid for the tender to hold, administer, and disperse the settlement monies, with Amalgamated Banks of South Africa (ABSA) the successful bidder. The local communities and Leigh Day lawyers got to know Phillip and Benny, the two ABSA representatives assigned to the project, well. "They were a striking pair," says Richard, not just because one was very short and the other very tall, but because of their genuine commitment to getting the payouts into the hands of the claimants.

Phillip (Robinson), the shorter of the two, was especially well liked. A devoutly religious Afrikaner, he invested tremendous efforts in making sure that the payouts were administered "fairly and the claimants treated with dignity," as Zanele Mbuyisa recalled. He organized a "road show" that traveled throughout the affected communities to explain the process, and he oversaw the establishment of bank accounts for the many who had none and provided deposit cards for people to access their payments.[64] On the other hand, the ABSA-branded bags that Phillip and Benny enthusiastically distributed to everyone they met were less well appreciated. "They were crap," remembers Richard, "but they kept bringing more with each visit."

Before any payouts could be made to anyone, however, there remained the formidable task of verifying the nature and severity of claimants' illnesses, as measured against newly formulated eligibility criteria and payout schedules. Anticipating approval of the two settlements, work had already begun on building this ARD log-frame. The disease-payout schedule drawn up under the first, aborted, Cape settlement had been used as a starting point. But it had very quickly expanded into a far more complex template with some 600 permutations in total after all relevant considerations were factored in.

In a database of nearly 7,500 claimants, individuals had first to be separated into one of two groups according to their principal employer (Cape or Gencor/Gefco), followed by an assessment of their medical records. These ranged from substantial to almost non-existent and with varying degrees of documented exposure (long/short term; occupational and/or environmental) in order to establish the seriousness of their illness. Thereafter, account had to be taken of the claimant's age and length of employment, as well as the risk of future malignancy, an especially important factor for those exposed to blue asbestos. Altogether, a team of fifteen people spread across offices in South Africa and London working full time for a month was necessary to complete the job.

Zanele was a key player on the team, helping construct a points-based eligibility and entitlement matrix and applying it (via an algorithm devised by an inscrutable computer geek called Joel) to the specific circumstances of each claimant. As both she and Richard emphasize in retrospect, the aim was to be as dispassionate as possible, employing generous interpretations of often inadequate documentation, while being mindful of not "diverting money from deserving to less deserving claimants."[65] It was demanding work, emotionally as well as intellectually, especially as everyone agreed that it was imperative to distribute the money as speedily as possible. Errors were bound to occur, so they also created a "Fuck-Up Fund," as Zanele called it (officially labeled "Retention Fund"), of some £200,000 held back to deal with those who had been "mistakenly underpaid."[66]

As the settlement machine swung into action, it gave Richard cause to reflect on just how complicated and drawn out these class action cases can be—undeniably important, but with so many false summits along the way one couldn't help wondering when it would all end. For Richard and Leigh Day, the signing of the two settlement agreements in March 2003 had been a denouement of sorts. After dragging on for nearly eight years, involving some fifty lawyers and para-legals interviewing and engaging thousands of claimants, collecting evidence from hun-

dreds of sources, and poring over more than one million documents, the litigation stage was finally over.[67]

It would be another eighteen months, however, before the case
could finally be closed, with all payouts made and all the inevitable loose ends (including untraceable claimants) tied off. Only
then could Richard and everyone else involved begin to contemplate the case's legacy. What it had achieved. Where it had
failed. And how to build on its foundations.

CHAPTER 10

Legacy

—"It's Not Yesterday's Problem"—

GLADYS WITBOOI HAD JUST finished "matric" (final year of high school) when she began to care for her grandpa's brother, she tells me over tea in the leafy garden of a little café on the edge of Prieska.[1] In his early seventies, her great-uncle had worked for years in Cape's Koegas mine and been recently diagnosed with mesothelioma. "I nursed him 'til his death," she says, musing on whether that was the moment when she realized her vocation, or was it earlier? Gladys worked for nearly ten years as a nurse at Prieska Hospital from 1995 to 2004, coincidentally almost exactly the span of the Cape litigation.

Every year during that time, she reckons she saw three or four mesothelioma cases and twenty or so asbestosis cases out of the town's population of around 10,000, "but the true figures," she stresses, "were much higher." In those days, she explains, it was common practice to mark death certificates with such nonspecific labels as "natural causes" or "pneumoconiosis." Her own family tree is littered with victims of asbestos. Her mother and grandmother both died of asbestosis, as, probably, did her uncle, who "turned blue" the day before he died. (His death certificate stated "natural causes.")

In 2004, she watched a close friend die of mesothelioma (properly diagnosed) at thirty-seven, the same age as Gladys at the time. She remembers the two of them "rolling blue asbestos fibers from the mill into fake cigarettes," when they were still at primary school, aged ten. Her friend got no compensation from anyone, because her asbestos exposure was environmental rather than occupational, so she fell outside South Africa's occupational health compensation scheme, and her diagnosis had come too late to be included as a claimant in the case against Cape. "It seemed so unfair," Gladys says softly, "that Cape could get away with it."

Gladys is precisely the sort of nurse you'd want when you need one—caring, thoughtful, and smart, but perhaps above all, calm. She's plump with a perfectly symmetrical face, a buzz cut of copper-colored hair, and a beguilingly shy smile. From her generous, empathetic disposition, she has cultivated a strong Hippocratic ethic and a commitment to using health services in ways that help the marginalized (including trying to raise money for a mobile clinic she wants to drive around remote communities). She's not someone who is readily inclined to carp and complain, yet clearly, she's seen plenty to carp and complain about. At fifty-three, she's also quietly worried about her own health after all she has seen and done. When I ask her about what the next generation thinks of the town's blighted past, she replies that her daughter "likes the history," adding with a little huff, "because it is so dramatic."

It is indeed dramatic, but living and dying in it were often horrifyingly hopeless. Deceased relatives regularly refused to permit the removal of lungs for biopsies on cultural grounds, and, in any case, many thought "it was useless" doing so. Life and death then could also be sadly mundane. The most common advice dispensed by Gladys and her hospital colleagues to the families of asbestos patients was "just provide TLC; there's nothing we can do."

≈

Of all the many legacies of the Cape case, the most important are those experienced by the victims, their families, and the communities they come from. Gladys's story is unique, of course, but it shares elements with those of the many thousands who lived and worked in the towns where asbestos was mined, milled, and manufactured and it echoes how they are all coping today.

Like everyone in Prieska at the time, Gladys knew of the case, and while none of her close relatives was a claimant, many of her patients were. She'd seen and heard Richard but never met him. She knew people who'd received payouts and others, like her friend, who hadn't but who deserved to. She also knew that the money was never enough. The payments were modest, ranging from a few hundred to a few thousand pounds. Certainly, they paled in comparison to the millions awarded to US citizens in American courts and the hundreds of thousands in UK compensation payments. They were also far less than claimants would have received from the £100 million originally estimated as the total value of their claims. They were, unavoidably, a reflection of Cape's precarious financial circumstances, as Richard stresses, no matter how regrettable that was. Equally, while the subsequent dissatisfaction expressed by some claimants over their slice of the proceeds was understandable, it reflected the fact that the "compensation paid . . . was spent relatively quickly," as Richard frankly concedes.[2]

But neither were the payouts the sole measurement of Cape's atonement. Initially, nobody had really believed they'd be able to challenge Cape in any meaningful way, despite how much they had wished to. When Richard first came to town, people were happy to hear him but thought his ideas a little far-fetched. Taking on a big company like Cape in the courts was one thing; doing so successfully on its own turf—in English courts with English judges—seemed unlikely, to say the least. Still, they stuck with him through years of ups and downs. The payments, even if inadequate in monetary terms, nevertheless represented, in the claimants' eyes, a clear admission by Cape of its culpability. The legal subtleties of the settlement's "without prejudice" (or no fault conceded) status were, quite simply, beside the point. The fact that in the end there was no trial and therefore (for the lawyers) no establishment of a legal precedent of liability was for most people irrelevant and therefore ignored. "They paid up, didn't they?" many people now ask rhetorically.

The elation experienced when they had triumphed in the House of Lords in July 2000 was not forgotten by the claimants. Nor by South African politicians, who hailed it as a victory over Apartheid capitalism. Premier Manne Dipico of Northern Cape Province had written to Richard in the immediate aftermath of the judgment to tell him he was "over-joyed" with the "historic" outcome and offering his "sincere thanks and gratitude" for Richard's inspirational fortitude and his "steadfast belief and commitment" to fighting for justice on behalf of so many South African asbestos victims—though he added portentously that "the challenges ahead are enormous and daunting . . . for our people."[3] And following the settlement in March 2003, Premier Ngoako Ramathlodi of Limpopo Province put the litigation in an even broader perspective: "I would like to thank all those in the

UK who have stood alongside our struggle and hope that this solidarity and support will continue in the many similar cases involving underprivileged people across the world."[4]

Still, when today you talk to people in the two provinces about the case and its aftermath, their ambivalence is evident. "It helped us turn a corner," Cecil Skeffers from Prieska tells me,[5] but stresses, "we can't forget the effects Cape's operations had on thousands of people."[6] Charley Nkadimeng, who still lives and works in Limpopo, says much the same: "People appreciated getting some compensation, but it could never be enough. Their sense of loss lingers in their hearts and minds as they live and relive the experience daily."[7] Nor can these mining communities forget the 776 claimants who died during the many years of court battles raging half a world away and who were therefore denied the opportunity to see justice being done.[8]

Among those who survived, and no matter their initial satisfaction winning the case, it is this sense of being cheated that is most abiding. Cheated by a company that knew of the dangers and cheated of their own health, welfare, and livelihoods and, consequently, of securing their children's futures. And perhaps most of all, cheated of the truth. The earlier years of trauma and tragedy have given way to a lingering bitterness born of the wickedness that the case revealed.

In one of the very first documents he tendered in the Cape litigation, Richard stated: "The scale of the human tragedy of asbestos-related injury around the world is common knowledge. Nowhere has the human cost been greater than in South Africa."[9] While the country's political past ensured that asbestos's lethal touch was felt overwhelmingly by black and coloured communities, it spared no one.

As Jack Adams and I had been waiting for Gladys Witbooi to arrive for our meeting in the café, a big, bluff Afrikaner on the table next to us greeted Jack with a cheery "hello" and a bone-jangling handshake. Both long-time, Prieska locals, they'd worked together at a copper mine some years back. On hearing what I was doing there, he fell into a matter-of-fact story about both his parents playing in the asbestos stockpiles beside the mill when they were kids: "They'd no idea of the dangers back then" he says. "Mum died because of asbestos in 1992; she was fifty-five," he adds, as his young granddaughter slurps the last of her milkshake, having evidently heard the tale many times before.

What today unites people in places like Prieska and Griekwastad in the Northern Cape and Burgersfort and Mafefe in Limpopo are these shared and ongoing histories of sorrow and loss. Strong ties bind people together in these communities and the communities to their land, with people staying and helping one another precisely because of what they've all gone through rather than leaving, as one might expect many to do.[10]

South African social anthropologist Linda Waldman, who has written extensively on the Northern Cape's complicated social history with asbestos, believes these bonds are built on notions of "extended kinship" and "caring for each other" through which "ARD sufferers find solace and respite."[11] Waldman notes that while provincial and national governments have tried to help make staying an attractive option after (finally) banning asbestos mining, manufacture, and use in 2008[12] and by rehabilitating former asbestos mine and mill sites, these efforts have been perfunctory, doing "just enough . . . to allay people's fears . . . by covering visible fibres."[13]

Typically, according to the people I spoke to in Northern Cape and Limpopo, such rehabilitation entails spreading a thin layer of earth (approximately 300 millimeters) over exposed asbestos deposits, which is easily disturbed by wind and rain, as well as by grazing and burrowing animals. The acacia bushes planted with the aim of holding the topsoil in place often fail to take root, as was evident when Cecil, Jack, and I visited the abandoned Koegas mine site and the nearby Draghoender railhead, where patches of discolored bruise-purple grass signify poorly covered slagheaps of crocidolite asbestos ore.

Similarly, in Limpopo, re-exposed amosite asbestos dust is today seen blowing off the hillsides and flowing into rivers when it rains heavily.[14] And while asbestos tailings have been removed from Prieska's sports fields and school playgrounds and the asbestos cement roofing that used to be everywhere has now been replaced, there are still some "fifty kilometers of asbestos cement-lined water pipes under our feet," says Andrew Phillips, Prieska's mayor, pointing to the polished concrete floor of the KFC in which we are struggling to conduct an interview, suddenly surrounded by a mob of excited kids from the school next door.[15]

As lessons in legacy, these are vivid illustrations that certainly schooled me. One of the first places I visited when I first arrived in Prieska was the Siyathemba (local district) Municipality Office where I'd been told lumps of crocidolite asbestos were still on display. The uniformed and armed officer at the entrance was more than happy to show me the less-than-airtight glass cabinet where various rock samples from the region were haphazardly on show. The labels had been jumbled, and he wasn't quite sure which one was blue asbestos, "but Leonard can tell you," he offered, pointing across the road to where I'd find the office of the municipality's geologist. Leonard wasn't around, but I couldn't help wondering about the safety of the display cabinet. Realizing, in the weeks that followed, the smallness of my concern compared to what the townsfolk of Prieska had lived through and were now living with, helped put matters in perspective.

≈

The foundations of this dreadful legacy were laid decades ago by short-sighted design as well as monumental carelessness. While Cape, in the present story, may have played the part of principal villain, there were other supporting actors who played noteworthy roles. Tony Davies hinted at the role of his own profession in an early letter to Richard:

> All the existing evidence, imperfect though it may be, points to a failure to control the working environment and a neglect of vital research and follow up studies on the part of the industry. A major component of the failure of development in the rural areas of colonial Africa is the high level of epidemic and endemic disease, part of which is due to occupational lung disease.[16]

Whereas the asbestos industry may have been neglectful in its research efforts, it was the implicit and, at times, complicit, support it received from some medical professionals and scientists that helped pull a veil of respectability over the asbestos corporations' corruption of science. The cover-up revelations of the Cape case precipitated many difficult years of soul-searching among occupational health researchers in South Africa.

Delving into the lessons learned from this exercise, Leslie London, a public health specialist who heads up a Conflict of Interest in Health Research program at the University of Cape Town, identifies what he calls "the challenge of 'dual loyalty'" facing such researchers. This challenge arises from the need to "strike a balance" between the demands of an employer, on the one hand, and the welfare of employees (including in obtaining workers' consent that is properly "autonomous and informed"), on the other.[17] For a practical example of the dilemma, it is no surprise that London and his co-authors cite Lundy Braun and

Sophie Kisting's work on South Africa's "invisible epidemic" of ARDs. "Because [asbestos] company doctors owed their livelihood to the mine owners, there was little incentive to diagnose diseases with a longer latency than the worker's tenure in the mine," write Braun and Kisting.[18]

South Africa's medical and scientific community have also been tracking the progress of ARDs in the former mining communities, albeit imperfectly due to poor or nonexistent health records of so many coloured and (especially) black former asbestos workers and to the inherent difficulties in accurately diagnosing ARDs.[19] One 2014 update of a longitudinal study of a cohort of "crocidolite-exposed" births in Prieska between 1916 to 1936 recorded that still, many decades later, "the mortality rates of mesothelioma and lung cancer are . . . very high in this cohort." It then adds, "the town and surrounding area remain contaminated with asbestos," meaning that ARD levels among Prieska residents are very likely to remain high.[20] In Penge, the levels of asbestos contamination were found to be so high in 2008 that recommendations were made for the village to be declared unfit for human habitation and the entire population (of about 3,000) to be relocated.[21] The relocation never happened, and the population size is roughly the same today.

Subsequent studies show a steady increase in the incidence of mesothelioma diagnoses across the country. According to the Global Cancer Observatory, 296 new mesothelioma cases were recorded in 2020 in South Africa, alongside 270 mesothelioma deaths,[22] as against earlier calculations between 2003 and 2013 of annual mesothelioma averages of 178 diagnoses and 194 deaths.[23] When these figures might peak is a matter of some debate, given mesothelioma's long latency period (more than fifty years, according to some sources),[24] though at least one global mesothelioma study published in 2021 offers some hope that it may be sooner rather than later. "An analysis of temporal trends in mesothelioma incident cases in the 47 countries with complete asbestos bans from 1990 to 2017 revealed that mesothelioma incidence began to decrease after 20 years of a complete ban on asbestos use," the authors note.[25] South Africa will cross that twenty-year threshold in the late 2020s, but with unprecedented quantities of amosite and crocidolite asbestos fibers still loose in South Africa's environment and more being steadily released from old mines and mills, uncovered tailings dumps, public buildings, and people's homes, such a time-frame may be fanciful.

≈

With no funding for environmental clean-up coming from the Cape settlements or from settlements arising out of subsequent litigation against asbestos corporations, the burden has been shouldered mainly by South African governments. It is true that a few asbestos mine sites have been rehabilitated by their former owners after stricter environmental regulations requiring them to do so were introduced in the 1980s and 1990s. By then, most companies were shuttering their asbestos operations in the country.[26] Gefco, for example, which inherited Cape's South African asbestos mining operations when Cape sold them all in 1979, undertook rehabilitation work at the main Penge mine between 1986 and 1992 (when the mine was finally closed down).[27] Cape itself undertook no such work before it left, and while some of its satellite mine sites around Penge had been rehabilitated by 2022, many more, according to government records,[28] remain untouched or only minimally treated in both Limpopo and the Northern Cape.

To a large extent, therefore, given that all asbestos mining ceased in South Africa more than twenty years ago, the mess has been left for the state to clean up. The Department of Mineral Resources and Energy has developed a mine rehabilitation program, which supports the work of the South African Council for Mineral Technology in overseeing and monitoring the rehabilitation of abandoned mine sites. The task is immense, and the challenges unending.

Of the 261 recorded asbestos mine sites in South Africa, only 40 or so had been fully or partially rehabilitated by the end of 2018, at a cost to the government of some R800 million ($65 million).[29] That is despite the fact that the rehabilitation of asbestos mines (all of which are deemed "high risk") is prioritized among the more than 6,000 abandoned mine sites of all types that the government has on its books. While the number of *fully* rehabilitated asbestos mines had risen slightly by March 2021, a damning report published in 2022 by South Africa's auditor-general pointed out that at the current rate of roughly three mines per year, "it will take approximately 69 years to rehabilitate the remaining 229 derelict and ownerless asbestos mines."[30] Mind you, the same report also makes it clear that the main obstacle to any faster progress is funding. The department itself estimates that to rehabilitate the outstanding 229 asbestos mine sites by 2033 would cost R3.8 billion ($260 million).[31]

Such cost estimates are unsurprising (and very likely understated), given the scale of restoration is often far larger than initial projections, with both the wind in arid conditions and water in wet ones helping to spread asbestos fibers far beyond the mine heads or mill sites. The primary aim of the exercise, according to the official mine rehabilitation guidelines, is rightly ambitious. That is to "permanently eliminate the dispersion of asbestos fibres into the environment by wind and water . . . result[ing] in a self-sustaining, cost-effective solution to the problem that requires no or very little human after care."[32] But there remains a world of difference between the objective on paper and the reality on the ground,[33] which impressively enhanced methods of assessing levels of environmental asbestos contamination now make only too obvious.[34]

Stakeholder engagement and employment opportunities in the clean-up process are important features of the program, but even they can be undone in unexpected ways. Some mine sites have already been re-occupied by itinerant communities. Jack, Cecil, and I encountered goat herders and fisher folk living in old staff quarters associated with the Koegas mine near a bend in the Orange River. All were unimpressed by any proposal to kick them off the land for rehabilitation work, no matter the health dangers they currently face.

Similarly, at other sites, and "reflect[ing] the current economic reality in South Africa, where people are desperate for livelihoods,"[35] asbestos mines have been reopened by "zama zamas" (opportunistic artisanal miners) looking for ancillary minerals of value. One of these is the gemstone "tiger eye" (as locals call it), which is often found in the same banded ironstone as crocidolite asbestos. This is no mere coincidence, as it is believed that the gemstone is formed from the gradual degradation of crocidolite fibers and their replacement by a lustrous quartz in a process known as pseudomorphism.[36] Tiger eye, Jack tells me, is a valuable commodity in the hills around Koegas, and the old asbestos mines provide ready access for people to get at it.

≈

While the rehabilitation process in South Africa may be troubled, inadequate, and slow, it is at least dealing with commercial asbestos sites that are no longer operating. In other parts of the world, asbestos mining, milling, and manufacture are still thriving. Incredibly, more than 1.3 million metric tons of asbestos were produced globally in 2022. Russia is, by far, the largest producer (700,000 tons in 2022), followed by Kazakhstan (230,000 tons), Brazil (190,000 tons), and China (130,000 tons).[37] Asbestos consumption today is concentrated almost entirely in countries in Asia and the Middle East, most especially China and India, where its handling is poorly regulated.[38] Relatively small quantities of asbestos are also still imported by the United States every year for use mainly in brake linings and gaskets.[39]

Worldwide, the annual death toll from asbestos-related diseases is more than 255,000,[40] with asbestos-related illnesses on the rise in countries that have continued to mine or manufacture the mineral.[41] Nowadays, asbestos production and use are focused entirely on serpentine chrysotile asbestos, as amphibole asbestos varieties (notably crocidolite and amosite) are no longer mined anywhere.[42] While the International Chrysotile Association will have you believe that white asbestos is safe when handled correctly,[43] the prevailing view among scientists and medical professionals today is that there is no safe threshold level of exposure to any kind of asbestos. The World Health Organization states bluntly that "all forms of asbestos are carcinogenic to humans," adding that "currently, about 125 million people in the world are exposed to asbestos at the workplace [and that] approximately half of the deaths from occupational cancer are estimated to be caused by asbestos."[44]

The Cape litigation coincided with the emergence of a strong global movement to ban all asbestos use everywhere, and the formation in 1999 of the International Ban Asbestos Secretariat (IBAS). Headed by the indefatigable Laurie Kazan-Allen, IBAS has led the charge to secure a worldwide ban, alleviate the damage caused by asbestos, and counter the asbestos industry's continuing "control of the information stream."[45] It is an uphill battle with, for example, a succession of failed attempts to block international trade in chrysotile asbestos under the UN Rotterdam Convention governing hazardous chemicals.[46]

But there have also been successes. Canada—an erstwhile major producer of chrysotile and the only remaining Western nation to mine and manufacture asbestos, as well as formerly the poster-child country of the International Chrysotile Association[47]—was eventually persuaded to introduce a comprehensive asbestos ban in 2018.[48] For many inside the ban asbestos movement, the Cape case helped galvanize support for their cause by highlighting the appalling and extended exploitation of poor workers in developing countries by Western-based multinational corporations. IBAS and Laurie Kazan-Allen were, therefore, enthusiastic backers of Richard and claimants throughout the litigation and, after its conclusion, keen advocates for further "legacy cases" to be mounted against former asbestos companies wherever they now reside.[49]

Many years later, Richard was able to return the favor for Laurie and IBAS, after they became the target of an outlandish episode of industrial espionage. Between 2012 and 2016, IBAS was infiltrated by a spy working for a corporate intelligence company in London called K2 Intelligence. Codenamed "Project Spring," it was supposed to gather "sensitive material about the leading figures in the campaign, their methods, funding and future plans."[50] Posing as a journalist, the spy was a washed-up former comedy television producer called Robert Moore, who claimed that shortly after he joined the group, he became a double agent ("I was utterly motivated by what I saw," he said) and actively worked to help the anti-asbestos advocates.[51] As unlikely as that seems (Moore continued to provide K2 with material throughout the four years, for which he was paid £466,000), everyone at IBAS was taken in by the ruse, most of all Laurie, whom Moore had specifically targeted. "He was very polite, incredibly engaging and completely believable," she recalls.[52]

After Moore's cover was blown in 2016, Laurie went "through feelings of denial, confusion, emotional outrage, emotional upheaval, distress, shock, anguish and anxiety," noted Richard when acting for her and four others, in a breach of confidence suit brought against Moore, K2, and Matteo Bigazzi, Moore's "handler" and K2's managing director.[53] K2 eventually settled for an undisclosed sum, but not before being forced to reveal the identity of its clients: "Wetherby Select Ltd, a company in the British Virgin Islands, Nurlan Omarov, a Kazakh asbestos industry lobbyist, and Daniel Kunin, a figure in Kazakhstan's asbestos industry."[54] The asbestos industry, it seems, continues to do whatever it takes to preserve itself, no matter how scurrilous its methods or where in the world it employs them.

≈

The Cape settlement monies helped support asbestos victims in the absence or inadequacy of occupational health compensation schemes in South Africa. Most importantly, they provided some financial recompense for those victims of environmental exposure to asbestos who were excluded from the state-based compensation schemes. What the final settlement lacked was any provision for asbestos victims beyond the 7,500 or so claimants named in the group action. Provision for such additional and future claimants, it will be recalled—whose number is likely thousands more—had been made in the first aborted settlement with Cape in the form of a trust. The absence of any such arrangement in the second (final) settlement was a significant loss, especially as payments for occupational lung diseases under the South Africa's two statutory occupational health schemes continue to be very low, ranging from R28,000 to R105,000 (approximately $3,500 to $13,000), and remain restricted to injuries or diseases acquired through one's work, not those acquired by environmental exposure outside work.[55]

The Asbestos Relief Trust (ART) established under the Gencor settlement at the same time as the Cape settlement does provide a mechanism through which past and future claims can be handled, and it covers environmental as well as occupational exposure. In 2006 the ART was later joined by another trust—the Kgalagadi Relief Trust—established along similar lines as the ART by the Swiss corporation Becon AG for employees of former asbestos mining corporations within the Becon Group.[56] Together, these mechanisms mark a new chapter in handling the country's asbestos legacy, one that, though initially based on litigation (or the threat of it), is expressly intended to reach trust-based settlement outcomes rather than contentious pursuits through the courts. The ART has been touted as "a model of efficient occupational disease compensation in South Africa,"[57] the instigation and design of which owes much to the lawyerly zeal of Richard Spoor who had acted for the claimants against Gencor.

While the relationship between the two Richards has yet to recover fully since their falling out over the Gencor litigation that ran parallel to the Cape case in its latter stages, the two are nevertheless forever joined. Not just by their both being pioneers in mass occupational health litigation, redressing corporate wrongs, and finding ways to compensate victims, but also by the coincidence of their respective asbestos cases being brought against multinational corporations on behalf of South African claimants. Without Richard Meeran's stubborn determination to pursue Cape for years through the UK courts and eventually win before the House of Lords, corporations throughout the common law world would have continued to hide their histories of exploitation and destruction behind the shield of *forum non conveniens* and the veil of separate corporate liabilities between parent and subsidiary companies. By winning the right to sue Cape in Britain for negligence, Meeran tore away these defenses, exposing Cape's soft underbelly—namely, its vulnerability to the preponderance of evidence collected by Meeran and Leigh Day of Cape's abject neglect, which even Cape knew would very likely succeed at trial. Corporate obstinacy to defend and deny until the bitter end, to "never surrender" when faced with mass tort actions, was suddenly a much less viable option.

There seems little doubt that the combination of such hazardous legal exposure and the likelihood of some very dirty linen being washed in public helped induce Gencor to seek an out-of-court settlement rather than fight the claims made against it in court. Richard Spoor's subsequent negotiation of the generously proportioned settlement with Gencor, therefore, was to a significant degree made possible by the unappealing alternative reality facing Gencor, should it have chosen to defend itself in the same manner as did Cape. Spoor hinted as much when he told me that his preferred *modus operandi* today, when dealing with corporations accused of serious workplace malpractice, is to make clear to them both the potentially dire consequences of going to trial and his earnest intention of going there if need be. It is against that barely disguised threat that he then offers the alternative of negotiating a settlement built on straight-talking trust, which, he tells me, many companies are inclined to take.[58]

Reflecting broadly on the jurisprudential legacy of the *Lubbe v. Cape* case, it is fair to say that the jurisdictional victory it secured is now widely seen as pushing open the door to holding multinational corporations to account in their home courts for past and present environmental and human rights abuses arising from their overseas operations.[59] It established an important bridgehead between Richard Meeran's earlier landmark cases of *Ngcobo v. Thor Chemicals* and *Connelly v. RTZ*, which tested the boundaries of parent corporate liability and of *forum non conveniens*, and the subsequent lineage of UK tort cases (notably *Chandler* [2012], *Vedanta* [2019] and *Okpabi* [2021]).[60] These latter cases firmly established both the potential liability of parent corporations for actions of their overseas subsidiaries and that the United Kingdom can be an appropriate forum in which to try cases against UK corporations being sued by overseas litigants. It is no accident that Leigh Day represented the claimants in each of these landmark cases and that all of them, except *Chandler* (coincidentally another case against Cape, but instigated by a British litigant), involved African plaintiffs who'd suffered at the hands of UK-based mining corporations failing in their legal duties of care owed to the claimants.

Above all, what this lineage of cases has done in terms of law reform is to redefine the notion of the corporate veil. While the plaintiffs' arguments in both *Lubbe v. Cape* (1998) and *Chandler v. Cape* (2012) were emphatically *not* about "'piercing the corporate veil"—rather, they asserted in both cases that the parent corporation was *directly* liable for the harm caused, not indirectly through its subsidiary[61]—they nevertheless initiated a line of reasoning that challenges long-established assumptions of what can and cannot be hidden behind the veil. Thus, in both *Vedanta* and *Okpabi*, the courts took the view that the proper test of whether a parent company owes a duty of care to the employees of its subsidiaries is based on the "business realities" of its relationship with those subsidiaries. Forensic analyses of the presence and exercise of lines of control and authority in each of these cases led the courts to conclude that such parental liability did indeed exist. This includes (in *Vedanta*), when a parent company "holds itself out [in published materials, for example] as exercising . . . supervision and control of its subsidiaries, even if it does not in fact do so."[62]

That the root of such a sizeable shift in thinking about corporate liability can be found in the words of Lord Bingham in *Lubbe v. Cape* in the House of Lords twenty years earlier, when he referred to the need to inquire "into what part the defendant [Cape Plc] played in controlling the operations of the group," demonstrates the path-breaking significance of the case.[63] Richard Hermer KC, who was lead counsel for the plaintiffs in both *Vedanta* and *Okpabi*, believes that "the legacy of the Cape case has been profound in transforming our understanding of the practical use to which private international law can be put to secure remedies for victims of human rights abuses."[64] Similarly, Dan Leader, a colleague of Richard's at Leigh Day and the instructing solicitor in the *Vedanta* and *Okpabi* cases, credits the Cape case with providing "the legal tools we have today to combat corporate impunity; . . . [it] represented a watershed moment in the fight for corporate accountability."[65]

Such talismanic cases are often referred to as "strategic litigation," in the sense that their object is to challenge legal orthodoxy in the course of representing the interests of the plaintiff litigants. When, however, they do so across state borders, they run the risk of being seen as supplanting one legal system with another. This is especially problematic when—as with all the above cases—the supplanting jurisdiction is Western and the supplanted jurisdiction is in the developing world. Critics have called the process "chauvinistic" or "colonial," as it tends to denigrate the displaced legal system and directly hinder its development by removing a case from its grasp. There is some truth in these concerns. "But what is the alternative?" asks Richard when I put this awkward point to him. "To leave the victims of transnational human rights abuses with little or no hope of

redress in their own jurisdictions?" He answers his own question: "No. Surely it is to offer them an alternative route to reparation, even if that means fighting the case in UK courts rather
than African courts."

Others are inclined to agree, arguing that while pursuing
transnational torts in home-state courts cannot be a long-term
solution, in the interim it offers the possibility of "substantial justice" where otherwise none would be available.[66] "Strategic litigation," as Daniel Augenstein, a legal academic and adviser to
a strategic litigation outfit in Berlin, notes, "has brought some
relief to victims of corporate human rights abuse in the Global
South—in spite of persistent legal and practical barriers to access to justice in European [and US] courts."[67] At the same time,
and with an eye to the longer term, Richard has also been a
strong advocate for litigating cases locally where possible. Hence,
following significant developments in the South African legal
system post-Cape—most especially regarding the availability of
class actions and litigation funding—Richard has collaborated
with Zanele's law firm, Mbuyisa Moleele, on gold miners' silicosis cases against Anglo-American and a huge Zambian lead
poisoning class action (also against Anglo-American), all of
which have been litigated in South African courts.[68]

≈

Transnational litigation of this David-versus-Goliath ilk has also
contributed to the growth of corporate social responsibility and
environmental, social, and governance movements by providing
a much-needed hard-law option amid rafts of soft-law regulations, policies, and promises. Litigation alleging involvement in
human rights abuses tends, irresistibly, to focus the minds of a
corporation's board and management. For Cape, the prospect of
further litigation along these lines was enough to compel it to

take one final controversial rear-guard action as it negotiated the fine details of the December 2003 settlement.

Mindful of the possibility that the enormous quantity of documents amassed by both sides during the life of the case might be used to inform the bringing of future actions against the company, Cape insisted that all non-public documents held by Leigh Day be destroyed. This draconian condition was overkill, as UK Civil Procedure Rules already stipulated that such documents must be not disclosed by either party following a court-endorsed settlement. In making document destruction a non-negotiable condition of settling the case, Cape showed both how concerned it was about future litigation and how hard it was prepared to play to minimize any such prospect.

Though the settlement terms were confidential, the appended three-page memorandum detailing this specific condition was leaked to the media, creating a storm of protest aimed as much at Leigh Day for agreeing to it as at Cape for insisting on it.[69] As a consequence, and after being contacted directly by the Clydebank Asbestos Group representing Scottish workers with ARDs, Leigh Day managed to persuade Cape that instead of shredding the documents, Leigh Day would return them to Cape, provided it undertook to secure "all the original documents in a purpose-built archive in Doncaster."[70]

The importance of retaining such documentation was made abundantly clear some years later in another case involving Cape, asbestos victims, and Leigh Day. The company—by then renamed Cape Intermediate Holdings, specializing in industrial insulation including asbestos replacement products—was on the verge of destroying thousands of documents following a settlement reached between Cape and one of its former client companies. Concerned at this prospect, the Asbestos Support Group Forum applied for an injunction to halt the process. The forum was represented by Harminder Bains from Leigh Day, who, together with counsel acting pro bono, succeeded before the UK Supreme Court not only in preserving the documents, but doing so by way of establishing an important new precedent balancing the principle of open justice against rights to confidentiality.[71]

≈

To reflect on the full measure of the Cape case, it is tempting to see it as a grand opera, with a score based on the imperative to expose and repair historical injustices done to some of the world's poorest and most marginalized people. It has a cast of characters at once heroic, villainous, colorful, and benighted, and a conductor whose uncompromising resolve guides the players through to the end. And while the final curtain can never, really, fall on this saga so long as asbestos's shadow remains cast across the stage, we are—a quarter of a century later—able to view it in some perspective.

It is Richard's single-minded drive—never to still the conductor's baton, as it were—that defines the story's journey. He provided the impetus to forge new legal pathways, to galvanize a small community of lawyers to do the job and, above all, to offer and then deliver on the opportunity of redemption for thousands of African victims of the so-called miracle mineral. Along the way, his unrelenting dedication to the cause won many friends and allies, and turned skeptics into believers and strangers into admirers. But he also made implacable enemies, irritated more than a few, and drove some to exhaustion or exasperation. Lawyer Susannah Read, a vital cog in the wheel for much of the case, departed Leigh Day before it concluded, burnt out and discontented. And the pioneering Marianne Felix, another critical collaborator in the early days, "was somewhat left behind later on," concedes Richard, alluding to one of the casualties of his blinkered focus.

However unintended and regrettable, there are always costs associated with endeavors pursued so stubbornly and with such vigor. Yet, it is in their very intensity that results are achieved and where inspiration is found for others to join the fray. The magnitude of what's at stake, the weight of odds against you, and the demands and sacrifices it makes are, therefore, both burdensome and seductive. Wherever I went while researching this book, I saw this trade-off between people's outrage-fueled determination to fight and the heavy toll they paid doing so. Asbestos victims, their colleagues, friends, and relatives; medics and scientists; politicians, government officials, and activists; and financiers and lawyers—all bore scars as well as decorations from the battle. They all had stories to tell, many vividly recalled in ways that took me by surprise but that, on reflection, showed just how important the issue remains to them.

The Cape case and many similar ones following it also inspired a whole generation of young (and not so young) lawyers. From Leigh Day's humble beginnings, the firm now employs some 1,000 staff, including more than 200 lawyers and a steady stream of legal interns and apprentices from all over the world. These days the firm occupies offices throughout England, while its stylish new London headquarters boasts a team of door persons and artfully displayed hydroponic plants in the building's foyer. It has a strong industrial disease practice, with a specialized Asbestos Disease Team of nearly twenty lawyers, headed by Harminder Bains and Daniel Easton. The firm's international practice now comprises some forty lawyers, led jointly by Richard and Sapna Malik, and is considered preeminent in the field: "Few compare to them on tackling complex matters involving human rights abuses committed by UK companies operating in the UK and abroad," as Chambers' 2024 legal directory puts it.[72]

These days Richard is still embroiled in big human rights cases against multinationals and governments in Africa and South America but doing less of the legwork (which he misses), as he now has a whole team to do that. He remains passionate and unrelenting in confronting corporate abuse,[73] though perhaps a tad less feverishly than before. "I'm more considered these days; I take fewer risks," he confesses. His analytical intellect is still razor-sharp, his wit still desert-dry and mischievous, and his store of remembered moments—some profound and shocking, others absurd and comic—remains as rich and capacious as ever; an Aladdin's cave of treasures that I have liberally plundered in writing this book.

He's pleased to be able to give a legal voice to those who are often otherwise powerless; happy to have helped build new legal ways to bring corporations to account; and heartened to see so many others now committing themselves to the cause. Accolades bear testimony to his pioneering work. In 2002 he was awarded the Liberty/Justice Human Rights Lawyer of the Year and, in the same year, presented with a Certificate for Outstanding Achievement by eighteen asbestos victims' support groups worldwide. His counsel is today sought far beyond legal circles, by governments, international organizations, policymakers, activists, and academics. He's written more than sixty articles and edited a major book on corporations and human rights and is regularly asked to speak publicly on the subject.

Above all, however, perhaps the truest measure of his worth comes from his family. Jahan and Nadia, both now in their thirties, are unstinting in their praise of their father's work.[74] "Now that I'm almost the same age as he was when he took on the asbestos case, I look back and I'm very, very proud of my dad," says Nadia. His resilience and resourcefulness in taking on powerful entities "to redress historic injustices," says Jahan, "fills me with hope that there are people like dad willing to stand up and fight." Along the way, however, there were also many sacrifices made by everyone in the family, especially when Richard was often away overseas or working long hours or simply preoccupied with the case. But through it all, says Munoree, "We've remained very close; we all love him to bits." Even, she adds, when he breaks out his "daddy dance at family get-togethers."[75]

≈

Late one afternoon, while immersed in the book's research and desperate to escape the tyranny of boxes of files piled up in the room Leigh Day had kindly loaned me, I ventured into the firm's kitchen for a glass of water. A young lawyer was there, hovering over the coffee machine, seeking brief respite from her own stack of documents. We got talking and she asked me (very politely) who I was and what I was doing there. After delivering my standard twenty-second spiel on Cape, Richard, and the book, I asked her whether she knew of the case. "Oh yes," she replied, "I remember it from law school." She then added, "In fact, it was cases like *Cape* that saved me from dropping out—when I realized that the law could be part of the solution, not just part of the problem." It was a grand statement to make, but sincere and, I have to say, inspiring. Richard agreed and was pleased when I told him of the encounter. He then paused for a moment, staring out the window while interlocking his fingers in his trademark ruminative fashion, and murmured, "Yes, but not a perfect solution. A messy one. Always messy."

Acknowledgments

In researching and writing this book, I leaned heavily on gaining access to historical records and to people's recollections of past events that they witnessed or took part in. The process allowed me to reconstruct the story by drawing on a wide range of primary sources and materials that, I hope, reflect its gravity and drama. The process also left me with many debts to those who generously gave me their time, energy, and expertise. There are too many of these fine folk for all to be listed here, but the names and contributions of many of them are recorded throughout the book's text and endnotes. To all of them and to the others I interviewed, talked with, and asked favors of, I offer my sincerest thanks and gratitude.

That said, I must single out a number of people for specific mention. Foremost among these is Richard Meeran, without whom, quite simply, there would be no book. His immediate and enthusiastic embrace of its suggestion some five years ago was followed by his tireless recounting of the people, places, and incidents that now populate its pages. I remain not a little amazed that he never once bridled at my steady bombardment of questions and requests for details. On the contrary. Our hundreds of hours together trying to retrace his footsteps across the nine-year span of the case from 1995 to 2004 were always eye-opening, heartfelt, and often punctuated by Richard's wry wit. It was, for me, an inspiring and richly rewarding experience.

Alongside Richard, Graham Read, as junior counsel at the time, was the other constant throughout the entire period of litigation. And, like Richard, Graham was unstinting in his efforts to ensure that I got the law and legal strategy right in the book while, crucially, doing so in a way that helped highlight the human stories of the case rather than bury them in legalese. Zanele Mbuyisa did much the same regarding the legal legacy of the case in South Africa, punctuated by her trademark bonhomie and robustly ventured opinions that extended our scheduled one-hour interview to three.

My efforts tackling the steep learning curves of the medical, scientific, and occupational health dimensions of asbestos were eased somewhat by the patient and forgiving instruction offered by Rodney Ehrlich, Emma Livingstone, Judith Kinley, Sophie Kisting-Cairncross, Leslie London, Jill Murray, Gill Nelson, Jim teWaterNaude, and Anthony Zwi. The redoubtable Tony Davies was also instrumental in my education, not least by way of a six-hour interview in his home that he insisted upon despite being ill, and, as it sadly turned out, not long before he died. His characteristic passion and dedication to helping others was evident to the very end.

My thanks to the scientists and administrators of the National Institute for Occupational Health in Johannesburg, most especially its director Spo Kgalamono and archivists Angel Mzoneli and Simphiwe Yako, who kindly hosted me for a week as I tried to piece together the story as recorded by the institution lying at its heart. While embedded there I was also grateful to occupational hygienist Gabriel Mizan, pathologist Mark Keyter, and medical scientists Lihle Mayeza, Lucia Mhlongo, and Zee Ngcobo for guiding me through the intricacies of asbestos microscopy and analysis and for being so polite both before and after they realized that my astonishing scientific ignorance was due, in part, to my *not* being a professor of natural sciences.

My first and unforgettable close encounter with the destruction wrought on human tissue by asbestos fibers was by courtesy of Murat Kekic, curator of the University of Sydney's Ainsworth

Pathology Museum, who deftly escorted me around the museum's lung and heart specimens afflicted by ARDs.

I am grateful to Carol Stewart and her fellow archivists in the University of Strathclyde's library for permitting me access to the cornucopia that is the Laurie Flynn Papers, and to Laurie Flynn himself, who has done so much over his long journalistic career to expose the skulduggery of mining companies in South Africa and elsewhere. Also, my thanks to Gordon Hodges at the University of Sydney's library, who has fielded my periodic pleas for bibliographic help with skill and good humor for more years than we both care to recall.

Sydney Law School provided vital funding to undertake the empirical work in South Africa and London, as well as granting me a six-month research sabbatical during which time much of the writing was completed. Jesus College, Cambridge, offered me a visiting fellowship for that period, providing not only a most accommodating environment in which to write but also a delightful home away from home.

The lawyers and staff of Richard Meeran's firm, Leigh Day, were also warmly welcoming, with seemingly nothing being too much trouble. Most especially Sam Jones, whose research skills and organizational acumen saved me and the project more than once from despair when faced with yet another Byzantine paper trail.

To Charlie Smith, another light on the hill, my thanks for being a friend, wit, critic, and ally, for allowing your home to become my long-time London pied-à-terre, and for seeing and believing in the story's potential from the outset, "if you're up to it!" Nikki Goldstein and Rowan Jacob also saw where the story could go, albeit into realms beyond my competence. And to my wife, Catherine, my fondest embrace for her calm patience and unwavering support, which was matched by her eagle-eyed editorial scrutiny of the manuscript's multiple drafts and her gently insightful suggestions to perhaps rethink this word or that bit of hyperbole. Her offerings of French Cartesian rigor were gratefully received where the temptations of Irish craic led things astray.

Robin Coleman, my editor (for the second time) at JHUP, has been a rock of support, sage advice, and good humor, as indeed has been my agent and ofttimes brother in arms, Chris Newson. Thank you, gentlemen.

Finally, I'd like to express my sincerest gratitude to the people of South Africa who were most and directly affected by the scourge of asbestos, notably those in the asbestos communities of the Northern Cape and Limpopo provinces who opened their homes to me and told me their stories. I also thank Jack Adams and Cecil Skeffers in Prieska, as well as Zack Mabiletja and Charley Nkadimeng in Limpopo, for giving up so much of their time to help me negotiate my way around their neighborhoods. Most remarkable of all, it was they, together, who showed me that amidst all the darkness of the asbestos legacy, light still shines.

Notes

Prologue

1. Though had the House of Lords rejected the appeal, an appeal to the European Court of Justice on the specific point of the compatibility of the defence of *forum non conveniens* with the Brussels Convention would still have been possible. That point is discussed further in chapter 5.
2. Heidi Kingstone, "Street Justice," *Business Age*, February 2001, 52–54.
3. That said, from the outset Richard was very careful not to provide me with access to any privileged or confidential documents.

1. David versus Goliath

Regarding the subtitle of this chapter, the same trope was used by South African journalist Susan Segar in her exposé of Richard published in *Natal Witness* on August 22, 1997, entitled "Helping David Take On Goliath." It's a marvellous piece, engaging as well as informative.

1. Arthur Scargill, the charismatic leader of the NUM, had earlier floated the idea with Leigh Day of pursuing test litigation against British asbestos corporations regarding their overseas operations in a Joint Asbestos Initiative memo (dated April 14, 1994) between the International Mineworkers' Organisation (of which Scargill was president), the African Miners Federation, NUM (South Africa), and Leigh Day & Co. Scargill was a keen follower of the case against Cape, including in correspondence with Richard regarding its progress.
2. Ultimately, though, the House of Lords was to rule in Connelly's favor, permitting the case to be heard in the United Kingdom; see *Connelly v. RTZ* [1997] UKHL 30 (24 July 1997). The subsequent

trial foundered, however, for being out of time—that is, it was ruled time-barred by the High Court according to relevant Namibian and UK limitation statutes; see *Connelly v. RTZ* (No.3) [1999] CLC 533 (4 December, 1998).

3. As recorded over forty years by local Prieska doctor, André Pickard. See further chapter 2.

4. As noted by Maxone Salone, who worked at Cape's Penge mine from 1961 to 1992; see David Beresford, "Death from the Rock Exposes British Firms to South African Asbestos Claims," *The Guardian*, February 1, 1999.

5. Greg Dropkin, "Cape and Rio Tinto: 'They Must Give Back What They Took from the People,'" *The Namibian*, June 21, 2000. Matlaweng Mohlala, another lead plaintiff, said much the same thing; see "I Was Given No Warning by Anyone," *The Independent*, March 31, 1997.

6. Interview with Thabo Makweya, March 13, 2023, Johannesburg.

7. In the building of the bridge between the two NUMs, Gwede Mantashe—then a rising star within the South African union movement and now (in 2024) Minister for Mineral Resources and Energy—was instrumental, according to Thabo Makweya, March 13, 2023.

8. This is the metaphor Thabo Makweya used in describing to me the critical role played by Gwede Mantashe, then Assistant General Secretary of the NUM (SA), in bringing the two unions together on the issue.

9. Typically, this is the route to a law degree taken by graduates in another discipline. Unlike in the United States, law is taught predominantly as an undergraduate degree in the United Kingdom.

10. Richard Meeran, communication, April 8, 2020.

11. It was the first such case before the Industrial Tribunal to be brought by a solicitor against a law firm. It was eventually settled with the law firm paying a monetary compensation to Richard, issuing him an apology, and instituting an equal opportunities scheme within its recruitment process. The name of the firm and the precise terms of the settlement are confidential. Richard Meeran, communication, May 2, 2023.

12. Sir Goolam Hoosen Kader-Meeran was knighted in 2009.

13. *Adams v. Cape Industries Plc* [1990] Ch. 433 (27 July 1989). The Court of Appeal so held despite accepting the plaintiff's submission that

"Cape ran a single integrated mining division with little regard to the corporate formalities as between the members of the group" (at 537).

14. See, for example, Peter Pringle, *Cornered: Big Tobacco at the Bar of Justice* (Henry Holt, 1998), which documents tobacco litigation in the United States, where so much of this legal drama was played out.

15. Per Brian Doctor QC, Cape's lead counsel at the time; Richard Meeran, communication, April 14, 2020.

16. Under the Courts and Legal Services Act (1990), at section 58. By the mid-1990s litigation funding was also legal, but in such an attenuated form that it was seldom offered, still less used. Conditional fee arrangements were permitted in the UK only from July 5, 1995, under the Conditional Fee Agreements Order (1995). See "A Brief History of Litigation Finance: The Cases of Australia and the United Kingdom," *The Practice*, September–October 2019, Center for the Legal Profession, Harvard Law School.

17. For further details of the legal aid sought by and granted to the plaintiffs throughout the litigation, see chapters 8 and 9.

18. Richard Meeran, "'Process' Liability of Multinationals: Overcoming the Forum Hurdle," *Journal of Personal Injury Litigation* (1995): 170–84. Coincidentally, one of the cases he cited in support of his argument was an Australian case involving a mesothelioma victim who successfully persuaded the court to lift the corporate veil and hold the parent company liable (*Olson v. CSR and Australian Blue Asbestos Pty Ltd*, NSWCA [1994; unreported]), which itself built on an earlier Australian corporate veil-lifting case of *Barrow v. CSR Ltd*, WASC (1988; unreported) also involving a victim of an ARD (asbestosis).

19. These encounters had occurred just as the *Thor* and *Connelly* cases were commencing (and therefore just before the start of the Cape litigation). Rokison had in fact been opposing counsel in a previous case that Leigh Day had brought against British Nuclear Fuels, and Lord Justice May was the father-in-law of Richard's friend and colleague (in the *Thor* litigation), James Cameron.

20. Cape Plc, Annual Report 1997, 50; see also similar sentiments expressed by Michael Langdon in his "Chairman's Statement," 2, immediately after noting that the company's operating profit had increased to £12.3 million. The annual report was published shortly after the first round of litigation (which Cape won) but before the plaintiffs' appeal to the Court of Appeal (which Cape lost).

21. Richard Meeran, communication, April 8, 2020.
22. *Merlin & Others v. British Nuclear Fuels Plc* [1991] 3 JEL 122; *Reay and Hope v. British Nuclear Fuels Plc* [1994] 5 Med LR 1. For a damning critique of these cases (and similar others), see Martyn Day, "The Environment: Modernising Justice?" *Energy & Environment* 11, 2 (2000): 127–33.
23. See chapter 4.
24. James Allenman and Brooke Mossman, "Asbestos Revisited," *Scientific American*, July 1997, 74.
25. For the United States, see Barry Castleman, *Asbestos: Medical and Legal Aspects*, 5th ed. (Prentice Hall Law & Business, 2004), and for the United Kingdom, see Geoffrey Tweedale, *Magic Mineral to Killer Dust* (Oxford University Press, 2000).
26. Allenman and Mossman, "Asbestos Revisited," 70.
27. Upon which points chapter 4 further expands.
28. For a potted history of UK asbestos regulation, see "History of Asbestos Law and Regulations," Oracle Solutions, undated, https://www.oracleasbestos.com/what-is-asbestos/asbestos-regulations/a-complete-guide-to-the-history-of-asbestos-law-and-regulations/. For US regulations, see Jennifer Lucarelli, "Asbestos Ban," Mesothelioma.com, undated, https://www.mesothelioma.com/lawyer/legislation/asbestos-ban/.
29. Cape Industries Limited, *Annual Report and Accounts for 1974* (1975), 4. Coincidently, it was also in 1974 that the US Environmental Protection Agency banned the use of spray-on asbestos in all buildings in the United States.
30. Over the years the company had operated asbestos facilities in London, Hebden Bridge, Uxbridge, Manchester, Glasgow, Newcastle, Liverpool, Belfast, and the Isle of Wight.
31. Jock McCulloch, *Asbestos Blues: Labour, Capital, Physicians and the State in South Africa* (Indiana University Press, 2002), 6.
32. On the long litany of unsuccessful litigation brought against Union Carbide in US courts, see Jayanth Krishnan, "Bhopal in the Federal Courts: How Indian Victims Failed to Get Justice," *Rutgers University Law Review* 72, no. 3 (2020): 705–48. While, in 1989, the Indian Supreme Court approved a settlement of civil claims for $470 million, a significant proportion of this amount failed to reach the estimated 70,000 dead or disabled victims. On this and the subsequent

extraordinarily lenient and much criticized criminal convictions of the corporation's executives in Indian courts, see Gopal Krishna, "A Litigation Disaster," *Outlook India*, February 3, 2022.

33. On the differences and relative difficulties of pleading *forum non conveniens* in UK and US courts, see Martin Davies, "Forum Non Conveniens: Now We Are Much More Than Ten," in Andrew Dickinson and Edwin Peel, eds., *A Conflict of Laws Companion* (Oxford University Press, 2021), 32–51.

34. Richard Meeran, "The Boots Mesothelioma Cases," in G. A Peters and B. Peters, eds., *Current Asbestos: Legal, Medical and Technical Research*, Vol. 12: *Sourcebook on Asbestos Diseases* (Butterworths, 1996), 273–83.

35. The specifics of which—most particularly how one determines the point when the clock starts ticking—are discussed in chapter 2 in regard to the Cape litigants.

36. See Meeran, "The Boots Mesothelioma Cases," 281, and Clare Gilham, Christine Rake, John Hodgson, Andrew Darnton, Garry Burdett, James Peto Wild, Michelle Newton, Andrew G. Nicholson, Leslie Davidson, Mike Shires et al., "Past and Current Asbestos Exposure and Future Mesothelioma Risks in Britain: The Inhaled Particles Study (TIPS)," *International Journal of Epidemiology* 47, no. 6 (2018): 1745–56, Table 1. It should be noted first, that the earliest birth cohort identified by the authors of this study was 1940–1945, which would likely be twenty years or so later than the estimated birth date of the woman to whom Richard refers, and second, that the mean fiber counts used in the study relate to milligrams of lung tissue (i.e., 18.3 per mg), equivalent to 1,830 per gram (i.e., "approximately 2,000").

37. Meeran, "The Boots Mesothelioma Cases," 281.

38. Meeran, "The Boots Mesothelioma Cases," 276. Owned by Australian conglomerate CSR, Wittenoom was the world's only other blue asbestos mine.

39. Being one of the two categories of asbestos types to which both crocidolite and amosite belong. Chrysotile asbestos belongs to the second category: serpentine. See Glossary for further details.

40. *Margereson v. JW Roberts Ltd* [1996] PIQR, P154 (27 October 1995). Incidentally, the lead plaintiff in this case was represented by the Manchester firm of John Pickering & Partners, which was later to

join Leigh Day in representing the final total of some 7,500 claimants in the Cape litigation.

2. First Encounters

1. When the NCOH joined the National Health Laboratory Service in 2003, it became the National Institute for Occupational Health (NIOH). From 1971 to 1979, the NCOH was known as the National Research Institute for Occupational Diseases (NRIOD).
2. Marianne Felix, "Environmental Asbestos and Respiratory Disease in South Africa" (PhD diss., University of Witwatersrand, 1997).
3. Marianne Felix, "Risking Their Lives in Ignorance: The Story of an Asbestos-Polluted Community," in Jacklyn Cock and Eddie Koch, eds., *Going Green: People, Politics and the Environment in South Africa* (Oxford University Press, 1991), 33–43.
4. Marianne has since established Yoga4Alex in Alexandra, Johannesburg, an organization dedicated to helping children through yoga, meditation, and relaxation.
5. Lynne Wallis, "The Obsession That Rules Your Life," *Daily Telegraph*, July 2, 1993.
6. As of this writing, Munoree Padaychee continues to work as a general practitioner in London.
7. He does, however, support Arsenal and shares two season tickets with three friends. Their outings may or may not classify as relaxing, depending on how well the team performs.
8. Tony was also professor of occupational health at the University of Witwatersrand from 1983 to 1996.
9. Gerrit Schepers, "Asbestos in South Africa: Certain Geographical and Environmental Considerations" *Annals of New York Academy of Sciences* 132 (1965): 246–47. Many years later Schepers elaborated on what he saw that day in an interview with journalist Laurie Flynn: "The conditions were unbelievable," he concluded. It's shocking reading (Laurie Flynn, *Studded with Diamonds and Paved with Gold: Miners, Mining Companies and Human Rights in South Africa* [Bloomsbury, 1992], 192–93).
10. Gerrit W. H. Schepers, correspondence with Richard Meeran, July 1, 1997. "Cobbing" refers to the process of separating asbestos fibers from their host rock, typically by women and children, who used small hammers and their hands. See chapter 4.

11. This distinction was made not just as a matter of practice but was sanctioned in legislation, according to Tony Davies, Affidavit, in *Lubbe & others v. Cape Plc* (undated), May 1997, para. 11. See also Leon Commission, *Report of the Commission of Inquiry into Safety and Health in the Mining Industry* (South African Government, 1995), 40–67.

12. James Mognie, Martin Rotsey, Peter Garrett, Robert Hirst, and Wayne Stevens, "Blue Sky Mine" (Sony/ATV Music Publishing LLC, 1990).

13. A. B. Zwi, G. Reid, S. P. Landau, D. Kielkowski, F. Sitas, and M. R. Becklake, "Mesothelioma in South Africa, 1976–84: Incidence and Case Characteristics," *International Journal of Epidemiology* 18, no. 2 (1989): 320–29.

14. For the original study, see G. Reid, D. Kielkowski, S. D. Steyn, and K. Botha, "Mortality of an Asbestos-Exposed Birth Cohort—A Pilot Study," *South African Medical Journal* 78, no. 10 (1990): 548–65. The updated and revised data were later communicated by Reid to Marianne Felix (in 1992) and summarized (including the quoted conclusion) in Marianne Felix, J.-P. Leger, and Rodney I. Ehrlich, "Three Minerals, Three Epidemics—Asbestos Mining and Disease in South Africa," in M. Mehlman and J. Upton, eds., *The Identification and Control of Environmental and Occupational Diseases: Asbestos and Cancer*, Advances in Modern Environmental Toxicology, Vol. 22 (Princeton Scientific, 1994), 265–86.

15. Zwi et al., "Mesothelioma in South Africa."

16. Tony Davies, correspondence with Richard Meeran, July 1, 1997. The survey was conducted between April and September 1996. Tony emphatically concludes his description of the survey, saying, "This series is so large that it can only be an accurate representation of the massive health damage attributable to the exploitation of the local asbestos deposits."

17. Davies to Meeran, July 1, 1997. It should be noted, however, that even these comparatively lower prevalence rates in gold miners are nevertheless likely due to their exposure to asbestos, because the kimberlite in which gold is typically found in South Africa is often encased in asbestos-bearing rock (notably in the Northern Cape) through which the gold miners must drill to get at their prize. Interview with Gill Nelson, March 15, 2023, Johannesburg.

18. As opposed to the serpentine (or twisted) filaments of chrysotile (white) asbestos, on which see chapter 3.
19. T. Vorster, J. Mthombeni, J. teWaterNaude, and J. I. Phillips, "The Association between Histological Subtypes of Mesothelioma and Asbestos Exposure Characteristics," *International Journal of Environmental Research and Public Health* 19, no. 1 (2020): 14520.
20. Marianne Felix, notes from her "Interview with Dr and Mrs Pickard," undated, but likely circa 1995.
21. In Pickard's estimation the contamination covered a 15-kilometer radius from the mill.
22. See Jock McCulloch, "Beating the Odds: The Quest for Justice by South African Asbestos Mining Communities," *Review of African Political Economy* 103, no. 32 (2005): 64.
23. That is under South Africa's Occupational Diseases in Mines and Works Act (1973) and its Compensation for Occupational Injuries and Diseases Act (1993), discussed further in chapter 10.
24. Details of each plaintiff are provided later in this chapter.
25. Susan Segar, "Helping David Take On Goliath," *Natal Witness*, August 22, 1997.
26. Namely, Lucas Phiri from Penge in Limpopo and "Strongman" Mpangana from Prieska in Northern Cape, regarding whom Richard later noted, whimsically, "I remember thinking how unwise it was to call a baby 'strongman' given the uncertainties how things will ultimately turn out" (Richard Meeran, communication, February 16, 2023).
27. Richard Meeran, communication, February 16, 2023.
28. Phone interview with Zack Mabiletja, April 6, 2023.
29. Penge was still considered "unfit for human habitation" in 2007 according to Steven Donohue, a community health specialist from the University of Limpopo. See Sheila Meintjes, May Hermanus, Mary Scholes, and Marcus Reichart, *The Future of Penge: Prospects for People and the Environment* (Centre for Sustainability in Mining and Industry, 2008), 4.
30. Richard Meeran, Affidavit; *Lubbe and Others v. Cape Plc* (June 2, 1997), at paras. 44–45. The affidavit refers to a statement Henri provided to attorneys in Pietermaritzburg in August 1992 shortly before he died, in which he details a litany of deaths from ARDs among his peer group in Prieska reminiscent of the devastation wrought by ARDs among Zack Mabiletja's peers in Penge.

31. André Pickard, correspondence with Richard Meeran, April 30, 1996.

32. Francois Loots, "The Killing Stone," *Guardian & Mail*, May 11, 2001. A staff reporter for the *Guardian & Mail*, Loots was a native of Prieska. He was compelled to write this story after returning to his hometown a few months earlier to visit his father who was dying of mesothelioma. "My father's body wastes away at an incredible speed. No flowers at my funeral, he asks; for him asbestos cancer was too bitter a reality to be adorned by beauty. He withdraws from the world and passes away. I feel exhausted and numb." It's a powerful and moving piece.

33. See *Lubbe and Others v. Cape Plc*, Transcript (QBD, before Justice Buckley), July 13, 1999 (Day 7, p.m.), at 67.

34. Interview with Fildah Bosman, March 8, 2023, Prieska.

35. These details come from an assortment of sources: various transcripts and judgments in the Cape litigation; statements and depositions as recalled by Richard; and my own interviews with former Cape employees and other victims, their families and friends, community leaders, activists and politicians, as well as local doctors and nurses.

36. As per section 11(4) of the Limitation Act (1980) and sections 11(d) and 12 of the Prescription Act (1969). Once the case got there, the House of Lords left open the question of whether English or South African law applied. Further, in respect of these five, as well as (and especially) Pauline Nel as the sixth plaintiff, Richard would have argued that this awareness included knowledge of the relevant acts and omissions of the parent company (as purported causes of the illnesses or deaths), which could not reasonably have been known until Leigh Day came on the scene less than three years previously. Richard Meeran, communication, June 7, 2024.

37. The watershed case of *Priestley v. Fowler* [1837] 150 ER 1030 had established that under tort law, employers owe a duty of care to their employees when engaged in their employ. (In this case Fowler, a butcher, was held liable for the injuries driver's companion Priestly sustained while delivering meat to London in an over-loaded horse-drawn cart that collapsed beneath him.) The challenge for Richard, however, was to show how and why such a duty extended to employees of a company's subsidiary entities as well. What is more, he "knew from the *Thor* and *Connelly* cases that Cape would contend

that as a matter of legal principle, the corporate veil precluded the imposition of a duty of care on a parent company save where the subsidiaries were sham companies or fraud was involved." Richard Meeran, communication, June 17, 2024.

38. These medical effects and other relevant scientific particulars are examined in detail in chapter 3.

39. See Morris Greenberg, "Cape Asbestos, Barking, Health and Environment: 1928–46," *American Journal of Industrial Medicine* 43 (2003): 110, quoting C. L. Williams, Medical Officer of Health, Barking Urban District Council, in his first annual report (1928).

40. W. J. Smither, *Visit to South Africa* (1962), 10, and which phrase I commandeered for this book's title.

41. Flynn, *Studded with Diamonds*, 177, 178.

42. Laurie Flynn, "South Africa Blacks Out Blue Asbestos Risk," *New Scientist*, April 22, 1982, 237–39.

43. Flynn, *Studded with Diamonds*, 333n8.

44. The report was dated May 4, 1962. Key extracts from the report are quoted in Richard Meeran, "Cape Plc: South African Mineworkers' Quest for Justice," *International Journal of Occupational and Environmental Health* 9, no. 3 (2003): 220. Remarkably, when I visited the offices of National Institute for Occupational Health (as the NCOH had become) in March 2023, Webster's report was still missing from its archives. A copy of the report, which Richard duly located and provided to me, had been exhibited in evidence during one of the court hearings. A copy was subsequently forwarded to the NIOH, so the report is now back where it belongs.

3. Breathless

1. Ian Webster, "The Effect of Dust on the Lung," undated (but likely mid-1960s), NIOH archives, Johannesburg, South Africa. The PRU was then part of the Council for Scientific and Industrial Research (South Africa). The PRU became the National Research Institute for Occupational Diseases (NRIOD) in 1971. See David Rees et al., "South Africa's National Institute for Occupational Health: From Phthisis to Occupational Health and Back Again," *Occupational Health South Africa* 12, no. 5 (2006): 5–7.

2. David Rees, "Obituary: Professor Ian Webster," *Occupational Health SA*, November–December 1998, 58. Webster was appointed professor

of Industrial Pathology at Witwatersrand University in Johannesburg in 1970.

3. Richard Meeran, communication, June 7, 2023.

4. Jock McCulloch, interview with Ian Webster, December 4, 1997, Johannesburg. When I asked Tony Davies about Webster, and specifically about McCulloch's interview notes, he told me that Webster "lacked confidence after being so beaten down. . . . He was treated appallingly as director of NCOH" (interview with Tony Davies, March 16, 2023, Kenton-on-Sea).

5. Flynn, *New Scientist* (April 22, 1982), in which he provides verbatim extracts from the interview, followed by the comment: "Unfortunately, this is not true" (238).

6. Richard Meeran, communication, June 7, 2023.

7. J. C. Wagner, C. A. Sleggs, and P. Marchand, "Diffuse Pleural Mesothelioma and Asbestos Exposure in the North-Western Cape Province," *British Journal of Industrial Medicine* 17 (1960): 260–71.

8. Pneumoconiosis Research Unit, *Report of the Progress of the Mesothelioma Survey as at 30th April 1962*, May 4, 1962, 2.

9. Ian Webster, "Asbestos and Malignancy," *South African Medical Journal*, February 3, 1973, 171.

10. Webster, "Asbestos and Malignancy," 171.

11. Ian Webster, deposition, in *Re: Asbestos Personal Injury Cases*, Jones County, Mississippi, November 12, 1996 (Johannesburg), at 190–93.

12. Webster added further weight to the possibility of such a causal break in an unpublished memorandum written in 1976 and entitled "The Health Hazards of Asbestos in True Perspective," in which he wrote: "Blue asbestos does cause a greater number of cases of one type of cancer, namely mesothelioma, but other people who are exposed to other types of asbestos do develop cancer, especially if they are smokers." Copy held in NIOH archives.

13. South African Medical Research Council, press release, August 24, 1970; the title was capitalized in the original. It is almost certain that the research on which the council draws in this statement is that of Ian Webster (as published two and half years later in the *South African Medical Journal* mentioned above in n9), such is the similarity of data cited and lines of argument pursued in each. Furthermore, it should be noted that the reasoning in both documents relies heavily on the contention that *if* crocidolite is *the* sole (or primary) carcino-

gen, then a certain number of mesothelioma cases should already have been found among the communities in Northern Transvaal where crocidolite was also mined (alongside amosite), in line with the mesothelioma cases documented among the crocidolite mining communities of the Northern Cape. It is true that apparently no cases had yet been found in Northern Transvaal, but to leap from there to the conclusion that crocidolite is not carcinogenic was peculiar, to say the least, when other reasons were just as, or more, likely explanations. Primary among these is the fact that the medical and post-mortem screening of black workers in Northern Transvaal was so inadequate—even compared to the poor, but nevertheless higher, levels provided to the mainly coloured workforce in the Northern Cape—that while mesothelioma cases almost certainly existed, they were simply not being picked up. Marianne Felix and colleagues labeled this a "hidden epidemic" and lamented that "the gaps in our epidemiological knowledge mean that the gravity of these asbestos epidemics will never be fully recorded" (Marianne Felix, J.-P. Leger, and Rodney I. Ehrlich, "Three Minerals, Three Epidemics—Asbestos Mining and Disease in South Africa," in M. Mehlman and J. Upton, eds., *The Identification and Control of Environmental and Occupational Diseases: Asbestos and Cancer,* Advances in Modern Environmental Toxicology, Vol. 22 (Princeton Scientific, 1994), 274, 282.

14. H. A. Shapiro, ed., *Proceedings of the International Conference on Pneumoconiosis, Johannesburg, 1969* (Oxford University Press, 1971), 1–282, being the record of the conference proceedings for April 23, 24, and 25, 1969. Notably, Ian Webster was one of three members of the editorial committee of these published proceedings.

15. See Felix, Leger, and Ehrlich, "Three Minerals, Three Epidemics."

16. Including, P. H. R. Snyman, "Safety and Health in the Northern Cape Blue Asbestos Belt," *Historia* 33, no. 1 (1988): 31–52; A. B. Zwi, G. Reid, S. P. Landau, D. Kielkowski, F. Sitas, and M. R. Becklake, "Mesothelioma in South Africa, 1976–84: Incidence and Case Characteristics," *International Journal of Epidemiology* 18 (1989): 320–29; and Danuta Kielkowski, Gillian Nelson, and David Rees, "Risk of Mesothelioma from Exposure to Crocidolite Asbestos: A 1995 Update of a South African Mortality Study," *Occupational and Environmental Medicine* 57 (2000): 563–67. For an overview of

relevant literature from this era, see Neil White and Eric Bateman, "Mesothelioma and Exposure to Asbestos in South Africa: 1962–2000," in Bruce Robinson and Philippe Chahinian, eds., *Mesothelioma* (CRC Press, 2002), 93–110.

17. Jonathan Myers, *Asbestos and Asbestos-Related Disease in South Africa*, University of Cape Town, South African Labour and Development Research Unit Working Paper 28, June 1980, 2. See also his statement that for mesothelioma, "Asbestos exposure is practically the only known cause" (22).

18. Peter Hawthorne, "Fight of Their Lives," *Time*, August 7, 2000.

19. G. Miserocchi, G. Sancini, F. Mantegazza, and Gerolamo Chiappino, "Translocation Pathways for Inhaled Asbestos Fibers" *Environmental Health* 7, no. 4 (2008), https://ehjournal.biomedcentral.com/articles/10.1186/1476-069X-7-4.

20. Miserocchi et al., "Translocation Pathways for Inhaled Asbestos Fibers."

21. Yasunosuke Suzuki, "Erratum to 'Short, Thin Asbestos Fibers Contribute to the Development of Human Malignant Mesothelioma: Pathological Evidence,'" *International Journal of Hygiene and Environmental Health* 208 (2005): 439–44, which shows, by contrast, that with ultrafine fibers the dimensions are so minute as to minimize the significance of the difference in shape.

22. A biological half-life can be defined as the time required for a biological system (such as the human body) to eliminate half of the amount of a substance. Whereas chrysotile (serpentine) fibers have a half-life "measured in weeks and, at most, months . . . the half -life of amphiboles [crocidolite and amosite] in the human lung is measurable in terms of decades, if not a lifetime" (John Craighead, Allen Gibbs, and Fred Pooley, "Minerology of Asbestos," in John Craighead and Allen Gibbs, eds. *Asbestos and Its Diseases* [Oxford University Press, 2008], 26).

23. Miserocchi et al., "Translocation Pathways for Inhaled Asbestos Fibers."

24. In respect of the osmotic process, Miserocchi et al., "Translocation Pathways for Inhaled Asbestos Fibers," suggest that the key chemical involved in these differing concentrations is sodium, creating "gradients" against which the flow or absorption of water travels until an equilibrium is reached.

25. Interview with Gill Nelson, March 15, 2023, Johannesburg.

26. Richard Meeran, communication, June 7, 2023.

27. Such effusion results in part from the body's immune response to the presence of the foreign material and in part from an increase in the above-mentioned "pressure gradient" pushing fluid into the pleural caused by "asbestos-induced lung inflammation that increases pulmonary interstitial pressure" (Miserocchi et al., "Translocation Pathways for Inhaled Asbestos Fibers," 1).

28. Devon Freudenberger and Rachit Shah, "A Narrative Review of the Health Disparities Associated with Malignant Pleural Mesothelioma," *Journal of Thoracic Disease* 13, no. 6 (2021): 3809–15.

29. For those who might appreciate or prefer visual depictions of the grim impact if ARDs on lungs, see C. Norbet, A. Joseph, S. S. Rossi, S. Bhalla, and F. R. Gutierrez, "Asbestos-Related Lung Disease: A Pictorial Review," *Current Problems in Diagnostic Radiology* 44 (2015): 371–82.

30. Kipp Weiskopf and Irving Weissman, "Macrophages Are Critical Effectors of Antibody Therapies for Cancer," *Monoclonal Antibodies* 7, no. 2 (2015): 303–10.

31. Cooke published his findings in two articles: "Fibrosis of the Lungs Due to the Inhalation of Asbestos Fibres," *British Medical Journal* 2, no. 3317 (1924): 147, and "Pulmonary Asbestosis," *British Medical Journal* 2, no. 3491 (1927): 1024–25. Kershaw had worked in a factory operated by Turner and Newall.

32. See also Miserocchi et al., who describe the process as asbestos fibers being "dragged from the lung interstitium by pulmonary lymph flow" ("Translocation Pathways for Inhaled Asbestos Fibers," 1).

33. For a compelling account of how macrophagal and lymphatic drainage systems combine when trying (and often failing) to eliminate asbestos fibers that penetrate deep into the lung and beyond, see Ronald Dodson, "Analysis and Relevance of Asbestos Burden in Tissue," in Ronald Dodson and Samuel Hammer, eds, *Asbestos: Risk Assessment, Epidemiology, and Health Effects*, 2nd ed.(CRC Press, 2011), 52–59.

34. See J. Huang, N. Hisanaga, K. Sakai, M. Iwat, Y. Ono, E. Shibata, and Y. Takeuchi, "Asbestos Fibers in Human Pulmonary and Extrapulmonary Tissues," *American Journal of Industrial Medicine* 14, no. 3 (1988): 331–39.

35. By way of their microvascular filtration *out* of blood vessels (capillaries) into the extravascular spaces occupied by these organs, as dictated by the "specific conditions of interstitial fluid dynamics"; see Miserocchi et al., "Translocation Pathways for Inhaled Asbestos Fibers," 1.

36. What the American Lung Association calls "the ultimate relationship"; see *Your Heart and Lungs: The Ultimate Relationship*, February 13, 2023, https://www.lung.org/blog/heart-lung-relationship.

37. Myoung Soo Kim, Ha Yeon Lee, and Eun-Jung Jung, "Brain Metastasis of a Malignant Pleural Mesothelioma: A Case Report and Review of the Literature" *Interdisciplinary Neurosurgery* 23 (2021): 101033, who note: "Typically, MPM [malignant pleural mesothelioma] is locally aggressive, and among those that undergo distant metastasis only 3% are found in the brain," 1.

38. Gill Nelson and Jim teWaterNaude, "Epidemiology of Malignant Pleural Mesothelioma in South Africa," in Tommaso Claudio Mineo, ed., *Malignant Pleural Mesothelioma: Present Status and Future Directions* (Bentham Books, 2016), 95.

39. Wagner, Sleggs, and Marchand, "Diffuse Pleural Mesothelioma and Asbestos Exposure in the North-Western Cape Province," 262.

40. Wagner, Sleggs, and Marchand, "Diffuse Pleural Mesothelioma and Asbestos Exposure in the North-Western Cape Province," 262, 265.

41. Wagner, Sleggs, and Marchand, "Diffuse Pleural Mesothelioma and Asbestos Exposure in the North-Western Cape Province," 262–67.

42. Interview with Charles Schoeman, March 9, 2023, Prieska Hospital. He also told me that such was the town's reputation for harboring an epidemic of ARDs that upon being offered a job there, all his medical school colleagues warned him: "Don't go!" He went anyway, on April Fool's Day 1990, and remained there until his retirement in 2024.

43. Reflecting the dignity and grace of all the victims I met and interviewed, Shirley was happy to allow me to take a photograph of the two of us together at the end of our meeting, but only after she rushed off to take out her curlers and put on a nicer dress.

44. The serendipitous circumstances under which du Plessis came to compile his photo-documentary are discussed in chapter 7.

45. Interview with Shirley Celanto, March 8, 2023, Prieska.

46. Michael Gochfeld, "Chronological History of Occupational Medicine," *Journal of Occupational and Environmental Medicine* 47, no. 2 (2005): 96–114.

47. Ramazzini's pathbreaking *De Morbis Artificum Diatriba* (Diseases of Workers) covering fifty-two different occupations, was published in 1700. See Giuliano Franco and Francesca Franco, "Bernardino Ramazzini: The Father of Occupational Medicine," *American Journal of Public Health* 91, no. 9 (2001): 1380–82.

48. In Agricola's *De Re Metallica* (1556), as quoted by George Kazantzis, "Occupational Disease," *Encyclopaedia Britannica*, https://www .britannica.com/science/occupational-disease#ref364085.

49. As the World Health Organization puts it, "Health and safety problems at work . . . should be prevented by using all available tools—legislative, technical research, training and education, information, and economic instruments," *Declaration on Occupational Health for All* (1995), article 6.

50. The Occupational Diseases in Mines and Works Act (1973).

51. *Leon Commission of Inquiry into Safety and Health in the Mining Industry*, Vols. 1 and 2 (Government of South Africa, 1995).

52. Leslie London and Sophia Kisting, "Ethical Concerns in International Occupational Health and Safety," *Occupational Medicine* 17, no. 4 (2002): 587, 588. Sophie was still stressing the cardinal importance of stronger ethical standards in the profession when I interviewed her in Cape Town, March 6, 2023. Note that while everyone (including Kisting herself) refers to her as "Sophie" in conversation and correspondence, she retains "Sophia" in her published works.

53. Lundy Braun and Sophia Kisting, "Asbestos-Related Disease in South Africa: The Social Production of an Invisible Epidemic," *American Journal of Public Health* 96, no. 8 (2006): 1386, 1394.

54. See Royal Society for the Prevention of Accidents (UK), "Occupational Health and Safety: Timeline," undated, https://www .historyofosh.org.uk/timeline.html. For a summarized timeline of asbestos medical events and regulation in United Kingdom, see Anthony Newman Taylor, "The Asbestos Story: A Tale of Public Health and Politics," *Imperial Medicine Blog*, February 2, 2018, https://blogs.imperial.ac.uk/imperial-medicine/2018/02/02/the -asbestos-story-a-tale-of-public-health-and-politics/.

55. Lucy Deane, "Report on the Health of Workers in Asbestos and Other Dusty Trades," in *HM Chief Inspector of Factories and Workshops, Annual Report for 1898* (Her Majesty's Stationary Office, 1899), 171–72.

56. E. R. A. Merewether and C. W. Price, *Report on the Effects of Dust on the Lungs and Dust Suppression in the Asbestos Industry* (Her Majesty's Stationery Office, March 1930).

57. Geoffrey Tweedale, "Science or Public Relations? The Inside Story of the Asbestosis Research Council, 1957–1990," *American Journal of Industrial Medicine* 38, no. 6 (2000): 723, 727.

58. Which did effectively prohibit the use of crocidolite in British factories by setting the maximum permissible airborne fiber count so low that the massive amounts of miniscule fibers produced during manufacture using crocidolite asbestos would almost always exceed that limit; see Andrew Webster, Conor Douglas, and Hajime Sato, "Emergence of Asbestos-Related Health Issues and Development of Regulatory Policy in the UK," in Hajime Sato, ed., *Management of Health Risks from Environment and Food* (Springer, 2010), 72. The authors lay bare the extent to which the British government (and its scientific advisory bodies) was subverted by the asbestos industry throughout these early decades of asbestos regulation in the United Kingdom.

59. Webster, Douglas, and Sato, "Emergence of Asbestos-Related Health Issues and Development of Regulatory Policy in the UK," 63, citing P. W. J. Bartrip, "History of Asbestos Related Disease," *Postgraduate Medical Journal* 80, no. 840 (2004): 74.

60. Richard Meeran, communication, July 21, 2023.

61. Decades later, the full extent of the sector's malign influence over the government's regulatory policy on asbestos during that period was discovered when, following another court case against Cape in 2019 (*Dring v. Cape Intermediate Holdings Ltd* [2019] UKSC 38), the company was forced to disclose documents regarding its political activities at that time. This case and its implications are discussed further in chapter 10.

62. Deane, "Report on the Health of Workers."

63. Webster, Douglas, and Sato, "Emergence of Asbestos-Related Health Issues," 67, 77.

64. He was right, as we shall see as the story progresses, and yet Cape's response when the initial writ was filed in February 1997 was interesting. Michael Pitt-Payne, Cape's company secretary at the time, said that the company no longer used asbestos in its products, having "sold the companies that were doing the [asbestos] mining in

South Africa in 1979 and as such we have got very few people here who had anything to do with that business at the time." He then added that the matter was now in the hands of the company's lawyers, while betraying little of just how hard the company would fight the case over the next seven years. See "I Was Given No Warning by Anyone," *The Independent*, March 31, 1997.

4. Mining the Miracle Mineral

1. Details drawn from anonymized claimant questionnaires, completed January 22, 2001. "Mmele" is a pseudonym.
2. Details drawn from a further anonymized claimant questionnaire, dated January 24, 2001, completed by another worker at the Penge mine. The advice regarding drinking milk seems to have been widespread as both Jack Adams and Cecil Skeffers told me the same recommendation was often heard around Prieska and Koegas.
3. See generally, for this paragraph, Malcolm Ross and Robert Nolan, "History of Asbestos Discovery and Use and Asbestos-Related Disease in Context with the Occurrence of Asbestos within Ophiolite Complexes,, *Geological Society of America*, Special Paper 373 (2003): 447–70, in which the authors suggest that asbestos was first used by humans "perhaps as long ago as 5,000 years."
4. See "Mechanical Properties of Asbestos," *Encyclopedia of Building and Environmental Construction, Diagnosis, Maintenance and Repair*, undated, https://inspectapedia.com/hazmat/Asbestos _Properties_Mechanical.php, which indicates that the average tensile strength of crocidolite asbestos has an upper limit of 300,000 pounds per square inch (psi), whereas that of carbon steel is 155,000 psi.
5. "A single strand weighing less than an ounce [28.3 grams] can be spun out for three hundred feet and a square yard of woven cloth will weigh less than eight ounces," notes Jock McCulloch, *Asbestos Blues: Labour Capital, Physicians and the State in South Africa* (Indiana University Press, 2002), 1.
6. *Cape Asbestos 1893-1953: The Story of the Cape Asbestos Company Limited* (Harley Publishing, 1953), 15. Lichtenstein's discovery is recorded as being between 1803 and 1806, and Oates's in 1890. It was not until 1835 that the mineral was labelled 'crocidolite' drawing on two Greek words for woolly stone.

7. *Cape Asbestos*, 15.

8. *Cape Asbestos* portrays the encounter as follows: "The African agreed to show Ward [the farmer] where he had obtained the asbestos in return for sufficient cattle to pay for *lobala*, or dowry, to enable him to procure a wife. Ward consented" (30).

9. Most notably nary a mention (nor even a hint) of the health or medical concerns of asbestos is made in the booklet's concluding pages summing up the company's past, present, and future, the focus of which is entirely on commercial matters.

10. Kevin Burwick, "The Snow in The Wizard of Oz was 100% Pure Asbestos," Movieweb, accessed December 30, 2023, https://movieweb.com/wizard-of-oz-snow-asbestos/.

11. For all these figures, see United States Geological Society (USGS), *Worldwide Asbestos Supply and Consumption Trends from 1900 through 2003* (2006), table 4.

12. USGS, *Worldwide Asbestos Supply and Consumption Trends*, table 4. See also John Harington and Neil McGlashan, "South African Asbestos: Production, Exports, and Destinations, 1959–1993," *American Journal of Industrial Medicine* 33 (1983): 321–26.

13. USGS, *Worldwide Asbestos Supply and Consumption Trends*, 9. Australia was the only other major producer of crocidolite, albeit at a fraction of South Africa's output. At its peak in 1962 Australia produced 16,707 metric tons of predominantly crocidolite asbestos before declining precipitously after the Australian Blue Asbestos Pty closed its Wittenoom mine in 1966. While significantly larger quantities of asbestos were mined in Australia thereafter (notably 92,418 tons in 1980), they comprised almost exclusively chrysotile, but even that dried up completely after an effective ban on asbestos mining in Australia was imposed in 1983.

14. Jonathan Myers, *Asbestos and Asbestos-Related Disease in South Africa* (University of Cape Town, South African Labour and Development Research Unit Working Paper 28, June 1980), 9–10. Cape was one of three major asbestos producers in South Africa, the other two being General Mining (later Gencor) and Everite, both of which mined similar quantities of crocidolite as did Cape. In presenting the data, Myers notes that obtaining "the relative production figures of the different companies [was] quite difficult as only General Mining gives production figures in their annual reports." Myers therefore

turned his forensic eye to disaggregating the overall production figures provided by the Department of Mines for the whole country.

15. *Cape Asbestos*, 80–81.
16. By one estimate "at least 18,000 articles are made of it," as cited in an excerpt in Jakob Gottschau's documentary, *The Evil Dust*, Danish Film Institute (2006). The term "magic mineral" was coined by Paul Brodeur in his ground-breaking 1968 article, "The Magic Mineral," *The New Yorker*, October 12, 1968. Many, including medical scientists, have since riffed on the label; see, for example, David Gee and Morris Greenberg, "Asbestos: From 'Magic' to Malevolent Mineral," in Paul Harremoes, David Gee, Malcom MacGarvin, Andy Stirling, Jane Keys, Brian Wynne, and Sofia Guedes Vaz, eds., *The Precautionary Principle in the 20th Century* (Routledge, 2002), 52–63.
17. *Cape Asbestos*, 25.
18. "Penge Asbestos Mine," Cape Plc pamphlet (undated, but probably circa 1965); copy on file with author.
19. See *Cape Asbestos Company Magazine* 6, no. 3, 1957 (Summer): 10–13.
20. Truly! It comprised six stanzas, the first of which read:

Mr Cape Asbestos say build me please
A nice fire-house, 14 foot to eaves
So I can stack it with timber and set it on fire
For to show my new curtain to de British Empire.

The calypso's author is cited as A. S. Crook.
21. *Cape Asbestos Company Magazine* 6, no. 3, 1957 (Summer): 10–13. Alongside a long list of "leading industrialists, architects, building contractors, fire prevention officers, Government officials and representatives of insurance companies," whose presence underscored the serious commercial intent behind the show.
22. *Cape Asbestos Company Magazine* 6, no. 3, 1957 (Summer): 10–13.
23. As excerpted in Gottschau, *The Evil Dust* (2006).
24. "Special Report on Asbestos," *The Times*, November 18, 1967.
25. "Number of Licensed Vehicles by Tax Class, 1950–2010," *Transport Statistics 2011* (Department of Transport, 2011), 1.
26. Douglas Henderson and James Leigh, "The History of Asbestos Utilization and Recognition of Asbestos-Induced Diseases," in Ronald Dodson and Samuel Hammar, eds., *Asbestos: Risk Assessment, Epidemiology and Health Effects*, 2nd ed. (Taylor & Francis, 2011), 14.

27. Letter from W. J. Smither to S. Holmes of the United Kingdom's Asbestos Research Council, December 30, 1968.

28. Ian Webster, "The Health Hazards of Asbestos in True Perspective," Memorandum, May 7, 1976; copy held in NIOH archives. Webster was then director of the National Research Institute for Occupational Diseases (NRIOD), the forerunner to the National Centre for Occupational Health (NCOH).

29. Burwick, "The Snow in The Wizard of Oz." As Bolger was also in the above-mentioned "it's snowing" scene, his significant exposure to asbestos throughout filming of the movie was guaranteed.

30. Richard Meeran, communication, August 17, 2023.

31. See Richard Meeran, Affidavit, in *Lubbe & Others v. Cape* (June 2, 1997), para. 19(f). The company dropped the word "asbestos" from its title in 1974, becoming simply Cape Industries Plc (later, Cape Plc). Cape UK refers to each of these companies.

32. Namely, Egnep (Pty) Ltd. and Amosa (Pty) Ltd. (focused on operations in Northern Transvaal), Cape Blue Mines (Pty) Ltd. (focused on operations in the Northern Cape), and Cape Asbestos Insulations (Pty) Ltd. (a manufacturing plant located in Benoni, a few miles east of Johannesburg).

33. Even here Cape would seek to rely on *forum non conveniens* as a defense, claiming that as the alleged tortious harm was sustained in South Africa, it was in South Africa, not the United Kingdom, that any litigation should be pursued.

34. Cape Asbestos Company, *Annual Report*, 1948. CASAP's registration became effective on December 31, 1948. Coincidentally, it was also in 1948 that South Africa's National Party gained power and immediately implemented Apartheid rule, from which system mining companies like Cape were to profit enormously.

35. *Cape Asbestos*, 56.

36. J. S. Enslin, *Registration of Mines: Dust Survey, Cape Asbestos Company, Prieska Area (Koegas)*, Department of Mines, Memorandum, Ref. GME 48/9/8, xxxix, December 13, 1948, in which Enslin canvassed various options to deal with the high levels of airborne dust detected during his inspections.

37. Which work was to be published in various formats, most notably in Jock McCulloch, *Asbestos Blues*. Jock's commitment to the cause and to field-work research in South Africa and his native Australia was,

eventually, to cost him his life after he contracted mesothelioma and died in 2018. In an obituary written by his friend and fellow anti-asbestos campaigner Laurie Kazan-Allen, Laurie refers to an email exchange with Jock after his diagnosis in which he wrote: "The injury almost certainly occurred while I was researching Asbestos Blues in South Africa, which is all of twenty years ago" (Laurie Kazan-Allen, "In Memory of Jock McCulloch," International Ban Asbestos Secretariat, January 21, 2018, http://ibasecretariat.org/lka-in -memory-of-jock-mcculloc.php). Not for the first time such words prompt uncomfortable moments of self-reflection on asbestos's long reach over time and space, poisoning even those whose brief exposure comes from mere observation, as well as those whose whole lives were immersed in it.

38. McCulloch, *Asbestos Blues*, 52–54, drawing mainly on Cape's annual reports from 1957 to 1974.

39. For extensive analyses of which see Paul Brodeur, *Outrageous Misconduct: The Asbestos Industry on Trial* (Pantheon, 1985); Barry Castleman, *Asbestos: Medical and Legal Aspects*, 4th ed. (Aspen Publishers, 1996); Stephen J. Carroll, Deborah R. Hensler, Jennifer Gross, Elizabeth M. Sloss, Matthias Schonlau, Allan Abrahamse, and J. Scott Ashwood, *Asbestos Litigation* (RAND Corporation, 2005).

40. *Yandle et al. v. PPG Industries, Inc. et al.*, 65 F.R.D. 566 (E.D. Tex. 1974). The case involved sick claimants who had worked on the site of an old asbestos manufacturing plant in Texas to which Cape had supplied raw fiber. Thereby, Cape became a co-defendant to the action. The case was eventually settled with Cape agreeing to pay $5.2 million of the total settlement of $20 million. See further Geoffrey Tweedale and Laurie Flynn, "Piercing the Corporate Veil: Cape Industries and Multinational Corporate Liability for Toxic Hazard, 1950–2004," *Enterprise and Society* 8, no. 2 (207): 268–96.

41. Geoffrey Higham, deposition, *Yandle v. PPG*, June 4, 1975, at 62. Cape's first use of such warning labels was in 1972.

42. Richard Gaze, deposition, *Yandle v. PPG*, June 4–5, 1975, at 50.

43. Richard Gaze, deposition, at 50.

44. Copy on file with the author.

45. An excerpt of the interview is replayed in Gottschau, *The Evil Dust*. Under cross-examination at an asbestos trial in a Pennsylvanian court in November 1984, Mendelle noted: "We had a running total of

between 70 and 80 asbestosis cases on the premises in any one year," though this figure would appear to also include mesothelioma cases, which Mendelle knew existed but was unsure of exactly how many (Anthony Mendelle, testimony, *Smith v. Pittsburgh Corning Co. & Others*, Court of Common Pleas, Allegheny County, PA, November 13, 1984, at 11). It is estimated that some 10,000 people were employed at Cape's Barking plant during its lifetime (1913-1968); see Emily Dugan, "Asbestos: A Shameful Legacy," *The Independent*, November 22, 2009.

46. As Jock McCulloch and Geoffrey Tweedale put it in their "Double Standards: The Multinational Asbestos Industry and Asbestos-Related Disease in South Africa," *International Journal of Health Services* 34, no. 4 (2004): 663–79.

47. However modest, it was nonetheless "presented to all the company's employees and pensioners together with a commemorative medallion which has been struck by the Royal Mint," as declared in its introduction.

48. South African asbestos production peaked in 1977 (see n11); Jonny Myers calculated that Cape was responsible for approximately 36 percent of the country's total asbestos output in 1976 (Myers, *Asbestos and Asbestos-Related Disease in South Africa*, 10).

49. Interview with Munoree Padyachee, May 5, 2023, London.

50. Richard Meeran, communication, August 28, 2023.

51. See 'Reamended Statement of Claim' in *Lubbe v. others v. Cape Plc*, 1997 L No.250 (Queen's Bench Division), October 12, 1998, at para. 6.4.

52. *In re: Asbestos Personal Injury Cases*, Arrington Lead No 93-9-114, Circuit Court of Jones County, State of Mississippi, Second Judicial District, 1996.

53. Schalk Lubbe, depositions, *In re: Asbestos Personal Injury Cases*, November 7, 1996, at 123, 138.

54. Lubbe, depositions, November 7, 1996, at 115.

55. Lubbe, depositions, November 7, 1996, at 123–24.

56. Lubbe, depositions, November 7, 1996, at 198–200.

57. Lubbe, depositions, November 9, 1996, at 54–58.

58. Lubbe, depositions, November 7, 1996, at 127–31.

59. See Statement of Claim, in *Lubbe v. Cape Plc*, 1997 L No.250 (Queen's Bench Division), April 2, 1997, at paras. 4 and 5.

60. Richard Doll and Julian Peto, *Asbestos: Effects on Health of Exposure to Asbestos*, Health and Safety Commission (Her Majesty's Stationery Office, 1985).

61. J. Peto, J. T. Hodgson, F. E. Matthews, and J. R. Jones, J. R. "Continuing Increase in Mesothelioma Mortality in Britain," *The Lancet* 345, no. 8949 (1995): P535–539.

62. For example, "Killer Dust," *The Guardian*, May 8, 1993; Robert Winnett, "Homeowners Hit by Asbestos Clean-Up Costs," *Sunday Times*, June 25, 1995; Martin Wainwright, "Dying Asbestos Victim Recalls Lethal Games as Bitter Court Fight Ends in Victory," *The Guardian*, October 28, 1995; Charles Arthur, "The Quiet Epidemic," *The Independent on Sunday*, April 7, 1996.

63. For example, "Deadly Legacy," BBC 1, April 14, 1993; "The Shocking Story of Asbestos," BBC Radio 4, *Face the Facts*, October 6, 1993; "Asbestos and the Third World," BBC Radio 4, *Face the Facts*, October 13, 1993; "An Acceptable Level of Death," BBC 2, April 14, 1994; as well as earlier, especially hard-hitting documentaries: "Dust to Dust," *World in Action*, Granada Television, November 11, 1981, and "Alice—A Fight for Life," Yorkshire TV, July 20, 1982.

64. *Lubbe v. Cape Plc* (Judgment: January 12, 1998), at para. 17 (oral hearings, July 7–11, 1997)

65. *Lubbe v. Cape Plc*, at para. 19.

66. *Lubbe v. Cape Plc*, at para. 20.

67. This combination of stoicism and optimism in both the claimants and their lawyers is reflected in the maxim at the head of this book.

5. Apartheid Capitalism

1. Richard Meeran, communication, August 17, 2023.

2. Suzanne Alderete, correspondence with Laurie Flynn, August 30, 1996. My thanks to Suzanne for giving me permission to quote from her letter.

3. Established by the Promotion of National Unity and Reconciliation Act (1995), the commission's rationale was summarised in volume 1 of its *Final Report* in 1998: "The telling of the truth about past gross human rights violations, as viewed from different perspectives, facilitates the process of understanding our divided pasts, whilst the public acknowledgement of 'untold suffering and injustice' (Preamble to the Act) helps to restore the dignity of victims and afford perpetra-

tors the opportunity to come to terms with their own past" (The Truth and Reconciliation Commission of South Africa, 1998), at 49.

4. Desmond Tutu, *No Future Without Forgiveness* (Rider, 2012), 179.

5. Susan Segar, "Helping David Take On Goliath," *Natal Witness*, August 22, 1997. Hearings before the TRC, which had begun a little more than a year earlier, included examinations of the roles played by corporations during Apartheid, as discussed later in this chapter.

6. Interview with Sarah Leigh, May 30, 2023, Shoreham-by-Sea, West Sussex.

7. Charley Nkadimeng from Limpopo and Chris Matlhako from Northern Cape were two other regulars.

8. Interview with Thabo Makweya, March 13, 2023, Johannesburg.

9. Interview with Tommy Ntsewa, March 3, 2023, Johannesburg.

10. "Apartheid and capitalism are two sides of the same exploitative coin," as Nicoli Nattrass put it at the time (in "The Truth and Reconciliation Commission on Business and Apartheid: A Critical Evaluation," *African Affairs* 98, no. 392 [1999]: 376).

11. *Truth and Reconciliation Commission of South Africa Final Report* (1998), Vol. 4, at 58

12. Kadar Asmal, Louise Asmal, and Ronald Roberts, *Reconciliation through Truth: A Reckoning of Apartheid's Criminal Governance* (David Philip, 1996), 155–56.

13. A "Bantu person" was defined in the act as belonging to "aboriginal tribes or races of Africa, including Bushmen, Hottentots, Korannas and Natives," but excluding "American Negroes, Eurafricans, Eurasians" (Occupational Diseases in Mines and Works Act (ODMWA) 1973, section 1(iv).

14. ODMWA, section 15.

15. ODMWA, sections 25, 36.

16. ODMWA, section 38

17. See Jonathan Myers, *Asbestos and Asbestos-Related Disease in South Africa* (University of Cape Town, South African Labour and Development Research Unit Working Paper 28, June 1980), 18.

18. ODMWA, sections 79–85

19. ODMWA, section 106. The compensatory regime for coloured workers was similar to that for white workers, just less generous; see ODMWA, sections 86–93.

20. Myers, *Asbestos and Asbestos-Related Disease in South Africa*, 18.

21. Marianne Felix, "Risking Their Lives in Ignorance: The Story of an Asbestos-Polluted Community," in Jacklyn Cock and Eddie Koch, eds., *Going Green: People, Politics, and the Environment in South Africa* (Oxford University Press, 1991), 33–43.

22. Interview with Tommy Ntsewa, March 3, 2023, Johannesburg.

23. Ngoako Ramatlhodi, personal communication to author (via Thabo Makweya), March 15, 2023. At its height (in 1970), the Penge mine had a total workforce of some 7,000, reflecting just how pervasive the industry was throughout these small communities in Limpopo; see James Phillips, David Rees, Jill Murray, and John C. A. Davies, "Mineralogy and Malignant Mesothelioma: The South African Experience," in Carmen Belli and Santosh Anand, eds., *Malignant Mesothelioma* (InTech, 2012), 12.

24. Premier Manne Dipico, correspondence with Richard Meeran, dated July 26, 2000, just a few days after the (eventual) success of the House of Lords judgment delivered on July 20, 2000.

25. Interview with Jack Adams, March 9, 2023, Prieska.

26. Notably, David Johnson was another initial skeptic of the case's chances, but as Richard recounts, "Many years later I bumped into him at conference where he told me how moved he had been by the facts of the case"; Richard Meeran, communication, February 16, 2024.

27. Stretching back at least to the seventeenth-century case of *Vernor v. Elvies* (1610) 6 Mor Dict of Dec. 4788 (Scot. Sess. Cas. 2d Div. 1610), involving a dispute between two Englishmen before a Scottish court, which jurisdiction was (successfully) argued to be inappropriate in the circumstances to trial the case.

28. Despite being significantly dismantled in much of the rest of the common law world, it remains a powerful defense available to corporations in the United States. See Erin Foley Smith, "Right to Remedies and the Inconvenience of *Forum non Conveniens*: Opening U.S. Courts to Victims of Corporate Human Rights Abuses," *Columbia Journal of Law and Social Problems* 44 (2010): 145; Richard Meeran, "Perspectives on the Development and Significance of Tort Litigation against Multinational Parent Companies," in Richard Meeran, ed., *Human Rights Litigation against Multinationals in Practice* (Oxford University Press, 2021), 24–57.

29. In *Spiliada Maritime Corporation v. Cansulex* [1987] 1 A.C. 460, a pair of English-insured ships were damaged after they were loaded with wet sulphur in a port in British Columbia, Canada. The House of Lords determined that despite the availability of British Columbia as an alternative forum, the English courts were the more suitable forum in terms of serving the ends of justice; per Lord Goff at 477E.

30. *Spiliada Maritime Corporation v. Cansulex* [1987] 1 A.C. 460.

31. There are important differences between the roles of barristers (counsel) and solicitors in the UK legal system, typically necessitating that the latter engage the former as advocates in court, especially in cases being argued in the superior courts. See Glossary for further explanation.

32. European Community Convention on Jurisdiction and the Enforcement of Judgments in Civil and Commercial Matters (a.k.a. Brussels Convention, 1968).

33. See Case C-281/02 *Owusu v. Jackson* [2005] ECR I-1383, where the ECJ ruled in favor of restricting the defense of *forum non conveniens* even in cases involving non-EU plaintiffs.

34. Albeit to no avail, as Kallipetis determined that there existed—at that time—no obligation on him to refer the matter to the ECJ. His reasoning was based on a prior judgment of the Court of Appeal (*Re: Harrods (Buenos Aires) Ltd* [1992], ch.72) that effectively relieved English courts of such an obligation; see *Lubbe v. Cape Plc* (Judgment: January 12, 1998), paras. 5.6–5.8. The ECJ's later decision in *Owusu* in 2005 (above) quashed that line of reasoning, effectively ending English courts' discretion to deny jurisdiction on grounds of *forum non conveniens*.

35. Architecturally designated as Victorian Gothic Revival and officially opened by Queen Victoria in 1882, the nineteen court rooms within the building deal mostly with civil litigation matters.

36. *Margereson v. JW Roberts* [1996] P.I.Q.R. P154, in which Justice Holland determined that:

> the defendants must have known of the continuing presence of children and took no steps to reduce the potential for dust emission, nor to keep children away. At all material times there was knowledge sufficient to found reasonable foresight on the

part of the defendants, that children were particularly vulnerable to personal injury arising out of inhalation of asbestos dust. No responsible contemporaneous medical opinion could have discounted the risk of injury to such children through inhalation as a mere possibility which would not occur to the mind of a reasonable man. (at 155)

37. "He is widely regarded as one of the leading advocates of the 20th Century," according to his Brick Chambers profile, ("Sir Syndney Kentridge KC," Brick Court Chambers, undated, https://www.brickcourt.co.uk/our-people/profile/sir-sydney-kentridge-kc).

38. No matter Kentridge's freedom fighting lineage, his surprising presence on Cape's legal team was no doubt explained by the barristerial "cab rank rule," whereby barristers accept clients as they come, unless unavailability or certain other limited reasons preclude them doing so. That said, Kentridge took no further part in the Cape litigation after the case's first appearance before the Court of Appeal.

39. *Lubbe & Others v. Cape*, Court of Appeal, Transcript of Proceedings, May 14, 1998, at 3–4.

40. *Lubbe & Others v. Cape*, Transcript, May 14, 1998, at 5.

41. *Lubbe & Others v. Cape*, Transcript, May 14, 1998, at 5.

42. Indeed, Richard was building something of a reputation among Cape's lawyers for his aggravating strategic maneuvers, as revealed in correspondence between Sydney Kentridge and Brian Doctor as they prepared to make additional submissions in the case, spurred, as Doctor notes, by the fact that "Meeran has again given us a pretext to do so"; Brian Doctor, correspondence with Sydney Kentridge, May 19, 1998. This letter was disclosed by Cape during proceedings.

43. *Lubbe & Others v. Cape*, Court of Appeal, Transcript of Proceedings, May 13, 1998, at 7.

44. *Lubbe & Others v. Cape Plc* [1998] EWCA Civ 1351 (30 July 1998); [1998] C.L.C. 1559, at para. 62.

45. *Lubbe & Others v. Cape Plc* [1998] EWCA Civ 1351 (30 July 1998); [1998] C.L.C. 1559, at para. 36 per Sydney Kentridge QC (as quoted by Evans LJ).

46. *Lubbe & Others v. Cape Plc* 1998] EWCA Civ 1351 (30 July 1998); [1998] C.L.C. 1559, at para. 37.

47. *Lubbe & Others v. Cape Plc* 1998] EWCA Civ 1351 (30 July 1998); [1998] C.L.C. 1559, at para. 55 (emphasis added). For a forensic analysis of the interpretation and application of *forum non conveniens* in this and other related cases, see Peter Muchlinski, "Corporations in International Litigation: Problems of Jurisdiction and the United Kingdom Asbestos Cases," *International and Comparative Law Quarterly* 50 (January 2001): 1.

48. *Lubbe & Others v. Cape Plc*1998] EWCA Civ 1351 (30 July 1998); [1998] C.L.C. 1559, at para. 30, per Evans LJ paraphrasing Barbara Dohmann's submissions and adding, "These matters were determined at Board or a senior level in England as part of company policy and they were implemented by directors and senior personnel in England and elsewhere, including South Africa during regular visits there."

49. Regulations promulgated under authority of section 12(g) of the 1956 Act permitted 300 fibers per milliliter (f/ml) were reduced to 45 f/ml by 1971, whereas the corresponding limits in the United Kingdom for those years were 30 f/ml and 2 f/ml. See Marianne Felix, "Environmental Asbestos and Respiratory Disease in South Africa" (PhD diss., University of Witwatersrand, 1997), 27; note dated October 11, 1983 from C. Venter, deputy director of air pollution control in the Department of Mines in South Africa (cited in Richard Meeran's first affidavit in *Lubbe v. Cape* [June 2, 1997]), who referred specifically to these limits being "set" by the SAAPAC. For accounts of the evasion and lack of enforcement of these upper limits, see Jock McCulloch, *Asbestos Blues: Labour Capital, Physicians and the State in South Africa* (Indiana University Press, 2002), 125–41.

50. "Asbestos-Cancer Link Storm in a Teacup—De Wet," *Diamond Fields Advertiser*, September 25, 1967, 1.

51. *Lubbe & Others v. Cape*, Defence (November 30, 2001), "Annex 6: Koegas and Prieska," at para. 16.1

52. *Lubbe & Others v. Cape*, Defence, at paras. 15–22.

53. *Lubbe & Others v. Cape*, Defence (2001), "Annex 6: Penge," at paras. 10, 12, 16.1, 24.4.

54. *Lubbe & Others v. Cape*, Defence, at para. 17.4.

55. These very points had been made in the Court of Appeal by Lord Justice Evans, who'd stated: "Even if it is assumed that all South African regulations were complied with, and even that the operations

were in no way unlawful under South African law, the allegation of negligence remains. Where business is carried on in this country [the United Kingdom], the fact that statutory regulations [in South Africa] were not breached does not mean that the defendant was not negligent." What matters, he added, was whether "the defendants . . . situated in England . . . ought reasonably to have taken account of scientific knowledge that was available to them here" (*Lubbe & Others v. Cape Plc* [1998] EWCA Civ 1351 (30 July 1998); [1998] C.L.C. 1559, at para. 41).

56. Phone interview, Russell Levy, September 13, 2023.

57. Jock McCulloch, *Asbestos Blues*, 180. Wagner died on July 1, 2000, just three weeks before the House of Lords judgment in the Cape case, the latter being a legal apotheosis of the politics of asbestos.

58. Which had been the PRU in Wagner's day, subsequently replaced first by NRIOD in 1971 and then the NCOH in 1979.

59. Interview with Sophie Kisting, March 6, 2023, Cape Town. Coincidentally, the interview was conducted in the rather grand surroundings of the harborside terrace of the Radisson Blu Hotel (chosen by Sophie because it would be easy for me to find), with Somerset Hospital immediately behind us and Robben Island (now a tourist attraction) shimmering on the horizon in front of us.

60. Lundy Braun and Sophia Kisting, "Asbestos-Related Disease in South Africa: The Social Production of an Invisible Epidemic" *Public Health Then and Now* 96, no 8 (2006): 1387.

61. Braun and Kisting, "Asbestos-Related Disease in South Africa," 1387.

62. As per MBOD certificates supplied by claimants during questionnaire interviews conducted by the plaintiffs' lawyers (Leigh Day and John Pickering Partners). The descriptions and quotations that follow are drawn from a number of these anonymized certificates dated between 1994 and 1999.

6. Corporate Cover-Up

1. Joan Usack and Jim Zakzeski, correspondence with the North American Asbestos Corporation (addressed simply to "Gentlemen"), August 26, 1971.

2. The biographies of both asbestos characters on the Marvel database are as terrifically ridiculous as they are macabre. For Asbestos Man,

see https://marvel.fandom.com/wiki/Orson_Kasloff_(Earth-616); for Asbestos Lady, see https://marvel.fandom.com/wiki/Victoria_Murdock_(Earth-616).

3. While an asbestos substitute was used for superstructure insulation on the remaining floors of the North Tower and on all floors in of the South Tower, there were still thousands of tons of asbestos fiber suspended in the plumes of pulverised walls, floors, and various other structural elements that billowed from their collapse on 9/11. In addition to the hundreds of tons of asbestos insulation used in the towers' construction, there were thousands of tons of asbestos-containing floor tiles. Paul Brodeur, "The Cruel Saga of Asbestos Disease," *Los Angeles Times*, February 18, 2005. See also David Biello, "What Was in the World Trade Center Plume?" *Scientific American*, September 7, 2011.

4. Richard Meeran, communication, March 3, 2000.

5. *Dust to Dust*, Granada Television, November 11, 1981. The original transcript for the documentary is held in the Archives Collection of the University of Strathclyde Library. See also Laurie Flynn, *Studded with Diamonds and Paved with Gold: Miners, Mining Companies and Human Rights in South Africa* (Bloomsbury, 1992), chaps. 9, 10.

6. *Dust to Dust*.

7. Geoffrey Higham, deposition, June 4, 1975 (London), in the case of *Yandle et al. v. PPG Industries, Inc. et al.*, 65 F.R.D. 566 (E.D. Tex. 1974). The quotations that follow are at 60–62. See also chapter 4.

8. As per Marianne Felix, "Environmental Asbestos and Respiratory Disease in South Africa" (PhD diss., University of Witwatersrand, 1997), 27.

9. Richard Meeran, First Affidavit, June 2, 1997, in *Lubbe & Others v. Cape Plc*, 1997 L No.250 (Queen's Bench Division), at paras. 34 and 53, respectively. Even these latter figures are likely to be gross underestimates. According to historical data released by the government mining engineer, average dust concentrations in asbestos mills stood at 1,900 per c.c. in the period 1940–1942, 1,500 per c.c. in 1947–48, and 280 per c.c. in 1961; Asbestos Research Project, Engineering Sub-Committee, "Comments on Research Regarding Engineering Aspects of the Project," March 15, 1965.

10. Higham, deposition, at 62.

11. Meeran, Affidavit, para. 61.

12. Justin MacKeurtan, deposition, November 19, 1996 (Johannesburg), in the case of *Re: Asbestos Personal Injury Cases*, Arrington Lead No. 93-9-114, Circuit Court of Jones County, Mississippi, Second Judicial District, 1996.

13. MacKeurtan, deposition, at 351–22.

14. MacKeurtan, deposition, at 28–34; my emphasis. MacKeurtan himself used the word "bizarre" in explaining the event, adding, for good measure, that "I'll swear to the Bible" as to its veracity.

15. MacKeurtan, deposition, at 377.

16. Born in Durban in 1920, MacKeurtan attended Eton College but not, thereafter, university because, as he put it, "Hitler got in the way" (MacKeurtan, deposition, at 40). MacKeurtan's uncompromising scientific opinions were nevertheless actively supported by Cape UK's company physician, W. J. Smither, following the latter's report on his "Visit to South Africa" (Barking, August 1962). "Mr MacKeurtan's critique of the [mesothelioma] survey report has my full agreement," noted Smither, without clearly stating why he agreed. He was equally opaque when he then recommended that "the company should not support any future wide-ranging survey of the industry with a view to discovering asbestosis or mesothelioma [because] . . . the company is well aware of the problem and has already some idea of its extent" (10).

17. MacKeurtan, deposition, at 388.

18. MacKeurtan refers to £25,000 in his 1996 deposition (at 380), albeit that I could not find that amount reflected in records held by the NIOH. What I did find, however, were records showing Cape making annual financial contributions to PRU's research—for example, R3,499 (approximately, £1,750) in 1961, which for that year was by far the largest contribution of any asbestos producer (Pneumoconiosis Research Unit, "Mesothelioma Survey—Financial Statement for Period 11 November 1960 to 30 June 1961").

19. This incident is recorded in MacKeurtan's 1996 deposition (at 394–95), in which his lawyer objects to the imputation of "outraged" in the deposer's question. MacKeurtan also says he wasn't outraged, but then rather betrays himself by adding: "I've heard from various people that I was a bad boy" during the meeting, and "I'm not that sort of chap. I don't normally exhibit my feelings to that extent."

20. Asbestos Research Project, "Comments."

21. Asbestos Research Project, Engineering Sub-Committee, "Notes of First Meeting," October 23, 1962, 1.

22. Asbestos Research Project, "Notes," 3-4.

23. Namely, under the Occupational Diseases in Mines and Works Act (ODMWA, 1973); see chapter 5 for discussion. Notably, however, there existed no statutory displacement of common law claims made by environmentally exposed asbestos litigants.

24. The point is underlined in a subsequent Cape brochure, "Progress at Penge" (undated), which proclaims: "Largely at the instigation of the asbestos industry the Pneumoconiosis Act 1961 made provision for research into the problems associated with asbestos," with "no less than 80 per cent" of the research funding directed at "trying to solve the engineering problems."

25. See Ntombizodwa Ndlovu, David Rees, and Jill Murray, Naseema Vorajee, Guy Richards, and Jim teWaterNaude, "Asbestos-Related Diseases in Mineworkers: A Clinicopathological Study," *ERJ Open Research* 3 (2017): 00022-2017, who examine the extent of misdiagnosed ARDs in living patients by comparing them with histological autopsy results after their death.

26. Richard Meeran, communication, April 13, 2024; see also Meeran, First Affidavit, June 2, 1997, at paras. 8-10.

27. Asbestos Research Project, "Comments," 6-8.

28. I. J. Selikoff, J. Churg and E. C. Hammond, "The Occurrence of Asbestosis among Insulation Workers in the United States," *Annals of the New York Academy of Sciences* 132, no. 1 (1965): 139-55; M. Newhouse and H. Thompson, "Mesothelioma of Pleura and Peritoneum Following Exposure to Asbestos in the London Area," *British Journal of Industrial Medicine* 22 (1965): 261-69.

29. Asbestos Research Project, "Comments," 12-13.

30. Jock McCulloch, "Public Health Chronicles: Saving the Asbestos Industry, 1960 to 2006," *Public Health Reports* 121 (September–October 2006): 609-14.

31. Jock died of mesothelioma in January 2018, having been diagnosed with the condition nine months earlier. He was seventy-two years old. See further, chapter 4 above, at note 37.

32. Jock McCulloch, *Asbestos: Its Human Cost* (University of Queensland Press, 1986), 257. Many years later Jock summed up the idea in more prosaic terms in an interview at the Power Reporting 2014, African

Investigative Journalism Conference in Johannesburg: "Don't believe the official data; always question it!" (McCulloch, "Manufacturing Ignorance: Risk, Lies, and Gold Mining," https://www.youtube.com /watch?v=L2FRhl9ILzQ).

33. *In re: Asbestos Personal Injury Cases*, Arrington Lead No. 93-9-114, Circuit Court of Jones County, State of Mississippi, Second Judicial District, 1996.

34. H. E. G. Wilson, deposition, *In re: Asbestos Personal Injury Cases*, November 25, 1996 (Johannesburg).

35. McCulloch, *Asbestos Blues*, 198.

36. Richard Meeran, communications, February 27, 2020, and June 18, 2024.

37. As per Gaze's own words in his 1975 deposition, June 4–5, 1975, in the case of *Yandle et al. v. PPG Industries, Inc. et al.*, 65 F.R.D. 566 (E.D. Tex. 1974), at 46.

38. McCulloch, *Asbestos Blues*, 199, citing H. E. Whipple, ed., "Biological Effects of Asbestos," *Annals of the New York Academy of Sciences* 132, no. 1 (1965): 682.

39. McCulloch, *Asbestos Blues*, 199.

40. Gaze, deposition, at 55–56.

41. Gaze, deposition, at 55.

42. Gaze, deposition, at 48.

43. See Emily Dugan, "Asbestos: A Shameful Legacy," *The Independent*, November 22, 2009.

44. C. A. Sleggs, Medical Superintendent, West End Hospital, Kimberley, correspondence to the Director of the Institute of Medical Research, October 30, 1956.

45. On which see generally, Maria Roselli, "Medical Findings and Silencing Them," chapter 2 in her *The Asbestos Lie* (European Trade Union Institute, 2014). The assault on scientific and medical practice by the industry was not peculiar to South Africa. There was in fact a concerted global effort by asbestos corporations to obstruct and sully and research that documented the ill-effects of asbestos on people's health. See Jock McCulloch and Geoffrey Tweedale, in both *Defending the Indefensible: The Global Asbestos Industry and Its Fight for Survival* (Oxford University Press, 2008) and "Shooting The Messenger: The Vilification of Irving J.

Selikoff," *International Journal of Health Services*, 37, no. 4 (2007): 619–34.

46. The PRU became the NRIOD in 1971, which was itself succeeded by the NCOH in 1979; see the glossary for further details.

47. Neil White and Eric Bateman, "Mesothelioma and Exposure to Asbestos in South Africa: 1962–2000," in Bruce Robinson and Philippe Chahinian, eds. *Mesothelioma* (CRC Press, 2002), 96–97, 104.

48. Laurie Flynn, "South Africa Blacks Out Blue Asbestos Risk," *New Scientist*, April 22, 1982, 237–39.

49. Medical Research Council, letter to the editor of the *New Scientist*, signed by A. J. Brink, June 23, 1982; held in the Laurie Flynn Papers, University of Strathclyde Library Archives.

50. Webster's letter is dated July 24, 1978, but in a cover note dated October 31, 1978, he reveals he didn't send it to Irwig until then because, as he put it, "I have debated for a long time as to whether the enclosed letter should be sent." Held in NIOH archives.

51. Pneumoconiosis Research Unit *Report of the Progress of the Mesothelioma Survey as at 30th April 1962*, May 4, 1962, at 1. Though unsigned, the report appears to have been written by Webster, under authority of I. G. Walters, who was director of the PRU at the time.

52. As quoted in Richard Meeran, "Cape Plc: South African Mineworkers' Quest for Justice," *International Journal of Occupational and Environmental Health*, 9, no. 3 (2003): 219–20.

53. Gerrit Schepers, "Asbestos in South Africa: Certain Geographical and Environmental Considerations" *Annals of New York Academy of Sciences* 132 (1965): 246–47. Further details of Schepers's account of the conditions endured by these child laborers are found in chapter 2 above.

54. Richard Meeran, "Perspectives on the Development and Significance of Tort Litigation against Multinational Parent Companies," in Richard Meeran, ed. *Human Rights Litigation against Multinationals in Practice* (Oxford University Press, 2021), 32.

55. That said, a letter from E. W. Lowe, the acting director of native labor, to the secretary for native affairs on October 19, 1940 (cited by McCulloch, *Asbestos Blues*, 126), indicated that at that time Cape's Penge mine employed 447 children (under the age of 16) out of a total workforce of 1,625.

56. See "Asbestos Claimants Hold Vigil for Court Date," *Independent Online*, May 20, 2001. https://www.iol.co.za/news/south-africa /asbestos -claimants-hold-vigil-for-court-date-66171#google_vignette.
57. This is how Tommy Ntsewa put it to me; interview, March 3, 2023 (Johannesburg).
58. As confirmed to Jock McCulloch by Jacoba Schnyders, a former manager at the Prieska asbestos mill during the 1940s and 1950s; see McCulloch, *Asbestos Blues*, 134–36.
59. As Tony Davies wrote, with colleagues Jill Murray and David Rees, a "migrant labour system weakens incentives to control dust and diseases because the costs can be externalized from the . . . mining industry to communities and the [foreign] state" ("Occupational Lung Disease in the South African Mining Industry: Research and Policy Implementation," *Journal of Public Health Policy* 32 [2011]: S67).
60. G. B. Peacock, "Report on Health Conditions at Asbestos Mines at Pietersburg," cited by McCulloch, *Asbestos Blues*, 128–29.
61. White and Bateman, "Mesothelioma and Exposure to Asbestos," 104.
62. White and Bateman, "Mesothelioma and Exposure to Asbestos," 93.
63. As per Smither's "Visit to South Africa" report (1962) mentioned earlier in this chapter.
64. Financial reward is another possible reason, according to Jock McCulloch. His research unearthed a financial "arrangement" between Wagner and two US-based asbestos companies that "continued for more than 15 years [across the 1980s and 1990s], from which Wagner probably received in excess of $300,000;" see McCulloch "Saving the Asbestos Industry, 1960 to 2006," *Public Health Reports* 121, no. 5 (2006): 612–14. Whatever the reasons, there can be no doubting the bitter disillusionment of many of Wagner's fellow scientists in South Africa over his behavior. Sophie Kisting-Cairncross, for example, remains bewildered after all these years: "I find it difficult to understand the psychology of a man who made such a profound discovery," she told me when I interviewed her in March 2023, "and then to deny its importance!" she added, in exasperation (interview, March 6, 2023, Cape Town).
65. Jonathan Myers, *Asbestos and Asbestos-Related Disease in South Africa* (University of Cape Town, South African Labour and Development Research Unit Working Paper 28, June 1980), 25–28. Myers

was writing at a time when the asbestos industry in South Africa was still thriving.

7. Outrage

1. Later, during settlement negotiations following the House of Lords judgment in 2000, access to and use of these records were matters of conflict between Cape's lawyers (who claimed that the company still "owned" them) and Leigh Day (who claimed that the Cape had abandoned them).

2. Author notes from visits to Koegas and Draghoender, Northern Cape, March 9, 2023.

3. The Prieska office was the bigger and more established of the two, the office space in Burgersfort being merely borrowed, temporarily, from the National Union of Mineworkers.

4. This being symptomatic of chronically poor gas-exchange of the lungs' alveoli; see Coutts et al., "Significance of Finger Clubbing in Asbestosis" *Thorax (British Medical Journal)* 42 (1987): 117–19.

5. Hein du Plessis's photograph of Hendrik is among those reproduced in the middle of this book.

6. As quoted by Jason Burke, "UK Firm in Court over Lung Disease," *The Guardian*, May 27, 2001.

7. As quoted by Francois Loots, "The Killing Stone," *Guardian & Mail*, May 11, 2001.

8. "Memorandum from Victims of Asbestosis, Northern Province," March 7, 2000. Copy on file with the author.

9. Phone interview with Zack Mabiletja, April 6, 2023, Ga-Mafefe.

10. Interview with Andrew Phillips, March 12, 2023, Prieska.

11. Under its constitution the CPAA's objectives include "help[ing] members of the community with guidance in regard to the rights accorded to them by law" and ensuring that asbestos mining companies are held "accountable to people affected with asbestos." Copy on file with the author. For a lengthy discussion of the organization's work, see Jock McCulloch, "Beating the Odds: The Quest for Justice by South African Asbestos Mining Communities," *Review of African Political Economy* 103 (2005): 63–77.

12. Interview with Cecil Skeffers, March 8, 2023, Prieska.

13. As listed by the new trial judge, Buckley J, in *Afrika & Ors v. Cape; Lubbe & Ors v. Cape* [2000] CLC 45 (1999), at 46–47.

14. Interview with Angela Andrews and Steve Kahanovitz, March 7, 2023, Cape Town. Notably, Sydney Kentridge was a founder and the patron of the LRC and while, as noted earlier (chapter 5, n38), his position as lead counsel for Cape during earlier stages of the case is likely explained by the "cab rank rule," there is no doubting the awkward incongruity of his acting for a client against whom evidence compiled by the LRC was being filed by Richard and his legal team. The starkness of this paradox was apparently a key reason why Kentridge withdrew from the case after the first Court of Appeal hearings. Richard Meeran, communication, June 22, 2024, in which he noted that the LRC was especially keen for Kentridge to withdraw, as long-term LRC attorney Ranjit ("JP") Purshotam told Richard some time later.

15. Interview with Sapna Malik, May 2, 2023, London.

16. Interview with Zanele Mbuyisa, March 13, 2023, Johannesburg.

17. Constructed by the aptly named sociable weaver bird, these amazing structures—looking more like a grass sun hut on a tropical beach than a bird's nest—can house up to 200 birds at a time.

18. Author notes, March 9, 2023, Prieska and Koegas.

19. To which physical demands some were especially well suited. Richard recalls, for example, that during one of the fund-raising events organized by Leigh Day for the claimants (as described below), there was, bizarrely, a demonstration by a martial arts group involving one of "our quietly spoken paralegals, Margaret Durbal, who karate chopped a thick piece of wood in half." Clearly impressed, Richard added, "I was very careful how I spoke to her in the office after that." Richard Meeran, communication, April 13, 2024.

20. Self-styled as "The People's Lawyer and the People's Poet"; for Neita in action, see "David Neita—BAME Apprenticeships Awards 2021," https://www.youtube.com/watch?v=faMQU0Ji-8Q.

21. Interview with Dave Neita, May 4, 2023, London.

22. Per the audio file sent to me by the Neita, the first stanza reads:

Some dogs in South Africa are trained to attack,
But not just anybody, them just attack black,
Them named racist dogs, racist dogs.

23. Richard's assistant, Bridget Heapy, was the winning bidder.

24. The Legal Aid Board was replaced by the Legal Services Commission in 2000.

25. Nicolas Rufford, "South Africans Cost Taxpayers £9m in Legal Aid," *Sunday Times*, July 23, 2000. Today the Institute of Directors appears to sing from a different song sheet, being a vocal advocate of practices promoting sustainability ("it's not a choice: it's a responsibility"), inclusion and diversity, corporate social responsibility, and good environmental and social governance, all under the banner of "Better directors make a better world" (Institute of Directors, homepage, undated, https://www.iod.com/).

26. A fuller account of what costs were finally covered by the LAB (and later the Legal Services Commission) is provided in chapter 9.

27. Including one episode of the BBC's popular *Newsnight* program in December 1998 detailing Cape's past asbestos operations in South Africa and the then case against it, alongside the harrowing story of Amanda Burger (whom we encountered in chapter 6). The airing of this episode likely had the greatest single impact on the British public's critical attitude toward asbestos corporations like Cape, such that it prompted Cape to take the extraordinary step of engaging a public relations firm to hit back at Leigh Day, as discussed in the next chapter. Unfortunately, the episode is no longer publicly available and despite our concerted efforts to obtain a copy, the BBC declined to make one available either to Leigh Day or me.

28. The church (St. John's) on both occasions donated the use of its hall for free. The *Cape Dust* exhibition was later displayed at international asbestos conferences in Sao Paulo, Brazil, and Buenos Aires, Argentina.

29. Laurie is now co-ordinator of the International Ban Asbestos Secretariat (http://www.ibasecretariat.org/). A few years later in 2002, Laurie was also a key player behind Richard being awarded a Certificate for Outstanding Achievement by eighteen asbestos victims' support groups worldwide presented at the South African High Commission in London.

30. Richard Meeran, communication, October 17, 2023.

31. For an indication of some contemporaneous UK claims payouts, see David Flickling, "Asbestos Compensation Payouts Set to Be Cut," *The Guardian*, May 4, 2006. For the gargantuan number of payouts in the US (estimated to comprise approximately 730,000 claimants

receiving a total of $70 billion up to 2002), see Stephen Carroll et al., "Asbestos Litigation Costs, Compensation, and Alternatives," RAND Institute for Civil Justice, Research Brief (RAND Corporation, 2005). As for the sizes of these US payouts, Michelle White estimated that between 1987 and 2002 the expected compensatory damage award for a mesothelioma claimant was $2.34 million and $460,000 for an asbestosis claimant, though she added the qualifier that "most tort claimants receive much less, since claims are generally settled out of court, and settlement levels are much lower than damage awards." Michelle White, "Asbestos and the Future of Mass Torts," *Journal of Economic Perspectives* 18, no. 2 [2004]: 199–200.

32. See "Claimants' Skeleton Argument on Abuse Allegations" in *Lubbe, Afrika, Cocks, Mphahlele, Alexander & Others v. Cape* (undated), before Buckley J (Queen's Bench Division), being a rebuttal of the defendant's (Cape's) contention. Copy on file with author.

33. The recollections of all three are contained in their separate sworn affidavits: Obert Mahlo, June 1, 1999; Christa Smith, undated, June 1999; Cecil Skeffers, June 4, 1999. Copies on file with author.

34. ZAR is the international code for the South African rand.

35. Prieska's resident physician, Deon Smith, who was also interviewed around the same time by no less than three lawyers from WWB, labeled the attitude adopted by one of them, Stuart McCafferty, as "very aggressive" in pursuing a line of questioning that revolved around legal issues and the activities of Richard in particular, rather than on medical matters as Deon had (fairly) expected to be the case (Gideon Smith, Affidavit, *Afrika and 1538 others v. Cape Plc*, 1999-A-No. 40 [Queen's Bench Division], May 31, 1999).

36. Interview with Christa Smith, March 10, 2023, Prieska.

37. Phone interview with Zack Mabiletja, April 6, 2023, Ga-Mafefe.

38. For examples of pushback from the "commercial elite of the Northern Cape" (as related to him by Cecil Skeffers), see McCulloch, "Beating the Odds," 71.

39. Matthys van Rooyen, deposition, *Re: Asbestos Personal Injury Cases*, Arrington Lead No. 93-9-114, Circuit Court of Jones County, Mississippi, November 8, 1996 (Cape Town; by video), at 40–41.

40. Zack's diaries, he says, were "confiscated" by the local chief in 1997, apparently due to Zack's growing media presence (interview, April 6, 2023). Christa's conspicuous media presence was evident from her

being featured in various glossy magazine articles she showed me, including one by Fienie Grobler entitled "SA's Erin Brockovich: The Battle against a Mining Giant," *Style*, September 2001, 52–56.

41. Richard Meeran, communication, December 21, 2023.

42. Christa Smith, Affidavit, undated, June 1999. Copy on file with author.

8. Offensive Lawyers

1. Copies on file with the author.

2. At the time Tony Blair's Labour Government was two years into its first term in office. The Lord Chancellor (then Lord (Derry) Irvine) was the minister responsible for legal aid.

3. Notably, the principal authors of Media Strategy's two audits were both formerly advisers to Tory prime ministers—Wilf Weeks had been the head of Sir Edward Heath's private office and Charles Lewington had been communications chief under John Major; see Steve Boggan, "Tory Advisors Try to Sabotage Court Case," *The Independent*, February 4, 1999.

4. Which cases we encountered, briefly, in chapter 1.

5. Interview with Graham Read, April 26, 2023, London.

6. *Lubbe & Others v. Cape Plc*, QBENI 98/0192/1, Transcript, 30 July 1998 (Court of Appeal), at 9, per Mr Doctor. A Court of Appeal judge in the United Kingdom—officially, Lord or Lady Justice of Appeal—is referred to as "Lordship" or "Ladyship," these being the same titles that were formally used for judges in the House of Lords (who were, officially, Lords of Appeal in the Ordinary) and are still used today for judges in the Supreme Court of the United Kingdom.

7. *Afrika & Others v. Cape Plc*; *Lubbe & Others v. Cape Plc* [2000] CLC 45 (1999), at 62

8. *Afrika & Others v. Cape Plc*; *Lubbe & Others v. Cape Plc*, at 62–63.

9. *Afrika & Others v. Cape Plc*; *Lubbe & Others v. Cape Plc*, 62–64. It should be noted that His Honour had previously ordered that the various multi-party actions then commenced (of which *Afrika* was only one, albeit the lead case) be joined as one "group action" (at 47).

10. Interview with Tony Davies, March 16, 2023, Kenton-on-Sea, Eastern Cape.

11. Tony Davies, Affidavit, *Afrika & 1,538 Others* (June 3, 1999), at para. 13.

12. Tony Davies, Affidavit, at para. 13.

13. *Afrika & Others v. Cape Plc*; *Lubbe & Others v. Cape Plc*, 60–62 (Buckley J).

14. Tony Davies, Affidavit.

15. As per Richard Meeran, Fourth Affidavit, *Lubbe & Others v. Cape Plc* (June 7, 1999), para. 221(d).

16. Richard Meeran, communication , March 22, 2024.

17. Richard Meeran, communications, March 16, 2020, and June 19, 2024.

18. Thus, two of the five combined writs heard by Justice Buckley were issued by Pickering & Partners.

19. Specifically, the Court of Appeal had introduced a new and unprecedented limitation on the doctrine of *forum non conveniens*—namely that the other putatively available forum having competent jurisdiction (i.e., South Africa) must be one that can exercise jurisdiction according to its internal rules *without* the need for the defendant (Cape) to submit to the jurisdiction of that forum; see *Lubbe & Others v. Cape Plc* [1998] EWCA Civ 1351 (30 July, 1998); [1998] C.L.C. 1559, at paras. 8–10 (per Evans LJ). Demonstrating no resistance to hyperbole, DAC's David McIntosh countered the Court of Appeal's reasoning by asserting that its "decision will give rise to capricious results devoid of underlying justice" (David McIntosh, Affidavit, *Afrika & Others v. Cape Plc* [August 13, 1999], para. 60.2).

20. Richard Meeran, Seventh Affidavit in *Lubbe & Others v. Cape Plc* (September 20, 1999), paras. 27–28.

21. Richard Meeran, Fourth Affidavit, *Lubbe & Others v. Cape Plc* (June 7, 1999), para. 228(f).

22. Meeran, Fourth Affidavit, at para. 228(f)(iii).

23. Interview with Graham Read, October 3, 2023, London.

24. *Afrika & Others v. Cape Plc*; *Lubbe & Others v. Cape Plc*, 64 (Buckley J).

25. Which reasoning corresponds with that of the first Court of Appeal, whose members had found in favor of the plaintiffs.

26. McIntosh, Affidavit, August 13, 1999, para. 4.5(a).

27. Interview with Graham Read, May 29, 2024, London; Graham Read, personal communication to author, June 19, 2024.

28. The Court of Appeal's order stated, pointedly, that "the decision of Lord Justice Evans on 30th July 1999 that he preside over the claimants' appeal from the decision of Mr. Justice Buckley . . . be set

aside"; in the matter of *Afrika & Others v. Cape Plc* (unreported, August 24, 1999), copy on file with author.

29. Defendant's Case, signed by Brian Doctor, Charles Gibson and Richard Coleman (July 1, 1999), at paras. 88 and 85, respectively; produced originally for first instance hearing (before Buckley J) but resubmitted for the subsequent appeal before the Court of Appeal.

30. Interview with Graham Read, October 3, 2023, London.

31. Interview with Munoree Padayachee, May 5 and 12, 2023, London.

32. *Afrika & Others v. Cape Plc; Lubbe & Others v. Cape Plc*, at 78 (per Pill LJ), and at 81 (per Aldous and Tuckey LLJ). The reference to wasted time prompted Cape's lawyers to make an application in a subsequent costs hearing for "wasted costs" on Cape's part, in which it submitted that Leigh Day should pay. The application lapsed and was later rendered nugatory following Cape's loss before the House of Lords in July 2000.

33. See Transcript, *Afrika & Others v. Cape Plc; Lubbe & Others v. Cape Plc*, October 8, 1999, at 56; and Richard Meeran, Seventh Affidavit, *Lubbe & Others v. Cape* (September 20, 1999), at para. 28.

34. Correspondence from Barbara Dohmann to Lords Justices Pill, Aldous, and Tuckey, October 7, 1999. Copy on file with author.

35. Tony Davies, Affidavit, *Afrika & 1,538 Others* (June 3, 1999), para. 12.

36. *Afrika & Others v. Cape Plc; Lubbe & Others v. Cape Plc*, 45–46 (*per curiam*). Lord Justice Pill also referred approvingly to Buckley J's additional supporting argument that "public interest" concerns (a concept he borrowed from US jurisprudence) pointed toward South Africa as the better forum because it "should have the opportunity of dealing with the case if it . . . arose within its jurisdiction and caused widespread injury or loss to its own citizens" (at 63–65, *per* Buckley J, 72–75, per Pill LJ). On reaching the House of Lords, however, this line of reasoning was effectively rejected by Lord Hope (with whom his colleagues unanimously agreed), who restricted any such public interest concerns to only those that would otherwise fit with the "ends of justice" considerations of the second limb of the *Spiliada* test; *Lubbe & Others v. Cape Plc and Related Appeals* [2000] UKHL 41 (20 July 2000), at para. 50. On the (final) House of Lords judgment, see chapter 9.

37. Though, as indicated earlier, the file was eventually closed with no action being taken in November 2000, due, in part, to a strong

supporting letter from Graham Read to the Office for Supervision of Solicitors explaining the mitigating circumstances.

38. Such stoicism was characteristic of many claimants: "They had waited for so long [since Cape had left the country] and just accepted what came their way," says Charley Nkadimeng, who was head of communications in the Department of Health in Limpopo Province at the time (Zoom interview, December 13, 2023, Polokwane).

39. *Afrika & Others v. Cape Plc*; *Lubbe & Others v. Cape Plc*, at 46 (*per curiam*).

40. Richard Meeran, communication, December 21, 2023.

41. As introduced by the Contingency Fees Act 1997 (no. 66).

42. That is, specifically, there then existed no "after the event" insurance in South Africa, meaning that claimants would have no way to protect themselves from the financial consequences of a costs order against them should they lose the case and be ordered to pay the other side's legal costs as well as their own. Meeran, Fourth Affidavit, *Lubbe & Others v. Cape Plc* (June 7, 1999), at paras. 50, 62, 66.

43. Various correspondence between David Unterhalter, WWB, DAC, and Leigh Day dated from September 30 to November 23, 1999, copies of which were duly communicated (by Richard) to all three Court of Appeal judges.

44. Letter addressed to Leigh Day, from the South African Legal Aid Board, signed by A. J. Brits, acting chief executive officer, October 14, 1999.

45. Richard Meeran, communication, March 13, 2024.

46. That is according to a friend of Richard's who'd meet Navsa many years later and to whom Navsa made clear his continuing irritation over the incident; Richard Meeran, communication, May 29, 2024.

47. Who by then was Lord Brennan, having been created Baron Brennan of Bibury on May 2, 2000.

48. Graham Read, correspondence with Anthony Coombs, May 17, 2000.

49. As noted above, the essence of this public interest factor, according to the second Court of Appeal, lay in South Africa having both "the opportunity of dealing with the case" (*Afrika & Others v. Cape Plc*; *Lubbe & Others v. Cape Plc*, at 64 and 73) *and* the capacity to deliver a just outcome. So presented, these two conditions invited refutation, thereby providing Richard with the foothold for appeal.

50. As argued by Lord Justice Pill, who stated: "I am entirely unper-
suaded by arguments that the South African High Court would be
unable to handle these actions efficiently" (*Afrika & Others v. Cape
Plc; Lubbe & Others v. Cape Plc*, at 73).

51. Ronnie Morris, "SA to Intervene in Asbestos Lawsuit," *Cape Times*
March 30, 2000. "The Republic's primary submission," the government told the House of Lords, "is that a trial of this action in England
is consistent with its perception of public policy requirements. In the
particular context of this litigation against an English domiciled
company, there is no public interest, certainly no *clear* public interest,
which points to a South African forum in preference to the normal
forum of the Defendant's domicile." It also asserted: "The allegations
against Cape did not take place in a legitimate legal system, and the
new South African government cannot afford to determine every
wrong of the old regime through its judicial system" (Statement of
Case on Behalf of the Republic of South Africa, in *Lubbe & Others v.
Cape* [House of Lords], May 26, 2000, at paras 2.3 and 5.5).

52. Richard Meeran, communication, March 13, 2024.

53. *Lubbe & Others v. Cape Plc and Related Appeals* [2000] UKHL 41
(20 July 2000), at paras. 27–28. The evidence included affidavits
from leading South African counsel (such as Jeremy Gauntlett SC)
and academics (such as Shadrack Gutto).

54. *Lubbe & Others v. Cape Plc* (2000), at para. 28.

55. In dismissing the claimants' appeal, the Court of Appeal had held:
"The court would not refuse a stay on grounds that legal aid was not
available in South Africa or that the South African courts were not
able to deal properly with the actions. Contingency fees were lawful
in South Africa and the court could not conclude that legal representation would not become available in South Africa;" *Afrika & Others
v. Cape Plc; Lubbe & Others v. Cape Plc*, at 46 (*per curiam*).

56. Lords Bingham, Steyn, Hoffmann, Hope, and Hobhouse. Notably,
both Lords Steyn and Hoffmann are South African.

57. *Lubbe* (2000), at para. 28 (per Lord Bingham). As David Pallister, a
legal correspondent with the *Guardian*, said of Lord Bingham's
words: "In judge-speak, that is pretty damning" (Pallister, "Poor
Law," *The Guardian*, July 28, 2000).

58. *Lubbe* (2000), at para. 36. The award of costs against it clearly stung
Cape and its lawyers. The next day DAC revealed to journalist

Nicolas Rufford that the plaintiffs' solicitors had indicated in court that the cost of litigating the case was in the region of £9 million, which was "far more than their clients [Cape] could afford." And as Leigh Day and John Pickering & Partners were seeking legal aid for their clients, DAC left it for Rufford to leap to the sensationalist conclusion that legal aid (and therefore the British taxpayer) would be on the hook for all that amount. See Rufford, "South African Cost Taxpayers £9 Million in Legal Aid," *Sunday Times*, July 23, 2000. Legal aid's contribution was, in the end, only £2.5 million.

59. Though there exists no transcript for the hearings, Richard remembers these incidents very clearly; Richard Meeran, communication, March 22, 2024.

60. Lord Bingham effectively dismissed concerns that additional claimants somehow tainted considerations of the United Kingdom as the forum best suited to deliver a just outcome by simply noting that provided "any new claimants are admitted to the group only upon their binding themselves by the undertaking of the present plaintiffs," then "the refusal of a stay will not expose the defendant to a significant risk of prejudice" before the UK courts. *Lubbe* (2000), at para. 31.

61. Richard Meeran, communication, June 7, 2024.

62. Jo Prince, a plaintiff suing on behalf of her husband, Richard, who had died of mesothelioma after working at Cape's manufacturing plant in Benoni outside Johannesburg, was later to present Richard with a two-volume scrapbook containing many dozens of articles she had collected throughout the litigation's long history, including the huge coverage following the House of Lords' decision.

63. Interview with Thabo Makweya, March 13, 2023, Johannesburg.

64. As Smiths of Smithfield, a favorite watering hole for lawyers and other city types in London's Square Mile, is fondly known.

9. Redemption

1. Built in the 1970s and situated on the outskirts of the city, the building was referred to as a "death trap" before all asbestos was finally removed in December 1998; Adele Baleta, "Power Station Becomes Asbestos Death Trap," *Independent Online*, June 24, 2001. For a description of the hazardous working conditions during its operation, see "Death Hangs in the Athlone Air," *Mail & Guardian*, October 1, 1997.

2. Interview with Liziwe McDaid, March 6, 2023, Cape Town. As Liziwe recalls, the industry representative was from Canada. She added that by then, South African asbestos industrialists were less bullish, as "they knew the end was nigh."

3. Richard Meeran, communication, April 14, 2023. See also Richard Meeran, "Cape Plc: South African Mineworkers' Quest for Justice," *International Journal of Occupational Environmental Health* 9 (2003): 218, 224.

4. See Meeran, "Cape Plc," 224.

5. Richard Meeran, communication, June 18, 2024. Also, Charles Bourne, correspondence with Mr Justice Wright, June 6, 2001, commenting on Ndelu's earlier letter, while seeking both to explain his and Nic Alp's presence in the MBOD that day and to express his embarrassment "to have been a part of yet a further incident of controversy in this case." Bourne's letter also notes the arrival during the incident of Sophie McMurray (a no-nonsense Australian lawyer with Leigh Day then stationed in Johannesburg), who had, apparently, wasted no time telling Cape's lawyers what she thought of their snooping around the MBOD.

6. Interview with Graham Read, April 26, 2023, London.

7. See Julian Peto, John Hodgson, Fiona Matthews, and Jacqueline Jones, "Continuing Increase in Mesothelioma Mortality in Britain," *Lancet*, 345 (March 4, 1995): 535–39; J. Peto, A. Decarli, C. La Vecchia, F. Levi, and E. Negri, "The European Mesothelioma Epidemic," *British Journal of Cancer* 79 nos. 3–4 (1999): 667.

8. Under the UK Asbestos (Prohibitions) (Amendment) Regulations (1999).

9. Fran Abrams, "Asbestos Miners Win Right to Sue in Britain," *Independent*, July 21, 2000; David Pallister, "SA Mine Victims May Sue in Britain," *Guardian*, July 21, 2000.

10. The House of Lords (as a court) was replaced by the formation of the Supreme Court as the United Kingdom's highest court in 2009.

11. Interview with Audrey Van Schalkwyk, March 10, 2023, Prieska. As is the case with nearly everyone in Prieska, Afrikaans is her first language.

12. Interview with Thabo Makweya, March 13, 2023, Johannesburg.

13. As quoted by Alex Duval Smith, "Heat and Dust," *Independent*, June 16, 2000.

14. Peter Hawthorne, "The Fight of Their Lives," *Time*, August 7, 2000: BBC, "The Fatal Fibre," *The Money Programme*, April 16, 2002.

15. Johnathan Freedland, "In Place of Violence," *Guardian*, May 2, 2001.

16. This theme continued when six months later a group of fifty MPs tabled a motion in the House of Commons, noting that "since Cape's AGM in May 2001, 150 claimants have died" (UK Parliament, *Early Day Motion 394*, November 9, 2001).

17. Richard Meeran, communication, May 14, 2023. Leigh Day's estimates of its legal costs were £9 to £10 million, and while at that stage it was unclear how much of that would be covered by UK legal aid, Richard's best guess was about half, with the remainder potentially being drawn from the settlement offer, in which case roughly £1 million would have been left for compensating the claimants.

18. Meeran, "Cape Plc," 225.

19. Meeran, "Cape Plc," 224.

20. Meeran, "Cape Plc," 224. Turner & Newall was by then owned by Federal-Mogul. See Saeed Shah, "Federal Mogul Files for Protection over Asbestos Liabilities," *Independent*, October 2, 2001, who notes that at the time, the company had 365,000 pending claims against it.

21. After declaring that the company will "vigorously contest" the action, the chairman's statement noted that "an exceptional charge of £7.0 million has been made in this year's accounts, bringing the total provision to £8.3 million for the estimated costs of defending the action" (Cape Plc, *Annual Report and Accounts 2000* [March 21, 2001], 5).

22. Cape Plc, *Annual Report*, 43.

23. See M. W. Janis, "The Doctrine of *Forum non Conveniens* and the Bhopal Case," *Netherlands International Law Review* (1987): 192–204.

24. Richard Meeran, communication, May 14, 2023,

25. Cape Plc, *Annual Report 2000*, 1; and Geoff Gibbs, "Cape Takeover Talks Fail," *Guardian*, July 6, 2001.

26. Cape's offer also precipitated the formal withdrawal of legal aid funding (on the basis that it was a genuine offer and the significant risk that the claimants might not do better), which had a serious effect on Leigh Day's own financial circumstances over the coming three years. See further at n36 and accompanying text.

27. He—or rather Montpellier—was also coming under political pressure to act. Another motion was tabled in the House of Commons urging Montpellier (among other major Cape shareholders) to "use their influence to encourage Cape to act responsibly and ethically towards the victims" (UK Parliament, *Early Day Motion 237*, 15 October 2001).

28. Paul Sellars (Montpellier's managing director), personal communication with author, November 22, 2023.

29. Sellars to author.

30. Richard Meeran, communication, November 29, 2023.

31. As Richard remembers Sellars telling him immediately after the meeting; Richard Meeran, communication, December 21, 2023.

32. Zoom interview with Paul Sellars, November 28, 2003, United Kingdom.

33. In an office building dubbed a "miserable dungeon" by one of DAC's own clients; as reported by *The Lawyer* in its entry for DAC Beachcroft (as it is now called), undated, https://www.thelawyer.com/dac-beachcroft/.

34. Richard Meeran, communication, July 28, 2023.

35. Interview with Sapna Malick, May 2, 2023, London.

36. According to Richard, at the outset they had estimated the full potential value of the claim to be in excess of £100 million. At the time of the settlement negotiations, however, especially considering all of Cape's financial circumstances, "We took the view that a total settlement of £33 million would be reasonable," he says. Richard Meeran, communication, June 7, 2024.

37. This contribution was of critical importance to Leigh Day not only to offset the substantial costs it had already incurred over and above that which it had received in legal aid from the United Kingdom's Legal Services Commission (LSC), but also because the LSC had, as a consequence of Cape's firm settlement offer in October 2001, formally ceased any further legal aid payments. Thereafter and until the final settlement payments were all assessed and distributed more than two years later, Leigh Day (and JPP) effectively worked pro bono.

38. "South African Asbestos Victims Settle with Cape," ICEM News Release No.2/2002, undated, but archived on August 11, 2005.

39. As quoted (both Richard and Ngoako) by Clare Dyer, "South African Asbestos Victims Win £21m," *Guardian*, December 22, 2001.

40. Richard Meeran, communication, March 5, 2020.

41. As calculated jointly by Leigh Day and JPP. The breakdown was also reported in "South African Asbestos Victims Settle with Cape."

42. See Statistics South Africa, "Labour statistics: Survey of average monthly earnings," May 2002.

43. Interview with Sarah Leigh, May 30, 2023, Shoreham-by-Sea, West Sussex.

44. Richard Meeran, communication, April 30, 2020.

45. Richard Meeran, communication, April 20, 2020.

46. Sanchia Temkin, "Cape Asbestos: Company May Not Survive to Pay Claimants," *Business Day*, January 18, 2002. Unaware of Cape's financial position, Mkhonto was adamant that "the company owes me and my family." Having been offered R1,491 (about £870 at that time) by Cape when he was diagnosed with an ARD in 1983, he was now looking forward to a far bigger payout under the new settlement agreement, which might enable him "to send his youngest daughter back to school to complete her education."

47. Meeran, "Cape Plc," 225.

48. As Richard recalls it; Richard Meeran, communication, November 24, 2023.

49. See the entry for Cape Plc in Greenpeace, *Corporate Crimes* (August 2002), 104.

50. See *Aviva Plc Annual Report and Accounts 2003*, which states:

> Asbestos, pollution, and social environmental hazards—In the course of conducting insurance business, various companies within the Aviva Group [including GASA and its successor companies] receive general insurance liability claims and become involved in actual or threatened litigation arising therefrom, including claims in respect of pollution and other environmental hazards. Amongst these are claims in respect of asbestos production and handling in various jurisdictions, including the United Kingdom, Australia, Canada, and South Africa. (99)

See also Sanchia Temkin, "Asbestos Victims Widen Quest for Compensation," *Business Day*, November 23, 2003; Richard Meeran, communication, June 7, 2024.

51. That is, in most cases, they had worked for Griqualand Exploration and Finance Company (Gefco), a subsidiary of Gencor.
52. The exact figure was £10,679,691.81; Richard Meeran, communication, June 7, 2024.
53. Richard Meeran, communication, June 7, 2024.
54. In addition, Gencor provided £240,000 for Leigh Day's and JPP's legal costs and their processing of claims and distribution of payments to those Cape claimants who had also been employed (and sickened) by Gencor; Richard Meeran, communication, June 7, 2024.
55. See Nikki Tait, "UK law Firm Adds New Twist in South Africa Asbestos Case," *Financial Times*, September 28, 2002.
56. As related to me by both, separately: Richard Meeran, communication, February 28, 2023; phone interview with Richard Spoor, March 16, 2023, Johannesburg.
57. Sizwe Sama Yende and Justin Arenstein, "Lion's Share for Lawyers," *Mail & Guardian*, May 24, 2002.
58. "M&G Apology to Leigh Day & Co," *Mail & Guardian*, May 31, 2002, signed by the article's two authors and the newspaper's editor, Howard Barrell. The original article also appears to have been pulled from M&G's online archive.
59. Colloquially referred to as "clawback," this practice was based on the LSC's estimation of how many plaintiffs (in a class action) have succeeded or are likely to succeed and which groups the LSC would *not* fund or fund only partially (i.e., the LSC would clawback that portion of its original outlay). No clawback (or a much reduced one) would apply to unsuccessful plaintiffs. In the Cape case the LSC had assumed a failure rate of 42.5 percent of claimants, which benefited the claimants and Leigh Day by limiting the size of its (LSC's) clawback. Richard Meeran, communication, May 30, 2024.
60. GASA was part of General Accident which through mergers with Commercial Union and then Norwich Union became Aviva Plc in July 2002.
61. As recorded by Cape in its *Annual Report 2003* (2004), 48 (at 26(ii)); see also "End of Struggle for Cape Asbestos Victims," MAC: Mining and Communities, March 15, 2003, http://www.minesandcommunities .org/article.php?a=739. The trust established under the parallel Gencor settlement (signed on March 12, 2003), access to which the Cape claimants were now expressly excluded, was much larger (£37.5m),

reflecting Gencor's far greater wealth and financial security at the time; see Thompsons Solicitors (who, alongside Richard Spoor, were acting for claimants against Gencor), "Landmark Settlement Brings Justice for Thousands of former SA Asbestos Miners," March 13, 2003, https://www.thompsonstradeunion.law/news/news-releases/asbestos -disease-news/landmark-settlement-brings-justice-for-thousands-of -sa-former-asbestos-miners.

62. This process was then repeated some weeks later when claimants received notification of their individual payouts.

63. Richard Meeran, communication, May 29, 2024.

64. Richard Meeran, communication, November 15, 2023; interview with Zanele Mbuyisa, March 13, 2023, Johannesburg.

65. Richard Meeran, communication, June 7, 2024. Such "generous" interpretations were necessary because so many of the claimants' medical records (and death certificates) were marked "pneumoconiosis," a generic diagnosis that almost certainly masked more specific (and often more deadly) ARDs. As confirmed to me by Gladys Witbooi, who was a nurse at Prieska Hospital from 1995 to 2004, in an interview, March 11, 2023, Prieska.

66. After eighteen months any remaining balance in this fund was distributed by ABSA on a pro rata basis.

67. Richard Meeran, communication, November 25, 2023.

10. Legacy

The subtitle of this chapter comes from an interview with Sophia Kisting-Cairncross, March 6, 2013, Cape Town.

1. All references to Gladys in the pages that follow are drawn from my interview with her (accompanied by Jack Adams), March 11, 2023, Prieska.

2. Richard Meeran, "Perspectives on the Development and Significance of Tort Litigation against Multinational Parent Companies," in Richard Meeran, ed., *Human Rights Litigation against Multinationals in Practice* (Oxford University Press,2021), 36.

3. Premier Manne Dipcio, letter to Richard Meeran, July 26, 2000.

4. "Cape Caves In on South African Asbestos Case," *Mines and Communities*, March 13, 2003.

5. Interview with Cecil Skeffers, March 8, 2023, Prieska.

6. "Cape Caves In."
7. Zoom interview with Charley Nkadimeng, December 13, 2023, Polokwane.
8. Which number was certainly an underestimate as deaths were seldom speedily reported. Leigh Day has subsequently estimated the true figure to have been around 1,000. See Meeran, "Perspectives," 35.
9. Richard Meeran, First Affidavit, *Lubbe & Others v. Cape Plc* (June 2, 1997), para. 8.
10. Prieska's population has in fact grown and is set to grow further according to Mayor Andrew Phillips, who has plans for building hundreds of new homes to cater for the influx of workers he believes will result from new copper and zinc mines opening in the area. These plans, however, do not include the former mill site, which, despite sitting on prime land near the town center, is still too contaminated to be built on. Interview with Phillips, March 12, 2023, Prieska.
11. Linda Waldman, *The Politics of Asbestos* (Routledge, 2011), 65.
12. Effective from March 28, 2008, pursuant to the Regulation for the Prohibition of the Use, Manufacturing, Import and Export of Asbestos and Asbestos Containing Materials (2008), issued under authority of the Environmental Protection Act 73 of 1989. See further, Laurie Kazan-Allen, "South Africa Bans Asbestos!" International Ban Asbestos Secretariat, April 2, 2008, http://www.ibasecretariat.org/lka _sa_asb_ban_08.php#1. The last operational asbestos mine in South Africa had closed down six years previously, in 2002.
13. Waldman, *The Politics of Asbestos*, 61.
14. Interview with Tommy Ntsewa, March 3, 2023, Johannesburg. See also Gift Muzi Matsabatsa, *Post Asbestos Mining Environment, Penge, Limpopo Province South Africa* (LAP Lambert; 2016), where the author notes that "although the mine dumps in Penge were rehabilitated according to the [Department of Minerals and Energy] guideline recommendations, some areas showed limited success" (61).
15. Interview with Phillips.
16. Tony Davies, letter to Richard Meeran, July 1, 1997.
17. Leslie London, Godfrey Tangwa, Reginald Matchaba-Hove, Nhlanhla Mkhize, Remi Nwabueze, Aceme Nyika, and Peter Westerholm, "Ethics in Occupational Health: Deliberations of an International Workgroup Addressing Challenges in an African Context," *BMC Medical Ethics* 15, no. 48 (2014): 6.

18. Lundy Braun and Sophia Kisting, "Asbestos-Related Disease in South Africa: The Social Production of an Invisible Epidemic," *Public Health Then and Now* 96, no. 8 (2006): 1393.

19. Ntombizodwa Ndlovu, David Rees, Jill Murray, Naseema Vorajee, Guy Richards, and Jim teWaterNaude, "Asbestos-Related Diseases in Mineworkers: A Clinicopathological Study," *ERJ Open Research* 3 (2017), https://openres.ersjournals.com/content/3/3/00022-2017.

20. Gill Nelson, Danuta Kielkowski and Gwinyai Masukume, "Mortality of Crocidolite-Exposed Birth Cohort from South Africa: 2014 Update" (National Institute of Occupational Health and University of Witwatersrand, 2014).

21. Sheila Meintjes, May Hermanus, Mary Scholes, and Marcus Reichart, *The Future of Penge: Prospects for the People and the Environment*, final report (Centre for Sustainability in Mining and Industry, July 2008). See further, Kevin Davie, "Precious and the Asbestos Dump," *Mail & Guardian*, March 19, 2010, whose visit to the village prompted him to write, "Nearly 30 years after the Penge mine closed, it has yet to be properly cleaned up."

22. Global Cancer Observatory, *South Africa: Fact Sheet*, (International Agency for Research on Cancer, World Health Organization, 2022), 2.

23. Michel Muteba, "Mesothelioma Incidence and Mortality in South Africa from 2003 to 2013" (Research Report, University of Witwatersrand, February 2018), 49, drawing on data from South Africa's National Cancer Registry. The congruity of rates of diagnoses and death is notably morbid given the life expectancy of mesothelioma patients is typically between twelve and twenty-one months.

24. Mary Ellen Ellis, notes that "someone exposed in 1970 may not yet receive a diagnosis and die from mesothelioma at present," in reference to circumstances in the United States and drawing on data from the Centers for Disease Control and Prevention (Ellis, "Mesothelioma Death Rate," January 30, 2023, https://mesothelioma.net/mesothelioma-death-rate/).

25. Zhen Zhai, Jian Ruan, Yi Zheng et al., "Assessment of Global Trends in the Diagnosis of Mesothelioma from 1990 to 2017," *JAMA Network Open* 4, no. 8 (2021): e2120360,6. Against this suggestion, a study undertaken jointly by the International Labour Organization and the

World Health Organization indicates that between 2000 and 2016, mesothelioma attributable to asbestos exposure globally rose by 40 percent; *WHO/ILO Joint Estimates of the Work-Related Burden of Disease and Injury, 2000-2016*, September 17, 2021.

26. Namely, the Minerals Act 1991 (per section 38), since repealed by Minerals and Petroleum Resources Development Act 2002 (see especially sections 37–46).

27. Guy Freemantle, Deshenthree Chetty, Mapadi Olifant, and Stanley Masikhwa, "Assessment of Asbestos Contamination in Soils at Rehabilitated and Abandoned Mine Sites, Limpopo Province, South Africa," *Journal of Hazardous Materials*, 429 (2022): 127588, 3.

28. Ministry of Mineral Resources and Energy, Memorandum from the Parliamentary Office, National Council of Provinces: 688, undated, which states that "Uitkyk, Lagerdraai and Uitval asbestos sites [in Limpopo] . . . have been rehabilitated by 31 March 2022."

29. H. Cornelissen, I. Watson, E. Adam, and T. Malefetse, "Challenges and Strategies of Abandoned Mine Rehabilitation in South Africa: The Case of Asbestos Mine Rehabilitation," *Journal of Geochemical Exploration* 205 (2019): 106354, 1. Seemingly only about half of these forty had been fully rehabilitated by 2018; see Auditor-General, *Follow-Up Performance Audit: On the Rehabilitation of Derelict and Ownerless Mines* (2022).

30. Auditor-General, *Follow-Up Performance Audit*, 28. The report notes that thirty-two asbestos mines had been fully rehabilitated by March 31, 2021, albeit that there were disparities in the numbers of both total asbestos mines and total rehabilitated mines, which "the Department could not explain," as the Auditor-General sharply notes (27).

31. Auditor-General, *Follow-Up Performance Audit*, 19. See further, Tony Carnie, "6,000 Health and Environmental 'Time Bombs' Still to Be Defused—South African Govt Decades Behind Schedule," *Land Portal News*, June 9, 2022.

32. Department of Minerals and Energy, *Standard Protocol and Guidelines for the Rehabilitation of Derelict/Ownerless Asbestos Mine Residue Deposits in South Africa* (1999).

33. Cornelissen, Watson, Adam, and Malefetse, "Challenges and Strategies," 1–10.

34. Freemantle, Chetty, Olifant, and Masikhwa, "Assessment of Asbestos Contamination in Soils at Rehabilitated and Abandoned Mine Sites," 8–10.
35. Cornelissen, Watson, Adam, and Malefetse, "Challenges and Strategies," 9.
36. Among geologists this version of its creation is now challenged by Peter Heaney and Donald Fisher, "New Interpretation of the Origin of Tiger's Eye," *Geology* 31, no. 4 (2003): 323–26, who argue that instead "tiger's eye classically exemplifies synchronous mineral growth through a crack-seal vein-filling process," at 323. So now you know!
37. "Major Countries in Worldwide Asbestos Production 2022," Statistica, October 30, 2023. This is a drop in annual global output from a recent peak of 2.03 million tons in 2011.
38. China, apparently, is taking steps to reduce consumption and "protect the population from toxic asbestos exposures" (Laurie Kazan-Allen, "Opposition to Asbestos Use Accelerates—Even in China," International Ban Asbestos Secretariat, October 11, 2023, at http://www.ibasecretariat.org/lka-opposition-to-asbestos-use-accelerates-even-in-china.php).
39. According to the US Geological Survey, the United States imported 100 tons in 2022, an increase from 41 tons in 2021, but a significant decrease from 608 tons in 2018 (US Geological Survey, "Asbestos," January 2023, https://pubs.usgs.gov/periodicals/mcs2023/mcs2023-asbestos.pdf). After the failure of Environmental Protections Agency's (EPA) 1989 total ban on asbestos (it was successfully challenged and overturned in 1991), the EPA has made several further, unsuccessful attempts to ban all uses of the mineral. That said, in March 2024 the EPA did issue a final rule under the Toxic Substances Control Act banning the importation, manufacture, and use of chrysotile asbestos in the United States, albeit to be implemented over a twelve-year phase-out period. See Rules and Regulations, 21970, *Federal Register* 89, no. 61 (March 28, 2024); Joe Lahav, "Asbestos Ban in the US," May 13, 2024, https://www.asbestos.com/mesothelioma-lawyer/legislation/.
40. Sugio Furuyo, Odgerel Chimed-Ochir, Ken Takahashi, Annette David, and Jukka Takala, "Global Asbestos Disaster," *International Journal of Environmental Research and Public Health* 15 (2019): 1, of

which number it is estimated that nearly 9 percent (some 22,000 deaths) are caused by environmental exposure to asbestos.

41. Diana Arachi et al., "Trend in the Global Incidence of Mesothelioma: Is There Any Changing Trend after Asbestos Regulation and Ban?" in Takashi Nakano and Takashi Kijima, eds., *Malignant Pleural Mesothelioma* (Springer, 2021), 3–13.

42. Western Australia's Wittenoom crocidolite mine, which had been operated by CSR Limited since 1943, closed down in 1966.

43. See Chrysotile Institute and Quebec Asbestos Mining Administration, "Safe Use of Chrysotile," 1998, as cited by the International Chrysotile Association, https://chrysotileassociation.com/sfuse/manual.php.

44. World Health Organization, "Asbestos: Elimination of asbestos-related diseases—Fact Sheet," February 15, 2018.

45. See the IBAS homepage, http://www.ibasecretariat.org/about.htm.

46. UN Rotterdam Convention on the Prior Informed Consent Procedure for Certain Hazardous Chemicals and Pesticides (1998). See Laurie Kazan-Allen, "UN Convention Defiled," International Ban Asbestos Secretariat, May 15, 2023, http://www.ibasecretariat.org/lka-un-convention-defiled.php.

47. Even today, the ICA continues to highlight the *Safe Use of Chrysotile Asbestos Manual* produced by Canada's Asbestos Institute and the Quebec Asbestos Mining Association more than 30 years ago in 1993, at https://chrysotileassociation.com/sfuse/manual.php.

48. "The Government of Canada Takes Measures to Ban Asbestos and Asbestos-Containing Products," Government of Canada, press release, October 18, 2018.

49. See Laurie Kazan-Allen, "The War against Asbestos," *International Journal of Occupational and Environmental Health* 9, no. 3 (2003): 173–93. Laurie is also a key supporter of an ongoing campaign demanding that Cape donate £10 million to mesothelioma research in the United Kingdom; see "Cape Must Pay," March 29, 2022, https://www.change.org/p/cape-must-pay-we-demand-that-cape-donate-10-million-to-fund-mesothelioma-research.

50. Ian Cobain, "Corporate Spy Infiltrated Anti-Asbestos Campaign, Court Told," *Guardian*, December 9, 2016.

51. Barry Meier, "A Spy's Tale: The TV Prankster Who Says He Became a Double Agent," *New York Times*, April 27, 2018.

52. Meier, "A Spy's Tale."
53. Cobain, "Corporate Spy," quoting Richard Meeran.
54. Rob Evans, "Security Firm Pays Damages to Anti-Asbestos Activists It Spied On," *Guardian*, November 9, 2018. Moore's hubris was his own undoing when he offered himself as a double agent to another activist group, Global Witness, who didn't trust him and alerted the IBAS campaigners to the mole in their midst.
55. Namely, the Occupational Diseases in Mines and Works Act (1973) and the Compensation for Occupational Injuries and Diseases Act (1993). The compensation range comes from Ntombizodwa Ndlovu, Jim teWaterNaude, and Jill Murray, "Compensation for Environmental Asbestos-Related Diseases in South Africa: A Neglected Issue," *Global Health Action* 6 no. 19410 (2013): 83.
56. Namely, Danielskuil Cape Blue Asbestos (Proprietary) Limited and Kuruman Cape Blue Asbestos (Proprietary) Limited. See Maria Roselli, *The Asbestos Lie* (European Trade Union Institute, 2014), 72–74.
57. The process by which claimants are vetted against the trust's strict qualifying conditions can, however, be arduous and time consuming. In its first ten years the ART processed about 14,500 applications out of which 3,639 were successful, being paid a cumulative total of R250 million ($22.5 million). See Samantha Herbst, "Asbestos Relief Trust pays out R250 million to 3,600 claimants in Ten Years," *Mining Weekly*, May 17, 2013. By 2023 the cumulative total of payouts was R442 million, with R212 million remaining available. The trust is scheduled to fold in 2028, but with the possibility of a five-year extension; see Asbestos Relief Trust, *Annual Report*, February 28, 2023, 1.
58. Phone interview with Richard Spoor, March 16, 2023, Johannesburg.
59. None of this would have happened had a remarkably reactionary proposal floated in September 1998 by the Lord Chancellor, Derry Irvine, been followed through. In response to the 1997 judgment of the House of Lords in *Connelly*, Irvine's proposal was to introduce legislation "to make the availability of funding in any form (for example, legal aid, conditional fees and legal expenses insurance), irrelevant when a court decides whether to allow litigation to proceed in the English courts, or whether there is a more appropriate foreign venue for the litigation under the doctrine of *forum non conveniens*"

(Lord Chancellor Irvine, letter to Mark Stobbs, head of Professional Standards and Legal Services at the Bar Council, September 15, 1998). Such a provision, if it had eventuated, would have scuppered the Cape case. It seems clear, however, that the proposal found little support from within the legal profession (aside, perhaps, from some corporate lawyers), and so the idea was dropped. Some years later, Richard bumped into Lord Irvine at a conference and asked him about the proposal. "Don't believe everything you hear" was Irvine's coy response. Richard Meeran, communication, June 16, 2024.

60. *Chandler v. Cape Plc* [2012] EWCA Civ 525 (an English asbestos victim, formally employed by Cape in the United Kingdom); *Vedanta Resources Plc and Konkola Copper Mines Plc v. Lungowe & others* [2019] UKSC 20 (2,577 Zambian farmers harmed by pollution from Vedanta's copper mine); *Okpabi v. Royal Shell Dutch Shell Plc* [2021] UKSC 3 (more than 13,000 Nigerian villagers harmed by pollution from Shell's oil exploration operations). A neat summary of this lineage is to be found in Lord Justice Simon's judgment in the Court of Appeal in *Vedanta*, [2017] EWCA Civ 1528, at paras. 67–79.

61. See *Lubbe & Others v. Cape* [1998] EWCA Civ 1351 (the first Court of Appeal judgment), at para. 20, and *Chandler v. Cape Plc* [2012], at paras. 69–70, and 79, where Lady Justice Arden establishes in precedent that which was promised (but not fulfilled because ultimately there was no trial) in *Lubbe & Others v. Cape Plc*—namely, that in certain circumstances parent corporations do owe a duty of care toward their subsidiaries' employees and others.

62. See *Vedanta* [2019] at para. 49 (per Lord Briggs) and *Okpabi* [2021], at paras. 65, 156–57 (per Lord Hamblen).

63. *Lubbe and Others v. Cape Plc and Related Appeals* [2000] UKHL 41 (20 July 2000), para. 20.

64. Richard Hermer KC, personal communication to author, December 4, 2023. In "private international law" Hermer is here referring to litigation between *non-state* actors across national boundaries. Hermer was appointed Attorney-General for England and Wales and Advocate General for Northern Ireland on July 5, 2024.

65. Daniel Leader, personal communication to author, December 8, 2023. See also Daniel Leader, "Human Rights Litigation against Multinationals in Practice: Lessons from the United Kingdom," in

Richard Meeran, ed., *Human Rights Litigation against Multinationals in Practice* (Oxford University Press, 2021), 58–84.

66. See Tibisay Morgandi, "Parent Company Liability, *Forum non Conveniens* and Substantial Justice," *Cambridge International Law Journal* 11, no. 1 (2022): 118–127.

67. Daniel Augenstein, "Towards a New Legal Consensus on Business and Human Rights: A 10th Anniversary Essay," *Netherlands Quarterly of Human Rights* 40, no. 1 (2022): 47. Augenstein is a consultant to the Institute for Legal Intervention in the European Center for Constitutional and Human Rights.

68. See further, Meeran, "Perspectives on the Development and Significance of Tort Litigation," 54–57; Jason Brickhill and Zanele Mbuyisa, "Multinational Company Litigation—South Africa," in Richard Meeran ed., *Human Rights Litigation against Multinationals in Practice* (Oxford University Press, 2021), 85–91. Notably, the pursuit of the Zambian lead-poisoning class action in South African courts reflects the jurisdiction (South Africa) in which the relevant Anglo American corporation is domiciled.

69. Barrie Clement, "Lawyers in Asbestos Case Agreed to Destroy Evidence," *Independent*, September 27, 2004; Kevin Maguire, "Law Firm Agreed to Shred Vital Data," *Guardian*, September 28, 2004.

70. Maguire, "Law Firm Agreed to Shred Vital Data."

71. *Dring v. Cape Intermediate Holdings Ltd* [2019] UKSC 38. The full set of Cape documents released after the case is maintained online by the Asbestos Forum at https://asbestosforum.org.uk/cape-documents/.

72. "Leigh Day," in Chambers and Partners, *UK Guide 2024: UK-Wide Civil Liberties & Human Rights*.

73. Financed, these days, mainly by litigation funders or through conditional fee arrangements.

74. Nadia Meeran, personal communication to author, December 15, 2023; Jahan Meeran, personal communication to author, December 16, 2023.

75. Interview with Munoree Padayachee, May 12, 2023, London.

Index

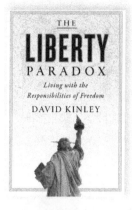
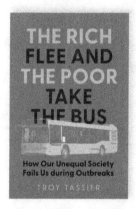
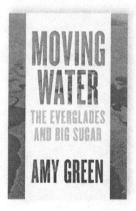